AM H^RVEY LIBRARY

fore th   st date shown below

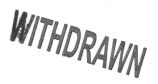
Introduction to Research in the Health Sciences

Dedication

To Sue, Sharon and Rebecca
To Colette and Liam

Commissioning Editor: *Mairi McCubbin*
Development Editor: *Veronika Watkins / Clive Hewat*
Project Manager: *Shereen Jameel*
Designer: *Christian Bilbow*
Illustration Manager: *Jennifer Rose*
Illustrator: *Antbits Ltd*

Introduction to Research in the Health Sciences

SIXTH EDITION

Stephen Polgar BSc (Hons) MSc PhD
Senior Lecturer, School of Public Health, Faculty of Health Sciences,
La Trobe University, Melbourne, Australia

Shane A. Thomas PhD MAPS
Vice Chancellor's Professorial Fellow, Executive Director and Associate President
(International Academic Development), Office of the Vice Chancellor,
Deputy Dean (International); Professor of Primary Health Care Research,
Faculty of Medicine, Nursing and Health Sciences, Monash University,
Melbourne, Australia

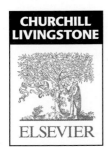

CHURCHILL
LIVINGSTONE

ELSEVIER

Edinburgh London New York Oxford Philadelphia St Louis Sydney Toronto 2013

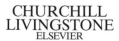

© 2013 Elsevier Ltd. All rights reserved.

First edition 1988
Second edition 1991
Third edition 1995
Fourth Edition 2000
Fifth Edition 2008

ISBN 978 0 7020 4194 5

British Library Cataloguing in Publication Data
A catalogue record for this book is available from the British Library

Library of Congress Cataloging in Publication Data
A catalog record for this book is available from the Library of Congress

---

Notices

Knowledge and best practice in this field are constantly changing. As new research and experience broaden our understanding, changes in research methods, professional practices, or medical treatment may become necessary.

Practitioners and researchers must always rely on their own experience and knowledge in evaluating and using any information, methods, compounds, or experiments described herein. In using such information or methods they should be mindful of their own safety and the safety of others, including parties for whom they have a professional responsibility.

With respect to any drug or pharmaceutical products identified, readers are advised to check the most current information provided (i) on procedures featured or (ii) by the manufacturer of each product to be administered, to verify the recommended dose or formula, the method and duration of administration, and contraindications. It is the responsibility of practitioners, relying on their own experience and knowledge of their patients, to make diagnoses, to determine dosages and the best treatment for each individual patient, and to take all appropriate safety precautions.

To the fullest extent of the law, neither the Publisher nor the authors, contributors, or editors, assume any liability for any injury and/or damage to persons or property as a matter of products liability, negligence or otherwise, or from any use or operation of any methods, products, instructions, or ideas contained in the material herein.

---

 your source for books, journals and multimedia in the health sciences

www.elsevierhealth.com

  Working together to grow libraries in developing countries

www.elsevier.com • www.bookaid.org

The Publisher's policy is to use **paper manufactured from sustainable forests**

Printed in China

Last digit is the print number: 10 9 8 7 6

Contents

Preface vii

Section 1 Methodological foundations of health research 1

  1 Foundations of health research 3
  2 Quantitative and qualitative methods 11
  3 The research process 17

Section 2 Research planning 25

  4 The formulation of research questions 27
  5 Sampling methods and external validity 33
  6 Ethics 43

Section 3 Research designs 51

  7 Experimental designs and randomized controlled trials 53
  8 Surveys and quasi-experimental designs 63
  9 Single case (n = 1) designs 71
  10 Qualitative research 77

Section 4 Data collection 83

  11 Questionnaires 85
  12 Interviewing techniques 91
  13 Observation 99
  14 Measurement 105

Section 5 Descriptive statistics 113

  15 Organization and presentation of data 115
  16 Measures of central tendency and variability 125
  17 Standard scores and normal distributions 133
  18 Correlation 139

Section 6 Data analysis and inference 147

19 Probability and confidence intervals 149
20 Hypothesis testing: selection and use of statistical tests 159
21 Effect size and the interpretation of evidence 171
22 Qualitative data analysis 181

Section 7 Evaluation and dissemination of research results 189

23 Critical evaluation of published research 191
24 Synthesis: systematic reviews and meta-analyses 199

Glossary of research terms 209
References and further reading 217
Appendix A: *z* scores and associated areas between *z* and mean
and beyond 219
Appendix B: *t* distribution 223
Appendix C: Chi-square (χ^2) 225
Index 227

Evolve Resources (evolve.elsevier.com/Polgar/research):

- MCQs
- True/false questions
- Short answer questions

Why do I need to know about research in order to be an effective health professional?

Welcome to our text! In this book our goal is to give you an effective working knowledge of health research needed to support high quality clinical practice. A key foundation of clinical practice is the use of research evidence concerning what works and with whom in health care settings. This evidence is generated by health research. Hence a basic knowledge of research methods is needed to be an effective clinician. The specific reasons you need to have a working knowledge of health research include the following.

Advancements in clinical knowledge: the health research explosion

Health and medical sciences knowledge is being generated and changing clinical practice at a very high rate. What you have learned in your clinical training will inevitably become out of date. You need to know about new research and research methods so that you can make sound decisions about integrating the major volume of new clinical knowledge into your practice and also discontinuing old less-effective practices. A sound knowledge of clinical research methods and how to evaluate evidence concerning clinical therapies is a foundation for the lifelong learning process that is required to deliver contemporary clinical practice.

Bloom's (2005, p 380) frequently cited review of the benefits of continuing (medical) education upon clinical quality and outcomes notes that:

> The objective of physician continuing medical education (CME) is to help them keep abreast of advances in patient care, to accept new more-beneficial care, and discontinue use of existing lower-benefit diagnostic and therapeutic interventions.

There is an explosion of new clinical knowledge that must be assessed by clinicians to be effective in their practice. How to best train health professionals to cope with the explosion of new knowledge that emerges post initial graduation is itself a whole field of enquiry sometimes with its own specific journals and accreditation systems for journals. Many clinical journals now have continuing education columns devoted to continuing clinician education and exercises relating to reading research and research critique that attracts credits under the profession's registration bodies. This is a big business and one that clinicians now interact with on a daily basis. As a practising clinician you will do this.

Figure P.1 shows the number of new entries to Medline made in each decade from the 1950s to the 2000s. Medline is the best known and largest indexing service for scientific publications in health and the medical and clinical sciences. During the decade of 1950 to 1959, 1.05 million new publications were added to Medline. Yet, in the decade 2000 to 2009, the corresponding figure was 6.23 million (see http://www.nlm.nih.gov/bsd/licensee/baselinestats.html and Figure P.1). The intervening decades showed strong growth in the numbers of new clinical research publications.

The rapid growth in publications reflects the corresponding growth in investment in health and medical research over the same period. In 1970 in the US the total investment in medical research across all federal agencies was USD 543 million. In 2001, the corresponding figure was USD 6585 million, a more than ten-fold increase. The strong acceleration in investment in health and medical research is a global phenomenon across most countries. Many countries now have major investments in medical research and these investments and the corresponding research outputs continue to grow strongly. As a health professional you are the key consumer of this work. You need to be an educated consumer.

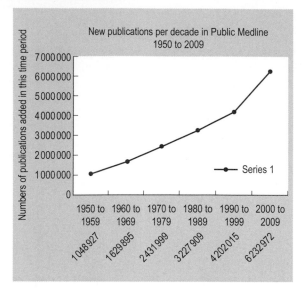

Figure P.1 • New publications per decade in Public Medline 1950–2009. Source: National Science Foundation/ Division of Science Resources Statistics, Survey of Federal Funds for Research and Development: Fiscal Years 2001, 2002 and 2003.

Continuing clinical education: the need to remain up to date

The consequence of this investment in health and medical research is a strong growth in new knowledge and hence a requirement for new approaches to health problems to be taken by clinicians. However, the mere numbers of publications, although impressive, do not reflect the major changes in practice that have occurred over the last few decades. Clinical practice has changed substantially in every field every decade in the 1900s and 2000s and this trend seems to be accelerating. There are new diagnostic technologies and interventions that are replacing the less-effective and outdated ones. This is why most registration bodies for clinicians have such strong requirements for continuing education and training to maintain current knowledge amongst the workforce. Many such bodies include clinical and scientific journal reading and research critique activities as a requirement for maintenance of current clinical knowledge of practitioners. Effective practice requires lifelong learning so that practitioners are up to date. This is a universally accepted principle in all countries. Thus all practitioners require basic research skills to enable them to properly interpret the research presented in the clinical and scientific journals to keep their practice up to date. This is what this text is all about.

Clinical practice guidelines and basic research skills

Many health professionals undertake their practice according to clinical guidelines. Clinical guidelines identify, summarize and evaluate the highest quality evidence about prevention, diagnosis, prognosis and therapy. The purpose of clinical guidelines is, through the standardization of evidence-based care, to improve quality, reduce risk and to maximize clinical effectiveness and efficiency. Adherence to guidelines has been consistently shown to achieve optimal outcomes for patients. Typically a guideline involves the critique of the systematic review and of the relevant research evidence described in Chapters 23 and 24 and then the synthesis of the reviews into recommended actions for clinicians.

Yet it is very important that guidelines are not followed slavishly and unintelligently. A key part of intelligent use of guidelines is to understand the evidentiary basis for them and how they are constructed. Our book provides you with the basic knowledge of the research methods that are the foundations for guideline construction so that you may use them intelligently to support the quality and effectiveness of your clinical practice.

The growth in consumer health knowledge: you need to be up to date because your patients will be!

One of the interesting phenomena associated with the widespread dissemination of medical and health sciences knowledge on the Internet is the extent to which many patients now research their own health problems and those of their family members. This means that patients are often (sometimes not exactly correctly!) very well informed of clinical knowledge concerning their and their family members' conditions. Practitioners need to know what is being currently discussed in the consumer forums in order that they are prepared to advise their patients. Many national health agencies go to significant efforts to provide their citizens with easily accessible advice concerning health problems. There are hundreds of such websites. The National Health Service in the UK has invested significantly in such

services. The SHALL network (see http://www.lib
raryservices.nhs.uk/shall/shallgroups/consumerhea
lthinformation/) makes the following points about
consumer health information:

> Access to appropriate, relevant and quality health
> information is a critical component of building indi-
> viduals' confidence to care for themselves, to maintain
> good physical and mental health and well-being and to
> seek help when they need it.
>
> Consumer health information encompasses the range
> of information services and resources needed by
> individuals, on their own behalf or on behalf of others,
> to enable them to:
>
> - make informed choices about health and
>   well-being
> - make informed choices about treatment and care
> - improve adherence to treatments
> - manage conditions
> - access services
> - navigate their way through the complexity of the
>   health and care system.

Similarly, the US National Institutes of Health has
a massive consumer information library. (see http://
health.nih.gov/see_all_topics.aspx).   Consumers
are now much better informed than in the past
because of the Internet and information revolution. Clinicians need to have a working knowledge
of research methods and evidence synthesis to help
their patients better evaluate and understand the
information they may obtain from these sources.

Advanced professional training and research skills

Finally, there is another reason for becoming adept
at clinical research. Most advanced clinical training
also requires research skills. To obtain a Masters or
PhD in your clinical discipline generally requires
advanced research skills training. The first step in
gaining these advanced skills is provided by completing a basic course of training such as that provided
by this book. So, although only some clinicians
will go on to become researchers, all require basic
research skills. This is what this book is intended to
provide to its readers. Good luck with your journey!

Melbourne, 2013   **Stephen Polgar**
                                       Shane A. Thomas

Acknowledgements

We would like to acknowledge our colleagues who
have contributed in various ways to the development
of the sixth edition: in particular, Melissa Buultjens,
Dr. Leila Karimi, Dr. Paul O'Halloran and Dr. Jane
Pierson. We are particularly grateful to Joanna Ng for
her hard work and dedication in organizing the text
for this sixth edition. We would also like to thank
Kate Williams for helping us to finalize the text. We
would like to thank all our readers, students and
reviewers for making this book relevant for introducing students to health research. Finally, special
thanks to our editor, Clive Hewat, for his support.

Section 1

Methodological foundations of health research

1 Foundations of health research 3

2 Quantitative and qualitative methods 11

3 The research process 17

In this section we will examine some of the basic characteristics of the scientific method. A 'method', in the present context, refers to a system for acquiring knowledge and establishing its truth. Health providers justify their theories and practices on the grounds that they are 'scientific', that is, based on scientific methodology. The scientific method is essential for conducting research and evaluation aimed at producing evidence, improving the effectiveness and cost-effectiveness of health services.

A common view of the scientific method is that it enables us to describe, predict and explain events in the world. In Chapter 1 we will discuss the fundamental principles for conducting health research and examine how these principles are applied to conduct health research. We will look at the meaning of constructs such as facts, hypotheses and theories and how these are used in constructing knowledge.

In Chapter 2 we discuss the elementary characteristics of both quantitative and qualitative methods of health research. The position taken in the present book is that the scientific method, as applied to health care, must include both quantitative and qualitative methods. These methods are used to produce evidence for solving health-related problems. Regardless of controversies regarding the nature of science and its methodology, there is a broad consensus concerning the principles and rules for producing scientific evidence. Our goal is to convey these principles and rules to our readers.

In Chapter 3 we will apply the basic methodological principles to the conduct of health research. The chapter outlines the stepwise problem-solving approach to research adopted in this book. We will also relate the problem-solving approach to the structure of publications reporting the results of health research.

Foundations of health research

1

CHAPTER CONTENTS

Introduction 3

Knowledge and methods 4

   Tradition 4

   Reasoning 4

The scientific method 4

Positivist paradigm 5

   Observations, description and measurement .5

   Generalization and induction 6

   Hypotheses and laws 6

   Theories 6

   Deduction 6

   Controlled observation. 7

   Verification and falsification 7

   Research and the advances of health care . .7

Post-positivist paradigms. 7

   What constitutes falsification? 7

   The theory-dependence of observation 8

   Science in a social context 8

Pragmatism: the combined use of quantitative
and qualitative methods 9

Summary. 9

Introduction

Health research is a systematic and principled way of obtaining evidence (data, information) for solving health care problems and investigating health issues. Research is *systematic* in that researchers follow a sequential process (see Ch. 3) and *principled* in that research is generally carried out according to explicit rules. These rules or principles constitute the method. The term '*method*' derives from the Greek word '*methodoi*', meaning a 'way of travelling' or 'the path which we follow'. It is the application of appropriate methods which guarantee the validity of the evidence and the truth of knowledge. In health research, 'method' refers to a set of rules which specify:

- How knowledge should be acquired.
- The form in which knowledge should be stated.
- How the truth or validity of knowledge should be established.

Strictly speaking, the terms '*method*' and '*methodology*' have different meanings. Method refers to the rules of evidence followed for collecting data in a project. Methodology refers to the critical discussion, comparison and application of methods. The present chapter is concerned with methodology. Later chapters in this book are concerned with specific methods used in health research.

The primary aim of this chapter is to examine the philosophical foundations of scientific research methods. Emphasis is placed on method as a means of conducting applied research and producing the best possible evidence for solving health problems.

The general aims of this chapter are to:

1. Examine the relationship between knowledge and methods.
2. Outline what constitutes the scientific method.
3. Examine positivist and post-positivist approaches.

Knowledge and methods

Two concepts drawn from philosophy are relevant to our discussion: *ontology* and *epistemology*.

Ontology refers to the question of what exists in the world, what is 'real'. Different knowledge systems take diverse positions on what constitutes reality. In contrast to the natural sciences, various traditional interpretations hold different views on what constitutes the reality. For example, the notion of life force or qi/chi, a central concept in traditional Chinese medicine, is absent in contemporary Western medicine. Of historical interest, is the classical Greek belief in humors that was once central to Western medicine. The balance of humors was thought to determine mental and physical wellbeing; however humors are no longer seen as 'real' in Western medicine.

Epistemology is a field of philosophy concerned with the nature, source and legitimacy of knowledge. In the domain of health research we are interested in knowledge as *applicable* to:

- Selecting and implementing practices.
- Producing and interpreting evidence.
- Constructing and applying theories to practice.

Before we begin discussion of scientific knowledge and research it is useful, as a means of contrast, to look at some other epistemological approaches.

Tradition

Western health care is one of many approaches; it is erroneous to believe that it is always the best option for preventing, treating and managing diseases. The World Health Organization (WHO 2010) defines traditional medicine as 'the knowledge, skills and practices based on the theories, beliefs and experiences indigenous to different cultures, used in the maintenance of health and … treatment of physical and mental illness'.

There are hundreds of different medical traditions. They are based on distinct ontological and epistemological positions, ranging from shamanism to empirically oriented components of traditional Chinese medicine (TCM). The beginnings of TCM can be traced back thousands of years, well before the introduction of Western medicine. The principles of TCM were, in part, based on the experiences of practitioners, successfully treating diseases using natural methods such as acupuncture and herbal remedies. This practical knowledge was combined with Chinese philosophy to formulate holistic theories of physiology, pathology and treatment (Lu et al 2004). These theories emphasize the close relationship between the human body as a system integrated with the natural and social environment. The prevention or treatment of disease is contingent on the re-establishment of a dynamic balance between the energy flows within the body, the mind and the environment.

Reasoning

Reasoning is commonly used to arrive at true knowledge. It is assumed that, if the rules of logic are applied correctly, then the conclusions are guaranteed to be valid. As an example, let us look at the following syllogism:

1. All persons suffering from heart disease are males.
2. Person X has heart disease.
3. Therefore, person X is a male.

Logic guarantees that the conclusion (3) is true, provided that the syllogism is in a valid form and the premises (1) and (2) are true. Clearly, the limitation of formal (that is, 'content-independent') reasoning is that it works in practice only if we have means for establishing the factual truth of the premises. In the above example, conclusion (3) might be empirically false, given that the premise (1) is factually false.

The origin of modern science originates from 'natural' philosophy. Reasoning and logic are very much a part of science. However, we require reliable evidence to support conclusions based on logic and mathematical operations.

The scientific method

Science and the scientific method evolved over a period of thousands of years (Fara 2009). Great civilizations, such as Babylonia, China and India, devised written languages and symbols for numbers, to permanently record observations and speculations about the world. This was an essential step in the development of formal science. Disciplines such as astronomy, mathematics and medicine were further developed by Greek and Roman philosophers and physicians. For example, the Roman physician Galen worked as a surgeon treating injured gladiators and used experimental methods to test hypotheses about physiology and anatomy. Much of the classical knowledge was lost during the dark ages, but an important fraction was preserved and expanded upon by Muslim and Christian scholars (Fara 2009).

The beginnings of modern Western science are generally traced to the beginning of the 16th century, a time in which Europe experienced profound social changes and a resurgence of great artists, thinkers and philosophers. Gradually, scholars' interests shifted from theology and armchair speculation to systematically describing, explaining and attempting to control natural phenomena. These changed circumstances enabled philosophers such as Descartes and Francis Bacon to challenge tenets of medieval thinking, and scientists such as Galileo, Newton and Harvey to propose new ways of conducting research and building knowledge.

The following points represent the essential characteristics of the early scientific world view:

- *Realism:* a position which holds that the world exists independently of our beliefs. For example, the planets are large objects which circle about the sun, regardless of what observations astronomers make about their orbits.
- *Determinism:* the assumption that events in the world occur according to regular laws and identifiable causes.
- *Empiricism:* the conviction that discovery ought to be conducted through observation and the truth of knowledge verified through evidence.
- *Scepticism:* an attitude which fosters questioning the truth of any proposition; even those made by great authorities. All aspects of knowledge, including methods, became open to questioning, critique and revision.

These approaches to knowledge remain an integral part of contemporary health sciences; however, there are several interpretations of what constitutes the scientific method (Chalmers 2007). The problem is that there is no stone tablet on which has been inscribed the permanent axioms of the scientific method. Rather, they are a set of rules devised and debated by philosophers and researchers. They are not eternal truths, but conventions believed to

be useful for conducting research. The interpretation of what constitutes the scientific method is an activity pursued by philosophers of science as well as researchers.

Positivist paradigm

The term *paradigm* has multiple meanings depending on the context in which it is used (Chalmers 2007). Here we are using the term to refer to basic belief systems, which include the fundamental ontological, epistemological and methodological positions adopted by the researchers (Guba & Lincoln 1994). Guba & Lincoln (1994) define paradigms as:

> …a worldview, that defines, for its holder the individual's place in it, and the range of possible relationships to that world and its parts, as, for example, cosmologies do.

(Guba & Lincoln 1994, p 207)

Positivism is an influential interpretation of the science and its methodology. It was initially described by the 19th-century philosopher August Comte. Currently, there are numerous versions of what is meant by positivism. Figure 1.1 represents our point of view.

Observations, description and measurement

Considering Figure 1.1, let us start with observations. The description of phenomena involving the precise, unbiased recording of observations of aspects of persons, objects and events forms the empirical basis of all branches of science. Observations can be expressed as either verbal descriptions or sets of measurements (see Section 4). The perceptions of the investigator must be transformed into descriptive statements and measurements that can be understood and replicated by other investigators. Some research is based on observation made with instruments (such as recording electrodes,

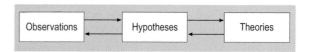

Figure 1.1 • The scientific method.

microscopes and standardized clinical tests), while other research calls for observation unaided by instruments. Although advances in instrumentation have contributed enormously to scientific knowledge, the use of complex instrumentation is not a necessary feature of scientific observation. Rather, the key attributes of scientific observation are accuracy and replicability by other scientists. When observations are appropriately summarized and are confirmed by others, they form the factual bases of scientific knowledge.

Generalization and induction

Statements representing observations or measurements are integrated into explanatory systems called hypotheses and theories. The logic underlying scientific generalizations is called induction. Induction involves asserting general propositions (hypotheses, theories) about a class of phenomena on the basis of a limited number of observations of select elements. For example, having observed that penicillin is useful for curing pneumonia in a limited set of patients, we make the generalization 'the administration of penicillin cures pneumonia (in all patients)'.

Hypotheses and laws

'The administration of penicillin cures pneumonia' is an example of an hypothesis. Scientific hypotheses are statements that specify the expected relationship between two or more sets of variables. In this instance, the first variable relates to the administration of penicillin and the second set of variables relates to beneficial changes in patients with pneumonia. As we shall see in subsequent sections, an important feature of scientific hypotheses is that the terms used must have clear-cut, observable referents. For example, the 'beneficial changes in the symptoms of patients with pneumonia' will include a reduction in temperature in degrees centigrade. When hypotheses acquire strong empirical support, they may be called laws. Therefore the statement, 'the administration of penicillin cures pneumonia', can be considered a law on the grounds that many patients with pneumonia have been effectively treated. Nevertheless there are problems concerning the universal truth of this statement (see 'Verification and falsification', below.)

Theories

Scientific theories are essentially conjectures representing our current state of knowledge about the world. Hypotheses are integrated into more general explanatory systems called theories. A theory will clarify the relationships between diverse classes of observations and hypotheses. For example, a theory to explain why drugs called antibiotics are effective in curing some infectious diseases integrates evidence from diverse sources such as microbiology, pharmacology, cell physiology and clinical medicine. Other examples include the DNA theory of genetic inheritance, and the neuronal theory of central nervous system functioning. It is an essential feature of scientific theories that they are statements based on the correct use of language and logic. Some theories entail a model which is a mathematical or physical representation of how the theory works. In this way, theories specify the causes of events and provide conceptual means for predicting and influencing these events. In health care, theories are important for explaining the causes of health and illness and predicting the probable effectiveness of treatment outcomes. For example, the theory of AIDS is based on the assumption that signs and symptoms of the disease are caused by the HIV retrovirus, which is transmitted by bodily fluids (e.g. blood, semen). This theory guides practices such as screening of blood and promoting safe sex to control the pandemic.

Deduction

A scientific theory will lead to a set of empirically verifiable statements or hypotheses. In addition to being generalizations based on evidence, hypotheses are also deduced logically from the statements and/or models which specify the causal relationships postulated by the theories. For instance, if we hold the theory that the patterns of activity of a set of neurones in the occipital lobe mediate visual sensation in humans, then the hypothesis follows that the activation of these neurones (say, by electrical stimulation) will lead to the report of visual sensations. Such hypotheses have been the bases for subsequent spectacular clinical advances such as artificial vision through cortically implanted electrodes.

Controlled observation

It is desirable that hypotheses are tested under controlled conditions. The aim of control is to discount other competing hypotheses for explaining the predicted phenomenon. For example, if we intend to show that occipital lobe stimulation causes the visual sensations, we must show that we are controlling for any type of brain stimulation causing such changes. Conversely, we would need to show that occipital lobe stimulation does not lead to a host of other types of sensations. Only by discounting alternative explanations through control can we have confidence in the relevance of our observations for our research hypothesis.

Verification and falsification

After the evidence has been collected, the investigator decides whether or not the findings are consistent with the predictions of the hypothesis. If the hypothesis is supported by the evidence, then the theory from which the hypothesis was deduced is strengthened or verified. When the data are not consistent with the predictions, the theories from which the hypotheses were deduced are falsified. If a theory can no longer predict or explain evidence in its empirical domain, it becomes less useful and is usually later discarded in favour of new, more powerful theories. Therefore, scientific theories are not held to be absolute truths, but rather as provisional explanations of available evidence. An essential characteristic of a scientific proposition is that it should be 'falsifiable'. That is, there should be a clear empirical outcome that could, if found, show that the proposition was false. For example, consider the previous statement, 'the administration of penicillin cures pneumonia'. This statement is clearly falsifiable because there is the possibility that penicillin will not work.

Research and the advances of health care

The use of the positivist paradigm has contributed to the spectacular growth of scientific knowledge. Research relying on observation and measurement, facilitated by new instrumentation, resulted in the discovery of an enormous number of accurate and reproducible facts about health and illness. New facts both challenge existing theories and call for the creation of novel, more powerful theories. The new theories serve as impetus for more research, resulting in new instrumentation and observations. Advances in scientific knowledge have been applied to creating new technologies, which in turn contribute to new discoveries and advances in scientific knowledge. For example, the invention of computers was possible because of advances in electronics, chemistry and mathematics. In turn, the use of computers is now contributing to making and summarizing scientific observations or formulating explanatory models. In addition, the use of computers as information-processing systems has generated useful metaphors for theoretical advances, such as explaining the human brain and mental functioning. In this way, the scientific method contributes to advancing theory and practice, helping us to describe, explain, predict and sometimes control the world in which we live.

Post-positivist paradigms

The above description is not the only interpretation of the scientific method. Rather, there are compelling reasons why the positivist view was challenged in the second half of the 20th century. Advances in science contributed to changes to our methods and the ways in which we explain the world. For example 'quantum theory' and the 'theory of relativity' challenged the mechanistic, clockwork-like view of reality. Modern theories of physical reality are fuzzier and more probabilistic and the observers are not seen as being outside the phenomena they are studying.

What constitutes falsification?

It was stated earlier that, when new evidence is inconsistent with the predictions of a theory, the theory is 'falsified' and is eventually modified or discarded. Commentators (see Chalmers 2007) argued that theories are not, in practice, so readily modified or discarded by scientists. Rather, they are structures which have an inner hard core of propositions protected by an outer belt of auxiliary, modifiable hypotheses. Evidence inconsistent with predictions based on the theory results in the modification of auxiliary hypotheses, rather than discarding the 'core'. Consider, for example, the 'germ' theory of infectious disease, on the basis of which one would predict that penicillin (which kills 'germs') will cure bacterial infections. Suppose that we administer penicillin to a number of patients with an infectious disease and find, contrary to what was predicted, no clinically useful changes. On the basis of this falsification, will we discard the germ theory of disease? No. Rather, we will utilize an auxiliary hypothesis to explain our findings, such as 'the development of penicillin-resistant bacteria'.

The methodological issue which remains controversial is the logical basis for discarding one theory and accepting its rival. Researchers judge the outcome of a research program in the context of an overall pattern of related findings and theories. Judgements may be affected by considerations other than the state of the evidence. For example, the personal and social contexts in which the researchers work may influence what is said to be 'true' or 'false'.

The theory-dependence of observation

Critics argued that it is simplistic to believe that observations are made independently of theoretical notions held by the observer. The observer is selective with regard to what is recorded as evidence. Our observations and facts are 'theory-dosed'; that is, theories specify what observations are of importance and what aspects of these observations should be recorded or ignored. For instance, in observing the electroencephalogram (EEG) of an epileptic patient, our perception is guided by theories of the electrical activity of the brain and the nature of brain pathology. We will also hold ideas about how the EEG machine works (e.g. electrode sensitivity, amplification, etc.) and identify artefacts in the evidence. What is observed as evidence of epilepsy by an expert could be perceived as meaningless squiggles by a naive observer.

Also, we can assume that human participants are actively engaged in the research process. Criteria for conducting ethical research (see Ch. 6) require that participants are informed of the aims, risks and potential benefits of a research project. It follows that participants will have expectations regarding the processes and outcomes of the project. These expectations may be a source of bias and there are various ways for controlling for this (see Ch. 7).

Science in a social context

Health research is conducted in particular social settings, by individuals with personal aims and values. There are multiple perspectives from which researchers may view research problems. Professional affiliation is a particularly important factor in deciding which research questions will be investigated and how the evidence is applied. Consider the example of the growing problem of obesity in developed countries. A public health researcher would look at programs which would contribute to preventing/reducing obesity in a given population. The following programs might be devised and evaluated:

- Mandatory labelling of manufactured food, e.g. kilojoules, trans-fat, sodium, sugar, etc.
- Promotion of healthy eating, e.g. restrictions on the type of food sold in school canteens.
- Government-funded promotion of healthy living programs, e.g. tax incentives for joining gyms, community based sporting events, etc.

In contrast, a medical researcher would focus on the efficacy of therapeutic interventions, such as:

- Medically supervised diets and exercises for individual patients.
- Medication which suppresses appetite or inhibits the absorption of fats.
- Surgery for morbidly obese patients, e.g. gastric banding.

Until recently, the 'medical model', as exemplified above, was by far the most dominant approach to identifying and solving health problems. The role of the health professional is to identify the underlying pathology and to implement appropriate measures to correct the problem. The patient is assigned a rather passive role in this process, being the 'locus' of the problem, and is expected to comply with medical advice. The aim of medical research is to enhance the range and efficacy of treatments which can be offered to affected individuals.

The more holistic approach, which also informs health care research, is called the *psychosocial* or *biopsychosocial* model (Engel 2003) and currently has had considerable influence in how we conceptualize health care and how we plan and carry out research. At the same time, the medical model strongly based on positivist thinking remains influential in research aimed at understanding the workings of the human body and improving the technical aspects of health care. A post-positivist paradigm retains the realist ontology of positivism but emphasizes that reality is interpreted from different perspectives. These perspectives are essential and are best researched using qualitative methods (see Ch. 2).

Pragmatism: the combined use of quantitative and qualitative methods

A post-positivist paradigm recognizes different perspectives of reality. In this book, we will explore two of these approaches to conducting health research: *quantitative* and *qualitative*. Using a quantitative approach, we view our patients objectively, as natural objects, and attempt to identify and measure important variables which represent the causes and expressions of health problems. We develop models and theoretical frameworks which systematically explain how these variables are interrelated and undertake therapeutic actions which serve to diminish the values of the variables representing illness or disability. Our therapeutic actions are the technical applications for our scientific theories; their outcomes and effectiveness should be tested under controlled conditions. Using a qualitative approach to research and knowledge, we view our patients as individuals and attempt to gain insights into their subjective experiences and the reasons for their actions. We develop theories for interpreting personal points of view, and to inform our therapeutic actions so that they are meaningful and appropriate to our patients.

Not all scholars agree that qualitative and quantitative methods can be logically combined. It has been argued that these two methods are incommensurate in that an *objective* view of reality need not necessarily correspond with that of a *subjective* experience (Minichiello et al 2008). The controversy was resolved on pragmatic grounds, based on the argument that both methods are needed to solve problems in applied areas such as health care (McGartland & Polgar 1994, Minichiello et al 2008). *Pragmatism* is a system of philosophy that avoids speculation about nebulous abstractions such as 'The Truth'; rather it defines truth as what works. A pragmatic, problem-solving approach is followed in the present book, emphasizing the need for both qualitative and quantitative methods for effectively solving health problems. The introduction of a biopsychosocial approach has raised questions about the combination of methods relevant to health sciences research. We perceive patients or clients in two different but interrelated frameworks: first, as broken down or malfunctioning biological systems; and second, as persons, like ourselves, living in a society and who are attempting to make sense of and cope with their particular health care problems.

Summary

Methods are used for acquiring, stating and establishing the truth of knowledge. The scientific method underpins the validity of theory and practice in Western health care. The scientific method is concerned with applying a set of rules or conventions that will allow us to produce scientifically valid knowledge. These rules specify how observations should be made, and how theories and hypotheses should be stated and evaluated.

Theories and hypotheses obtained and verified through scientific enquiry are not held to be absolutely 'true'. An inherent part of the scientific approach is scepticism regarding both the contents of knowledge and the underlying methodology. We have pointed out that there are controversies concerning what constitutes scientific methodology. It was argued that the scientific method is directly applicable to conducting research in the health sciences. We have adopted a post-positivist paradigm which entails the use of both qualitative and quantitative methods. We will examine these methods in more detail in the next chapter.

Quantitative and qualitative methods

2

CHAPTER CONTENTS

Introduction 11

The social construction of reality 11

Contrasting qualitative and quantitative
methods 12

   Perception of subject matter 12

   Positioning of researcher 13

   Data and evidence 13

   Theories 14

   Theory testing 14

   Applications in health care delivery 15

The integration of quantitative and qualitative
methods 15

Summary 15

Introduction

In Chapter 1, we discussed the conceptual foundations of health research methods. It was suggested that contemporary health research follows a pragmatic paradigm which includes both quantitative and qualitative methods. In terms of the quantitative approach, health problems are conceptualized as impairments and dysfunctions in an organism. The aim for researchers is to accurately describe these problems and to identify their causes and consequences. Armed with accurate, evidence-based knowledge, practitioners can act to prevent illness or to repair or mitigate the associated damage and dysfunction. This type of approach may be considered to think of patients as if they are broken-down mechanisms in need of repair. However, ignoring personal values and experiences will undermine the efficacy and ethics of health services. This is why qualitative research is also essential in the clinical context; this method provides the evidence that enables us to understand our patients as human beings. Qualitative research gives a voice to research participants, allowing us to gain valuable insights into how health problems are viewed and experienced. In this chapter, we will examine these two methods in greater detail.

The aims of this chapter are to:

1. Outline different conceptual approaches to qualitative research.
2. Compare and contrast specific dimensions of qualitative and quantitative approaches to research.
3. Emphasize the importance of using evidence from both qualitative and quantitative research.
4. Discuss basic strategies used for ensuring the validity of qualitative research.
5. Examine the scope and limitations of qualitative research in the health sciences.

The social construction of reality

As discussed in Chapter 1, knowledge is acquired and applied from a particular perspective. It follows that there are a number of different ways of looking at and researching health problems. To illustrate qualitative and quantitative perspectives, let us look at an example outside health research.

Imagine that you are given a piece of paper. Say that it is a bank note and it has £100 printed on it. You can look at this object from a number of perspectives (qualitative and quantitative) depending on who you are and how you are positioned in relation to this object:

- If you are a person from a remote tribe with no exposure to the use of bank notes, you might see it as a decorative object and value it as a curio. (Qualitative.)
- If you are a person having financial difficulties, £100 would be seen as a means of improving your quality of life; for instance, allowing you to buy food or cover outstanding bills. (Qualitative *and* quantitative.)
- If you are an accountant, you would focus on the number printed on the bill for making fiscal calculations. (Quantitative.)
- If you are a counterfeiter (we hope not!), you would be intensely interested in the physical properties of the object, such as its length, width, colour, texture: details required for successful forgery. (Quantitative.)

Money is very much a social construct. It is 'real' enough; having it or not having it can influence all aspects of life, including the level of health services a person can access. At the same time, money is an abstraction; it can take virtually any physical form (e.g. coins, notes, or even a set of numbers representing your bank balance). Its reality is constructed through the actions of a number of institutions (e.g. banks, State treasuries, etc.), which determines its value for buying goods and services. Likewise, health researchers can look at a problem from different perspectives depending on the questions they are asking and the nature of the information they wish to acquire.

Contrasting qualitative and quantitative methods

In this section, we will identify and discuss the fundamental differences between quantitative and qualitative methods (see Table 2.1). One key difference is that these two methods have different historical and disciplinary backgrounds. Quantitative methods are based on the traditions of the natural sciences (physics, biology, etc.), whereas qualitative methods emerged from disciplines such as philosophy, anthropology and other social sciences (see Ch. 10).

Perception of subject matter

As discussed in Chapter 1, quantitative researchers favour a 'realist' ontological position. The associated research strategy is through discovery of novel

Table 2.1 Contrast between quantitative and qualitative methods

	Quantitative	Qualitative
Perception of subject matter	Reductionistic: identification and operational definition of specific variables	Holistic: persons in the context of their social environments
Positioning of researcher	Objective: detached observation and precise measurement of variables	Subjective: close personal interaction with participants
Database	Quantitative: interrelationships among specific variables	Qualitative: descriptions of actions and related personal meanings in context
Theories	Normative: general propositions explaining causal relationships among variables	Interpretive: providing insights into the nature and social contexts of personal meanings
Theory testing	Controlled: empirically supporting or falsifying hypotheses deduced from theories	Consensual: matching researcher's interpretations with those of participants and other observers
Applications	Prediction and control of health-related factors in applied settings	Interacting with persons in a consensual, value-consonant fashion in health care settings

Adapted from McGartland & Polgar (1994). Copyright (1994) The Australian Psychological Society Ltd. Reproduced by permission.

facts about the world. *Reductionism* is central to conducting quantitative research; this is the process of reducing complex phenomena to simpler, more fundamental elements. For example, the discipline of chemistry has been enhanced by reducing the immense variety of materials to the interaction and combination of elements, represented in the periodic table. Also, the enormous array of physical and mental symptoms has been compiled into taxonomy of illnesses. Good health can be differentiated from ill health along with a number of clearly defined factors, such as blood pressure or the presence or absence of infectious agents. For example, ischaemic heart disease can be attributed to diminished blood flow in the coronary arteries. This in turn can be linked to risk factors such as high cholesterol or high blood pressure.

Quantitative health research involves the discovery of relationships among a multitude of health variables. To identify causal associations, clearly stated hypotheses need to be tested (see Ch. 1). An important example of this is the relationship between factors or variables representing changes in signs and symptoms. For example, Lipitor® is effective in lowering blood cholesterol, reducing the incidence of heart attack.

By reducing health problems to specific disease processes and associated signs and symptoms, quantitative researchers lose track of the person with the health problem. An *holistic* perspective focuses on the person with the problem in the context of their physical and social environment. Qualitative researchers aim to understand how individuals experience health problems and the reasons for their actions to cope with these problems. For example, qualitative researchers investigating heart disease would consider the participants' experiences and understanding of their health issue. In understanding the interaction between a person and their environment, the person at risk of heart attack is no longer reduced to a failing mechanism, but rather as an active agent for positive health change. An important step in qualitative methods might include making participants aware of their predisposition to heart disease as well as encouraging involvement in healthy eating and living programs.

Positioning of researcher

Quantitative researchers follow a positivist paradigm: postulating an external world which exists independently of their awareness (Baggini & Fosl 2010). Research is conducted to discover more facts about the world, as discussed in Chapter 1. The fundamental positioning of the researcher is 'objective', aiming to perceive and record events dispassionately, without any personal bias or distortion. However, there is recognition of the possibility of error and bias entailed in collecting data. Therefore, quantitative health research has invested much effort in devising and evaluating accurate measuring instruments and tests (see Ch. 14). Also, research designs such as 'double-blind randomized controlled trials' (see Ch. 7) have been implemented to reduce both observer and participant bias.

The problem with highly structured data collection is that participants' true responses are limited. Qualitative researchers find standardized instruments intrusive, as they restrict self-expression and impede the understanding of the true ideas and emotions of participants. When conducting qualitative research, the researcher becomes a part of the phenomenon being investigated. To understand personal meanings and subjective experiences one has to become involved with the lives of the participants being studied. In this way, the researcher takes a subjective position, as some degree of empathy must develop between the researcher and the participant. By empathy we mean the ability to 'put ourselves in the other person's shoes' or to see things from their perspective(s).

It is essential in qualitative research that the reports of events should be truthful and not be confused with advocacy. The investigators should not allow ideological biases to distort or censor their observations, or deliberately lie to place research participants in a good or bad light. This is a particularly important point as, given the close personal interaction with the participants, one may be predisposed to report favourably.

Data and evidence

By 'data' we mean the results which are analysed to provide the evidence required for theory formation and evidence-based health care. In quantitative research, the database will consist of the statistically treated data which will enable us to see how specific variables are interrelated. The data obtained in quantitative research consist of sets of measurements of objective descriptions of physical and behavioural events. These are summarized and analysed in accordance with statistical principles outlined at an introductory level in Sections 5 and 6.

In qualitative research, the database is essentially a narrative (or a story, if you like) that reports what has happened to people, what they did or said in specific situations. This narrative should be adequately detailed so as to illuminate for the reader the personal meanings that the health-related events had for the informants.

The data in qualitative research are descriptive, a 'thick' or thorough description of what people said, their actions and activities, non-verbal behaviours and interactions with other people. An important aspect of qualitative research is keeping thorough, up-to-date field notes. These should be recorded as closely as possible to the time of occurrence of the phenomena under study. The field notes should contain direct quotations from the participants and the settings in which the statements and actions were recorded. Where possible (where it is appropriate and not overly intrusive), the researcher may use audio and video recordings. This helps to record interviews, and improves accuracy in conveying what was said and done in a given setting, since it is possible to review the obtained information (see Ch. 22).

Theories

Theories represent our current state of knowledge about the state of the world. Theories are abstract, coherent explanatory systems which integrate a broad range of research findings. Theories may be constituted of premises stated in everyday language, with particular attention paid to the appropriate use of concepts and the logical development of the premises.

Theories based on quantitative evidence integrate patterns of findings concerning the interrelationships among variables. Such theories often contain 'models', which may be mathematical and/or systems representations of the patterns of findings. Models of anatomical and physiological processes, such as those of the circulatory or nervous systems, are good examples of successful quantitative models. Quantitative theories are 'normative' in the sense that they aim to describe and explain, as closely as possible, how things actually work. They are assumed to be stable and

universally applicable. Conversely, theories integrating evidence from qualitative research do not address facts about how objects are constituted and interact, but rather are the overall interpretations of personal meanings emerging in specific social settings.

Some qualitative researchers contend that data collection and theory formation should be intrinsically integrated rather than being different stages of the research process (see Ch. 10). Others have suggested that personal meanings should be seen as unique and idiosyncratic, and thus no attempt should be made to integrate systematically diverse personal positions. Theory is seen essentially as the accurate presentation of the situation from a particular person's perspective.

More commonly, qualitative health researchers approach theory formation by attempting to identify common 'themes' or categories of meanings emerging from the data. The important point here is that the theoretical categories are developed from evidence expressing personal meanings, rather than 'facts' derived from the statistical treatment of objective measurements concerning variables. In this way, theory is said to be 'grounded' in the narratives of a group of individuals.

Researchers working from a critical framework stress the broad, culture-interpreting aspects of qualitative field research. *Critical theory* explains how personal meanings and actions emerge and are influenced by the person's social and cultural milieu. These theories identify the extent to which individuals' self-perception and freedom for action may become distorted and limited by the operation of power and coercion within a cultural setting.

Theory testing

Theories based on quantitative evidence are tested through precisely stated predictions or hypotheses logically deduced from the theories (see Ch. 1). The accuracy of a quantitative theory is judged by the extent to which the predictions generated by the theory match the evidence produced by methodologically rigorous research. However, as discussed in Chapter 1, theories are not easily discarded on the basis of preliminary, insufficient evidence.

Testing qualitative theories is somewhat different, as no causal mechanisms are included in the theoretical framework. The simplest verification of qualitative interpretations is to go to the participants themselves, in order to establish if the researcher's interpretations make sense to them. The extent to which a consensus develops between researchers and their participants is one of the important indications of the truth of qualitative theories.

Applications in health care delivery

The applications of quantitative evidence and theories are essentially technical, providing mechanisms in terms of which we can *predict* and *control* specific health-related variables. That is, we apply quantitative approaches for (i) discovering the causes of diseases and disabilities, (ii) predicting the burden of diseases and disabilities on individual populations, (iii) developing and validating assessment procedures and (iv) evaluating the effectiveness of interventions.

In contrast, qualitative research provides evidence and theories that enable us to better understand our participants as human beings. This research discloses how illnesses, disability and health care delivery affect people's lives interpreted from their points of view.

The integration of quantitative and qualitative methods

When used jointly, quantitative and qualitative research tools can be particularly powerful. One of the authors has conducted a study of how people evaluate primary health services (Thomas et al 1993). The first step in this process was to conduct focus group interviews with 20 groups of eight participants specifically selected from a wide range of ethnic backgrounds, ages and sexes. The groups were conducted by a facilitator who presented questions concerned with knowledge and opinions of, and satisfaction with, health services. The discussions were recorded and transcribed.

One set of analyses of the transcripts involved consideration of everything that had been said about the health services with regard to satisfaction or dissatisfaction. This resulted in a range of separate categories or themes. These themes, therefore, were directly derived from the participants' own words and interpretations of their experiences.

The themes were then framed in the form of questions that sought information from people about their satisfaction and dissatisfaction with health services. The questions were then incorporated into a questionnaire (see Ch. 11). When the questionnaire was piloted with a sample of 500 people who attended several doctors' surgeries over a period of three weeks, it was found that none of the participants nominated new factors that affected their satisfaction and dissatisfaction. Thus, the procedure used in developing the questionnaire had very effectively captured how people decided whether they were satisfied or dissatisfied with their health services. This study is an example of where qualitative and quantitative research methodologies can combine powerfully. There are many productive ways for combining quantitative and qualitative approaches to health research. Interested readers are advised to consult Tashakkori & Teddlie (2003).

Summary

Qualitative research is based on the assumption that reality is *socially constructed*. It entails disciplined enquiry examining the personal meanings of individuals' experiences and actions in the context of their social environment. By 'qualitative' we mean that the data consists of detailed descriptions based on language or pictures recorded by the investigator. The term 'discipline' indicates that the enquiry is guided by explicit methodological principles for defining problems, collecting and analysing the evidence, and formulating and evaluating theories. 'Personal meaning' refers to the way in which individuals subjectively perceive and explain their experiences, actions and social environments.

In contrast, quantitative research holds the view that reality is independent of personal views and social contexts. The role of the researcher is to discover the objects and processes as they exist in the world. Quantitative research also involves disciplined enquiry based on reducing issues and problems to defined variables. Data collection involves measurement and observation under controlled conditions, enabling researchers to generate mechanistic or systems theories for explaining how variables are interrelated. The data are presented in a numerical form and are analysed using statistical techniques.

Qualitative research strategies include data collection which is aimed at understanding persons in their social environments. Rather than generating numerical data supporting or refuting clear-cut hypotheses, qualitative research aims to produce accurate descriptions based on face-to-face knowledge of individuals and social groups in their natural settings. The role of the observer in this context is crucial and usually involves physical and social closeness between the participant and the observer. Data collection involves objective and accurate reporting of the activities and appearances of persons in their natural environments. As with other strategies of research, investigators must pay considerable attention to the external and internal validity of qualitative research. We briefly looked at some ways in which qualitative researchers can cross-check their descriptions in an attempt to ensure the validity of their reports and interpretations.

Different research designs may be used to generate evidence of the same processes, although from different perspectives. For instance, any complex clinical phenomenon, such as schizophrenia, may be studied using any of the research strategies outlined in Chapters 7–10. To understand the scope of the problems and the effectiveness of the appropriate treatments, it is desirable to use a variety of research strategies. Conversely, a comprehensive theory of a clinical problem should generate any number of hypotheses within the realm of the research strategies discussed in this book. We will look at the analysis of qualitative data in Chapter 22.

The research process

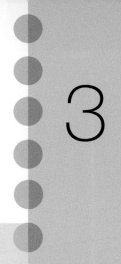

3

CHAPTER CONTENTS

Introduction 17

Sequential steps of the research process . . . 17

  1. Research problems and questions 18

  2. Planning. 18

  3. Design 18

  4. Data collection 18

  5. Organization and presentation of the data 19

  6. Data analysis 19

  7. Interpretation of the evidence 19

  8. Evaluation and dissemination
    of the results 19

The structure of a research paper 19

  Title and abstract 20

  Introduction 20

  Method. 20

  Results 21

  Discussion 21

  References and appendices 21

The style of research publications 21

The publication process 22

Research and evidence-based health care . . 22

Summary. 23

Introduction

The previous two chapters were concerned with conceptual and philosophical foundations of the scientific method. In this chapter, we will examine the method in a practical way, as it is applied to collecting research data and generating research evidence. Health research is conducted as a step-wise, problem-solving approach. The steps for conducting research are reflected in the way in which research is reported in professional journals (which you will be reading throughout your career as part of the process of keeping up to date). The central aim of this chapter is to enable you to read and understand original research. The specific aims of the chapter are to:

1. Outline the steps of the research process.

2. Describe the conventions for presenting published research.

3. Discuss the style and language used in publications.

4. Briefly outline the way in which research papers are selected for publication by journal editors.

Sequential steps of the research process

Although there are differences in how health scientists approach problems, Figure 3.1 shows the steps commonly followed in applied research. You might recognize this as an 'algorithm', a general way of solving problems. To illustrate the different steps, we will refer to a published research paper titled 'A qualitative study of GPs' views of treating obesity' by Epstein & Ogden (2005). You should access this publication from the *British Journal of General Practice* to enable you to follow the steps below.

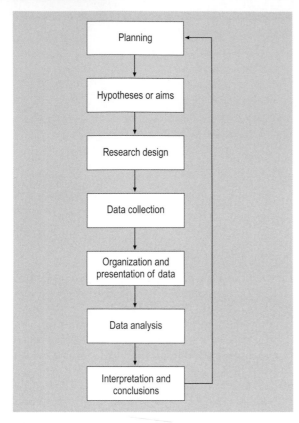

Figure 3.1 • The research process.

1. Research problems and questions

The first step in the problem-solving process is to state clearly and unambiguously the problem that we are intending to solve. Research problems reflect both the unmet health care needs of patients and opportunities created by new theoretical and technological advances for improving health care (see Chs 4 and 24). The problem must be realistic, one which can be solved with the resources at the researchers disposal. It is pointless, even unethical, to initiate research that cannot be completed (see Ch. 6).

Having identified a problem, our next step is to ask the 'right' research question (see Ch. 4). A well-formulated research question will guide the research project in producing the evidence required to answer the question and to solve the research problem. We will discuss in more detail

the way researchers formulate questions in Chapter 4. In the case of the paper by Epstein & Ogden (2005), the research problem was the lack of evidence concerning GPs' views of their treatment approaches to obesity. The research question is: *'How do general practitioners view the treatment of obesity?'* Therefore, the aim of the researchers was to obtain evidence to describe and understand GPs' views.

2. Planning

Research planning (see Section 2) involves selecting appropriate strategies and data collection techniques to answer research questions and to test the research hypotheses (we explain what these are in Chapter 4). Research planning relies on detailed knowledge of previous research summarized in a literature review. Also, the plan should take into consideration ethical and economic factors before the appropriate data collection strategies are collected and the precise research aims are stated. In addition, the planning process will take into account the target population and formulation of a sampling strategy to select the participants. In the present example, the population was defined as GPs working in London and the sample consisted of 21 GPs who consented to being interviewed for the study.

3. Design

Research designs are clear statements of how the research data are to be collected in the study. Appropriate research designs will guide data collection suitable for answering the research question (see Chs 7–10). In the study we are discussing, the design is described as *qualitative* research using semi-structured interviews. This design was appropriate for obtaining data pertinent to how GPs view the treatment of obesity.

4. Data collection

The next step in the research process is the collection of data. We will examine data collection methods employed in health research, including observation, measurement, in-depth interviews and focus groups, in Chapters 11–14.

5. Organization and presentation of the data

Descriptive statistics are used to organize and summarize quantitative data. Chapters 15–18 examine basic concepts in this area, outlining how graphs and various descriptive statistics are used to condense and communicate research and clinical findings. In qualitative research, the results are often presented in the form of direct quotations of what was expressed. In the study we are examining, the researchers provided a series of direct quotations of GPs' understanding and management of their patients' weight problems.

6. Data analysis

The analysis of quantitative data involves applying the principles of probability for calculating confidence intervals and testing the research hypotheses. Inferential statistics and decision-making is outlined in Chapters 19–20. The presentation and analysis of qualitative data involves identifying key themes which provide insights into participants' personal meanings of events and experiences. The way in which GPs conceptualized their responsibility in the management of obese patients and the role of the patients in this process were two key themes which emerged from the interviews.

7. Interpretation of the evidence

The next step in a research project is the interpretation of results (see Ch. 21). The evidence is used to answer the research question and may support existing theories or practices or suggest new techniques. It is rare that the findings from any single research project are completely definitive, and often the results may suggest the need for further investigation in related subject areas or contexts. In the discussion section, the authors reported that the GPs conceptualized obesity in terms of patient responsibility. It was suggested that future research was required to resolve an apparent conflict between the understanding of GPs and patients views of the management of obesity.

8. Evaluation and dissemination of the results

For research to be meaningful, investigators must present their results in professional journals and at conferences. Research findings become part of scientific knowledge only if they stand up to methodological critique and replication. We will outline steps for critically evaluating published research and demonstrate how evidence from various related publications can be synthesized for guiding evidence-based practices in Chapter 24. Epstein and Ogden disseminated their results by publishing their findings in the *British Journal of General Practice*. In doing so, the results of the study should generate further discussion and research.

The structure of a research paper

The format of a professional publication reporting health research generally reflects the stages of the research process discussed in this book. Table 3.1 represents the relationship between the stages of research and the commonly used publication format. This form is not exactly followed for all types of scholarly communications, such as for some

Table 3.1 Format of research publications and the research process	
Publication format	**Research process**
Title	
Abstract	
Introduction	Research planning
Method:	Design
Participants	
Apparatus	Measurement
Procedure	
Results	Descriptive statistics Inferential statistics
Discussion	Interpretation of the data
References	
Appendices	

qualitative research, theoretical papers or literature reviews, but it is used for most. In the subsections following, we examine in detail each of the components of a research report shown in Table 3.1.

Title and abstract

The *title* is a descriptive sentence stating the exact topic of the report. Many titles of quantitative research reports take one of the following two forms:

- *y* as a function of *x*
- the effect of *x* upon *y*.

In causal research, such as experiments, *y* refers to the dependent variable being measured and *x* refers to the independent variable being manipulated (see Ch. 7). For example:

- The incidence of alcoholism in health professionals as a function of work-related stress.
- The effect of major tranquillizers on the cognitive functioning of persons with schizophrenia.

For descriptive or qualitative research the title should inform the reader about the groups being studied and the characteristics being reported: for example, 'The experience of chronic pain in injured workers'. In general, titles should be concise and informative, enabling a prospective reader to identify the nature of the investigation. Immediately below the title should appear the name(s) of the investigator(s) and affiliation.

The *abstract* is a short (not more than 250 words) description of the entire report. The purpose of this section is to provide the reader with a general overview of the communication. It should provide enough details to enable the reader to decide whether or not the article is of interest. This section can be difficult to write because of its precise nature. When writing an abstract you should include:

1. A brief statement about previous findings that led you to conduct your own research.
2. The hypothesis and/or aim of your research.
3. Methods, including participants, apparatus and procedure.
4. A short description of what you found and how you interpreted your results.
5. What you concluded.

In some journals, this section may appear at the end of the manuscript in the form of a summary.

For our purposes, however, we will treat this section as an abstract.

The title and the abstract together are important and should contain *key words* that enable the efficient retrieval of the results.

Introduction

The introduction describes the planning stages of research, discussed previously. A good introduction sets the stage for the research question. It does this by discussing the theoretical background of the problem under consideration and describing and evaluating the relevant research previously completed. The introduction thus serves as a link between the past and the present knowledge.

Generally, all aspects of the previous research literature cannot be covered in a relatively brief research paper; therefore the review of past research is done with a bias towards only those aspects of the problem that are of direct relevance to your report. In this way the research question can be derived in a logical manner. For this reason, the introduction generally starts out by making a few general statements about the field of research, focusing logically to a narrow and specific set of statements which represent the research questions, aims or hypotheses.

Method

The purpose of the methods section is to inform the reader of exactly how the research study was carried out. It is important to remember that the method section should contain enough detail to enable another researcher to replicate your study. (Of course, replications may not be feasible for a unique event, such as a case study of a specific individual.) Conventionally, three subsections are used: participants, apparatus/tools and procedure.

Research participants

Three questions must be answered concerning the participants: who were they, how many were there and how were they selected? Specific information must be given concerning the participants, as results may vary from one sample to another. Ethical considerations are also to be discussed here.

Apparatus/tools

A description of all equipment, questionnaires and standardized tests used in the research must be provided. If it is commercially available, provide the reader with the manufacturer's name and the commercial identification of the equipment. Alternatively, if the equipment was privately made, provide the reader with enough information to allow replication. Measurements and perhaps a diagram will be necessary. In qualitative research, equipment often includes devices used to record interviews.

Procedure

Once again, this section should provide enough information for other researchers to replicate the study. Details of how the research was carried out should include how the research participants were assigned to groups, how many research participants per group, the experimental procedure and a description of how the data were collected.

Results

The results section presents the findings of the investigation and draws attention to points of interest. Raw data and statistical calculations are not presented in this section. Rather, we use the principles of descriptive and inferential statistics to present the summarized and analysed data: graphs, tables and the outcomes of statistical tests are presented in this section. It is essential that all the findings are presented and that the graphs and tables are correctly identified. Qualitative researchers will present original quotes from participants and describe how analysis was conducted.

Discussion

The discussion section restates the aim(s) of the research study and discusses your results with reference to the aims or research hypothesis stated in the introduction. Did you find what you expected? How do the present results relate to previous research?

It is important to remember that one study in isolation cannot make or break a theory or establish the effectiveness of a practice. Thus, the discussion should connect the findings with similar studies and especially with the theory underlying such studies. If unexpected results were obtained, possible reasons for the outcome (such as faulty design and controls) should be discussed. By this, the discussion will point the way to further problems that remain to be solved. Unconstructive, negative or unimportant criticism should be avoided, so that the report does not end with long discussions of possible reasons for the outcome. Brief, concise discussion is more appropriate.

In the conclusion, which is usually the last paragraph of the discussion section, the main findings are summarized and suggestions made for further research. For example, you may have demonstrated certain phenomena that may have implications for explaining broader concepts which can be empirically tested. You are therefore taking your findings and generalizing them to phenomena not directly tested in the present research.

References and appendices

It is expected that all the literature discussed in the paper is listed in the references section. This enables your reader to evaluate your sources. You should refer to appropriate style manuals for information on how references should be listed. Sufficient information must be provided for an interested reader to be able to identify and retrieve the sources. In addition, a report may include labelled appendices. These might include a full description of questionnaires or other measuring instruments, raw data or statistical calculations if required.

The style of research publications

It is essential that you read research publications in your professional area to gain a 'feel' for the appropriate style of writing research papers and reports. In general, the following points should be kept in mind when writing reports:

1. Avoid long phrases or complicated sentences. Short, simple sentences are far more easily understood by your reader. In other words, try not to posture but to communicate.

2. Use quotations sparingly; put ideas in your own words. Quotations are only used when it is necessary to convey precisely the ideas of another researcher, for instance while conducting a critique of a paper.

3. Use past tense when writing your research report.

4. Use an objective style, avoiding personal pronouns wherever possible.

5. Make sure you are writing to your audience; if the material is specialized or difficult, explain it clearly.

6. Make sure that you are concise and clear; do not introduce issues and concepts which are not strictly relevant to reporting your investigation. Raising interesting but superfluous issues might distract and confuse your reader.

In general, you should aim to improve your report writing and your ability to communicate your findings and ideas by seeking constructive criticism from your colleagues and supervisors.

The publication process

The formal knowledge representing the empirical and professional basis for your professional practice is in large part stored in journals, books and conference reports. Journals are published by appropriate professional associations, government departments or private companies. Having completed a research project, how does one publish it in a professional journal? After all, the value of research is negligible if it is not made public.

In general, the prospective author will:

1. Select a professional or scientific journal appropriate for the material.

2. Present the research report in a format required by the journal.

3. Send the completed manuscript to the journal's editor.

The editor is generally a person of high standing in a given scientific or professional area. If the article is judged as being appropriate for the journal, the editor will send the article to two or more peer reviewers and, on the basis of the reviewers' reports, publish or reject the manuscript. Sometimes the reviewers recommend certain additions or changes which have to be made by the author before the manuscript is judged to be publishable.

Therefore, when you read research publications in peer reviewed journals, you can be confident that the articles have been scrutinized by experts. However, as shown in the next section, this does not necessarily guarantee the truth of either the evidence or the conclusions.

Research and evidence-based health care

Research methods cover a wide variety of skills and techniques aimed at the methodologically valid investigation of questions of interest to the researcher. These methods of enquiry are not restricted to research laboratories, nor need they involve expensive equipment or large research teams. Rather, these methods imply an approach to stating and answering questions in any setting.

Research in the health sciences may focus on issues such as the prevalence and causes of illness, the usefulness and accuracy of assessment techniques, or the effectiveness of treatments. Applied research which is published aims at producing findings that are of general interest to groups of professionals working in the health sciences.

Research methods interact with health practices in multiple and mutually productive ways. An important general aim of this textbook is to discuss the relationships between theories, practices and the ways in which research methods contribute to improvements in health care. The term 'evidence-based medicine' has been defined by Sackett et al (2000) as '... the integration of best research evidence with clinical expertise and patient values'. Evidence-based health care is a contemporary movement aimed at ensuring that health services are based on the best available scientific and clinical evidence. The fundamental question that is explored in this book is 'what constitutes best research evidence to inform clinical practice?' The evidence is, of course, produced by health research conducted in accordance with the principles of the scientific method. Clearly if you expect to participate in the delivery of evidence-based health care you will need to understand research methods sufficiently for making informed and critical judgements concerning the quality of the available evidence to drive high quality and effective clinical practice.

Finally, we need to keep in mind that the research is produced by the hard work of men and women who were undergraduate students, just like you. Ultimately it will be up to you (as nurses, podiatrists, physiotherapists, speech pathologists and occupational therapists) to carry out the research that underpins the effectiveness, advancement and prestige of your profession. If not you, then who?

Summary

In this chapter we discussed the ways in which the scientific method is directly applicable to conducting research in the health sciences. The sequential steps of the research process follow a general problem-solving algorithm. Identifying these steps enables you to understand the rationale underlying the planning, conduct and interpretation of research. We outlined how the general format of a published research paper is associated with these steps. We also examined the style and structure of a research publication. The style involves clarity, accuracy and sufficient completeness for colleagues to understand or replicate the research project. Research is published in journals, which are generally edited by persons of high standing in the field. Every effort is made by editors to ensure the validity of the research published in their journals. The individual researcher is also ethically bound to report findings in an unbiased and truthful fashion. Although the format and style outlined in this chapter might seem rather arduous, poor presentation may destroy the intrinsic value of a research project.

Section 2

Research planning

4 The formulation of research questions 27
5 Sampling methods and external validity. 33
6 Ethics. 43

The first stage of research involves the detailed planning of the project. The plan for what is to occur in the project is written up in a document called the research protocol. Before the research project may proceed, the protocol is examined by ethics committees and funding bodies to ensure that it conforms with general methodological and ethical principles. The three chapters of Section 2 aim to outline the basic considerations for the successful preparation of a research protocol.

The primary reason for carrying out a research project is to obtain evidence that will advance theory and practice in the health sciences (see Ch. 4). Before all else, we must be sure that we are asking the right questions; that is, raising issues and problems which are central to progress in contemporary health care. We must convince the critical reader that our aims of the hypotheses which we are attempting to resolve are of central importance. Asking the right research questions depends on being creative; for example, identifying ignored patterns in data, or the construction of novel theories that predict new, as yet unobserved phenomena.

To justify the research proposal it is necessary to write a 'literature review'. The literature review is a summary and critical evaluation of previous research and theory relevant to the problem we are intending to investigate. In this way the literature review provides both a conceptual background for our proposal and justifies the need for further empirical evidence by identifying 'gaps' in our knowledge.

The way in which samples are selected is discussed in Chapter 5. Selection of an appropriate sample is crucial for the generalizability (or external validity) of your findings. Our aim is to select a representative sample of the population but this may not always be possible in health sciences research. We need a sample size which is sufficiently large to identify the phenomena in which we are interested, but not too large or we are simply wasting resources.

A project cannot proceed unless it is judged to be ethical by an appropriate committee (see Ch. 6). A research proposal is judged ethical if it conforms to our rules of conduct and values concerning caregiving. These rules and values are made explicit in documents representing the standards of professional groups and of institutions (e.g. hospitals, universities and research councils). The research protocol must be described in sufficient detail so that a decision can be made as to whether any harm might occur to participants in the research project.

Economic considerations, or the availability of resources, also have a strong influence on research planning. For example, you may have designed a qualitative research project which involves 100 'in depth' interviews with persons suffering from a disorder. Say you have only one year and a very limited amount of money to complete your project. You would be advised either to reduce your sample size, or, if this is not possible, change your topic. Ethics or funding bodies will only approve projects which can feasibly be completed with the available resources.

Thus, research planning is a process through which we transform our ideas into a well-planned, ethical and realistic research project.

The formulation of research questions 4

CHAPTER CONTENTS

Introduction 27

Identifying research problems . . . . , 27

   Environmental and social changes 27

   Demographic changes. 28

   Scientific and technological advances. . . . 28

   The cost-effectiveness of health services . . 28

Literature reviews and research 29

Formulating the research question 29

Methodological considerations 30

   Deciding between using qualitative
and quantitative methods in your research . 30

   Research participants and sampling. 30

   Study design 30

Ethical issues and procedures 31

Aims and hypotheses 31

Research proposals 31

Summary 32

Introduction

The planning of a research study begins with the identification of a research problem, followed by the formulation of a research question. In the introduction of a research paper you will find the research question guiding the investigation. The formulation of a research question is the outcome of a complex, iterative process. Researchers refine and focus the question, as they plan the stages of the research project, as shown in Figure 4.1. There is a close relationship between the process of conducting research and the way in which research questions are formulated.

The aims of this chapter are to:

1. Describe the process for identifying research problems.
2. Discuss the use of literature reviews for developing research questions.
3. Describe the relationship between formulating research questions and methodology.
4. Explain the relevance of ethics and resources to the statement of specific aims and hypotheses.
5. Describe what constitutes a research proposal.

Identifying research problems

In health research many research problems are often focused on identifying effective interventions for preventing or treating health problems. However not all research problems are concerned solely with treatment. There are numerous other research problems, including gaps in our knowledge of the causes and consequences of health problems and an opportunity to improve the quality of our practices. Let us look at some examples of some research problems.

Environmental and social changes

As the biological and social environment changes, new health problems may emerge. For example,

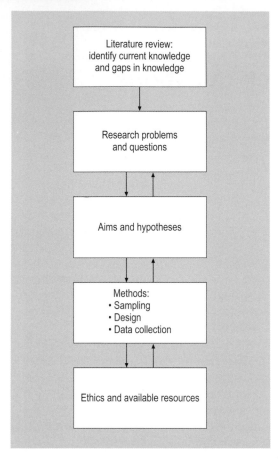

Figure 4.1 • Formulating the research question.

abundant food supplies and increasingly sedentary lifestyles have led to a high prevalence of obesity in some communities. Obesity is a serious risk factor for a numerous health problems including, type 2 diabetes and coronary heart disease. The research problem of interest to a researcher may be the lack of effective interventions for preventing and reducing obesity in the community.

Another example is the health impact of climate change, a process which is predicted to impact on population health. The environmental changes (in particular the prediction of global warming) act as impetus to identifying new research problems as further research is required to provide the evidence. Many countries have research priorities based on the prevalence of diseases as identified by epidemiological studies (see Ch. 8). Public and political concern of the 'burden of disease' in a community may result in funding bodies preferentially channelling resources to researchers in these

areas since the identified health problems are the most pressing and expensive to the communities in question.

Demographic changes

Changes in population characteristics, such as the increasing proportion of elderly people, have shifted the health needs of communities in most countries. There is increased research activity concerning the health problems associated with ageing and the ways of designing and delivering effective and efficient health services. Also, in many counties there now are immigrants and asylum-seekers who have health needs different to the rest of the population, as they may have language or socio-cultural barriers which prevent them from accessing the appropriate services. The research problems arise from the limitations of the current health services being offered to a population with changing needs.

Scientific and technological advances

There are continuing and remarkable discoveries in the biological, behavioural, social and information sciences that can be applied to improving the assessment, treatment and prevention of illnesses. Advances in electronics and information technology have created opportunities in a variety of health professions, devising new diagnostic techniques or data collection and management strategies. The research problems arise from the need to *translate* pure research into practical solutions. An example of this is stem cell research, which has led to spectacular discoveries in the biological sciences. Translational research aims to develop cellular therapies for the treatment of a variety of disorders such as heart disease, diabetes and Parkinson's disease.

The cost-effectiveness of health services

Economic pressures from increasing health costs require that service providers are accountable for the way in which they use available resources. Program evaluations for services are now routinely incorporated into service delivery. Evidence from this research is necessary to demonstrate that the resources are being used in the best way and that the services are meeting the needs of patients and the community. While often a source of stress for health professionals and administrators who participate in them, well-designed evaluation programs can contribute to the development of cost-effective, 'value for money' services to the community. For example, if you can demonstrate that program A and program B provide the same benefits but A costs half as much as B to deliver, then you will have made a significant contribution to health care. The money saved can be used to provide better services to other people.

We hope the above discussion demonstrates to you that there are innumerable research problems waiting for you when you graduate! Perhaps you will take up the challenge and by asking the right questions produce research which will contribute to the advancement of health care.

Literature reviews and research

Before embarking on the design and conduct of a research project, the investigator must review previous work and publications relevant to the aims of the intended project (the process of literature review is described in detail in Chapter 24). This process is essential, both for providing the appropriate background and context for the investigation, and for justifying the investigation in contributing to existing knowledge. It is potentially a waste of money to inadvertently duplicate very similar research (although deliberate replication of previous studies may be a legitimate activity if there are uncertainties about the validity of a previous research). Another reason for reviewing the literature is to examine how previous researchers have approached sampling, design, data collection and analysis decisions in their research. There are benefits in reviewing how previous researchers succeeded or failed in achieving their objectives.

There are several standard approaches to identifying research papers of interest to a specific research study or problem. An example is PICO (see http://pubmedhh.nlm.nih.gov/), an acronym for:

P = Target Population/Patients.
I = Intervention (or type of exposure).
C = Comparison (alternative intervention).
O = The Outcome measures.

By examining the keywords, title and abstract of a paper, you can see how the above criteria apply. Imagine that you are interested in identifying papers investigating the efficacy of neural transplantation for treating Parkinson's disease. Using PICO, you should be able to find the following paper by Olanow et al (2003) 'A double-blind controlled trial of bilateral fetal nigral transplantation in Parkinson's disease'. Here:

P represents patients with Parkinson's disease.
I refers to the bilateral fetal nigral transplants.
C refers to the placebo surgery group.
O refers to outcomes on standardized tests.

Literature searching may be carried out at appropriate research centres or libraries where scientific and professional journals are stored and, of course, by using the Internet. In health research, as opposed to historical research, almost all searches use Internet search engines and electronic journals databases. There are powerful web-based search methods that can simplify the search. The most widely used search tool for health research publications is probably PubMed, the web-based Public Medline (see http://www.ncbi.nlm.nih.gov/entrez/). Professional library staff can help you to locate the relevant literature. However, the critical evaluation of the literature depends on the application of research methods for the identification of controversies or 'gaps' in the available evidence (see Ch. 24). A detailed and critical review of the literature enables us to ask the questions most relevant to planning the kind of research that will enable us to address the research problem.

Formulating the research question

To formulate a research question, we need to investigate what is known and what is not known in the area (i.e. to identify what we know and what we do not know in the existing published literature). By stating the research problem and reviewing the literature, we are able to devise a research question. The research question will guide the investigation and guide us in producing the evidence required to solve the research problem. Inspiration for research questions may stem from direct personal experience as well as literature review and analysis. Exposure to an issue or problems may raise questions suitable for a research study. The identification of research questions is a creative act. It draws upon consideration of previous relevant work in the area under study. This work may be reviewed and the review may give rise to questions that have not been answered by previous work.

Methodological considerations

The precisely stated research question requires an examination of the proposed methodology of the project. To illustrate the methodological issues, let us look at an example based on a publication titled 'Ribavirin for Crimean-Congo haemorrhagic fever: systematic review and meta-analysis'. The health problem is the Crimean-Congo haemorrhagic fever (CCHF) which is a potentially lethal viral disease. There is a drug called ribavirin which has been approved by the World Health Organization (WHO) and has been used with apparent success to reduce the mortality rate associated with CCHF. A review by Soares-Weiser et al (2010), identifies a research question regarding the efficacy of ribavirin:

> No clear message of benefit is available from the current data on ribavirin as observational data are heavily confounded, and the one trial carried out has limited power. However ribavirin could potentially have benefits in this condition...

Let us imagine that we are scientists working in public health and that we want to contribute to solving this problem. The first thing to do is to formulate a precise research question and, if appropriate, a research hypothesis derived from the research question. To do this, we need to plan the data collection process for conducting the investigation.

Deciding between using qualitative and quantitative methods in your research

An essential consideration is whether we will use a qualitative or a quantitative research method. Quantitative research is normally structured so as to test a research hypothesis. Hypotheses are propositions about relationships between variables or differences between groups that are to be tested. Qualitative research does not usually test hypotheses. It is concerned with understanding the personal meanings and interpretations of people concerning specified issues. However, most qualitative researchers work with specified research aims and questions to guide their investigation. As we mentioned in Chapters 1 and 2, some research questions require both qualitative and quantitative methods (mixed methods).

For our hypothetical example, we would select a quantitative approach. The reason is that we intend to test a *causal* hypothesis that ribavirin, an anti-viral drug, is effective for treating CCHF. If we were investigating the experiences of patients undertaking this treatment, we would have selected a qualitative approach. The next step will be to refine our research hypothesis, taking into account the sample and proposed design.

Research participants and sampling

To focus our hypothesis, we need to define the population we wish to study. In the ribavirin example, our study population consists of people living in regions where CCHF is a public health concern. According to Soares-Weiser al (2010), recent outbreaks have occurred in Turkey and Iran. Due to pragmatic reasons (see following section), you might select people living in Turkey as your population of interest. We will look at details of sampling in Chapter 5.

Study design

In Section 3 we will look at research designs in detail. As discussed previously, we have selected a quantitative methodological approach for our hypothetical investigation. There are several types of research designs which fall under quantitative methods; the most basic distinction is whether they are *experimental* or *non-experimental observational* designs (see Section 3). In our example, we are investigating a causal hypothesis; therefore we would select an experimental design. As discussed in Chapter 7, a randomized controlled trial (RCT) would be the preferred design for establishing the efficacy of ribavirin.

In an RCT, the participants are assigned (by chance or random method) to a treatment (intervention) or control (non-intervention) group, and then given the intervention or, in clinical contexts, the treatment. In our example, the treatment is the quantity and administration of the ribavirin. We also need to make a decision about the type of control group we will use (i.e. no treatment, placebo treatment or current standard treatment other than ribavirin). The intervention and control groups are then observed and compared. At this point, we must consider how we are going to measure outcomes for enabling us to make a comparison. The selection of outcome measures is discussed in detail in Chapters 11–14. In this case, since CCHF is a potentially fatal condition, we should use mortality rates as our indicator of treatment efficacy.

Ethical issues and procedures

When conducting health care research, a primary concern is the wellbeing and dignity of the research participants (see Ch. 6). Ethical considerations will influence the sample selected, the design of a project and, ultimately, the research question which will be posed. In addition, the available resources such as time and money will determine the scope of the research project. In our present hypothetical example we have decided to:

- Select the sample only from Turkey for financial reasons.
- For ethical reasons, use a best-available treatment for the participants in the control group.
- Use mortality as an outcome measure.

All studies need to be ethically cleared by a properly constituted human research ethics committee (see Chapter 6 for a detailed discussion of ethics processes).

Aims and hypotheses

Having considered the methodology and ethics, we are able to refine our research question as follows: 'Is ribavirin more effective than best-available current treatment for reducing mortality in people with CCHF living in Turkey?' Our aim is to collect evidence showing the efficacy of CCHF. In general, the aims of a research project are to produce evidence for answering the research question. Both qualitative and quantitative research projects have clear-cut aims. Quantitative research may also test hypotheses. As mentioned previously, hypotheses are predictive statements about the relationship between the intervention and the outcome variables (see Ch. 1).

Because we have selected a quantitative method to investigate the question, we can also state a research hypothesis: 'Ribavirin treatment will reduce mortality more than best-available treatment in people with CCHF living in Turkey'. The obtained results will enable us to make a decision as to whether or not the research hypothesis is supported by the data we collect. This decision will enable us to answer the research question and contribute to solving the original research problem. You will recall that the research problem was an uncertainty regarding the efficacy of ribavirin. Figure 4.1 represents the steps that are followed to develop detailed and precise aims and hypotheses.

Research proposals

By the time we have stated our precise aims or hypotheses, we have also worked out in detail the way in which the data are to be collected. This information is written up as a research proposal. A research proposal is an explicit statement of how and why you intend to conduct a research project. A research proposal will contain the following information:

- Identification of the research problem.
- Literature review.
- Research aims and hypotheses must take into consideration the:
  - participants to be selected
  - data to be collected
  - research design/s
  - ethical considerations
  - estimated cost.

The research proposal is circulated to various individuals and committees in order to obtain critical feedback from supervisors, institutions and your fellow students concerning the practicality and quality of your research project. Most importantly, the research proposal is the basis for writing a detailed report to relevant ethics committees (see Ch. 6).

It is often desirable to carry out a small-scale preliminary study called a *pilot study*. This is an economical way of identifying and eliminating potential problems before you do the large-scale (and expensive) full study. Case studies and so-called safety and efficacy studies are often employed before randomized controlled trials are undertaken (see Ch. 9).

Summary

The planning of a research project requires the transformation of preliminary thoughts on solving a research problem into clearly stated research questions and aims. To achieve this, the researcher should review the relevant literature and evaluate ethical considerations and economic constraints in conducting the investigation. Next, an appropriate research strategy has to be formulated. Having considered the stages of the research project, the researcher is in a position to state precisely the aims or hypotheses being investigated. Before data collection begins, a research proposal must be scrutinized by an ethics committee to resolve methodological problems and to ensure the implementation of ethical research.

Sampling methods and external validity

CHAPTER CONTENTS

Introduction 33

What is sampled in a study 33

Basic issues in sampling 34

Representative samples 34

    Incidental samples 35

    Random and systematic samples 36

Sample size 37

    Sampling error 37

Sampling issues in qualitative research 38

Purposive sampling 39

External validity and sampling 40

    Ecological validity 41

Summary 41

Introduction

Research in the health sciences usually involves the collection of information from a sample of participants, rather than on the entire population in which the investigator is interested. Studies that involve an entire population or group are called census studies but these are relatively rare and generally expensive to perform. A sample drawn from the target population is studied because it is usually impossible or too costly to study entire populations. For instance, when individuals who have conditions such as diabetes, cerebral palsy or emphysema are being studied, it is not possible to study everyone because of the large size of such populations. Also because many people do not seek treatment or may be wrongly diagnosed, we may not be able to identify all members of the entire population in order to study them. Therefore, in most research, the researcher studies a subset or sample of the target population, and then attempts to generalize the findings to the population from which the participants were drawn. This general principle applies to both qualitative and quantitative studies.

The aim of this chapter is to examine ways in which samples can be drawn to permit the investigator to make valid generalizations from the study sample to the target population.

We will also consider the question of generalizing the findings of an investigation to other samples and situations. This is referred to as 'external validity' or 'generalizability'.

The specific aims of this chapter are to:

1. Define what is meant by sampling and representative samples.
2. Outline the relative advantages and disadvantages of commonly used sampling methods.
3. Discuss the relationship between sampling error and sample size.
4. Examine the concept of external validity for generalizing research findings to other settings.

What is sampled in a study

While this chapter will focus on the selection of the research participants in a study, many

Table 5.1 Examples of populations and samples

Population	Possible sample selection
All working podiatrists in a state	50 podiatrists selected for a study of job satisfaction
All working pathologists in a state	25 pathologists selected for detailed tax evaluation by an inspector
The temperature of a patient during a 24-h period	Hourly measurements of a patient's temperature recorded by staff
Stuttering in a child's speech	Number of stutters made during 5 min of reading a standard piece of material
All patients in a state with frontal lobe damage	30 patients with frontal lobe damage selected for evaluating a rehabilitation program
All surgical gauzes held by a given hospital	10 gauzes selected by a bacteriologist to test for sterility

other things are also selected or sampled. These include:

1. The information to be collected by the researcher.
2. The procedures used for the collection of the information.
3. Where the research is conducted, e.g. in a field setting or in a structured research setting.
4. The clinicians and researchers who are involved.

Many researchers focus on the selection of the research participants as the key or only issue in maximizing the generalizability of their research and they do not pay enough attention to the other factors they are sampling or the context in which the research is being conducted. It is not at all unusual to see studies that employ large and sophisticated participant samples yet with only one or two highly selected clinicians involved in the research in perhaps only one health setting. While the study sample may be highly representative the context in which the research is conducted may not be and it may be that the researchers and clinicians involved in the study have a particularly unusual or idiosyncratic approach to their work that is not reflective of others. It is our contention that, in many qualitative studies, there is strong consideration of the research context and its impact upon the research findings. However, there is often less emphasis upon sampling of research participants. This impacts upon the ability to generalize the findings more broadly from the actual research participants to other groups.

Basic issues in sampling

As we have discussed, often, because of the numbers involved, it is not within the resources of the researcher to study the whole target population. In any event, in most situations it would be wasteful to study all of the population. If a sample is representative, one can generalize validly from the sample's results to the population without going to the expense of studying everyone.

The population is the target group of individuals or cases in which the researcher is interested. Examples of valid study populations include: all English women under 25; all children with diagnosed spina bifida in the state of Alberta; all the students at a particular Australian college. The researcher defines the population to which he/she wishes to generalize. Note that a population need not consist of human participants or animal subjects. Objects or events can also be sampled, as shown in Table 5.1.

As can be seen from Table 5.1, a population is an entire set of persons, objects or events which the researcher intends to study. A sample is a subset of the population. Sampling involves the selection of the sample from the population.

Representative samples

There is a variety of different ways by which one can select the sample from the population. These are called sampling methods.

The ultimate aim of all sampling methods is to draw a representative sample from the population.

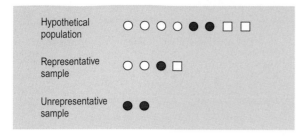

Figure 5.1 • A simple representative sample.

The advantage of a representative sample is clear: one can confidently generalize from a representative sample to the rest of the population without having to take the trouble of studying the rest of the population. If the sample is biased (not representative of the population) one can generalize less validly from the sample to the population. This might lead to quite incorrect conclusions or inferences about the population. This would mean that the results obtained in the study would not necessarily generalize to other studies using the same population. Figure 5.1 illustrates the concept of a representative sample.

Figure 5.1 illustrates a hypothetical population composed of three different types of study participants or categories of participants. A representative sample is a precise miniaturized representation of the population. An unrepresentative or biased sample does not adequately represent the key groups or characteristics in the population, and this may lead to mistaken conclusions about the state of the population.

The selection of the appropriate sampling method depends upon the aims and resources of the researchers. For instance, if someone is designing a very expensive health or social welfare program on the basis of a survey of clients' needs, it is imperative that the researcher uses a good sampling method and obtains a representative sample of the clients, so that appropriate conclusions may be reached about the population. Good sampling methods are somewhat more expensive and more difficult to implement than poor methods but they are worth it. The main sampling methods used in health research are incidental and random sampling.

Incidental samples

Incidental sampling

Incidental sampling is the cheapest, easiest and most commonly used sampling method in clinical studies. It involves the selection of the most accessible and available members of the target population. For example, a researcher who stands in the middle of a city street and quizzes people about their health status is practising incidental sampling. However, it is quite likely that this sample would not be representative of the general voting population. There would probably be an over-representation of businessmen and white-collar workers, and an under-representation of factory workers and housewives. The sample is likely to be unrepresentative and biased.

A further example of incidental sampling might involve a researcher surveying the needs of a group of spina bifida children at a local community health centre. Their measured needs may be representative of those of other spina bifida children but then again they may not if these children are not typical of the wider population of children with spina bifida.

Thus, incidental sampling is cheap and easy to implement but may give a biased sample that is not representative of the population.

Quota sampling

Sometimes it is known in advance that there are important subgroups within the population that need to be included in the sample. Two such important groups within the human population are males and females. Further, it is known that they occur in the ratio of approximately 49:51 in the general population. Our researcher might decide that it is very important that the sexes are proportionally represented in the sample. Thus, the researcher would set two quotas of 49 male and 51 female respondents in a sample of 100. This is still a form of incidental sampling but has some significant advantages over simple incidental sampling because the study sample's composition on this key demographic variable is guaranteed to match that of the target population.

More sophisticated examples involving more than two groups can be accommodated as shown in Table 5.2. We can see from Table 5.2 that, if our sample were to be representative regarding both sex and occupational status, in a sample of 100 people we would need 19 blue-collar males, 15 blue-collar females, and so on.

Quota sampling still has a number of shortcomings: before it can be used, one has to know which population groups are likely to be important to

Table 5.2 Distribution of percentages of gender and occupational variables in the general population

	Blue collar	White collar	Not employed 'no collar'	Total
Male	19	21	9	49
Female	15	15	21	51
Total	34	36	30	100

a particular question and the exact proportions of the various groups in the population. Sometimes we may not know these proportions. Also, the members of the sample within the quotas are still incidentally chosen. The blue-collar males, for example, selected in a city centre on a weekday may still be quite different from those working elsewhere. However, quota sampling is better than simple incidental sampling.

Random and systematic samples

Random sampling

This is one of the best but probably more expensive sampling methods to implement in drawing a study sample. A random sample is one in which all members of the population have an equal chance of selection. Thus a random sample is more likely to be representative of the relevant population than an incidental sample.

The procedure for drawing a random sample involves:

- The construction of a list of all members of the population.
- Using a method such as dice, coins, hat or random number tables to select randomly from the list the number of members required for the sample.

A simple example of a random sample is provided by a common raffle, where names on (preferably!) equal size papers are put in a hat, shaken and selected 'blind'. Many national and state lotteries use numbered balls that are drawn randomly from a barrel. Another way to draw a random sample is to construct a list of all the members of the population and assign a number to each element. Then a table of random numbers, generated by a computer, could be used to select a random sample.

Cases that are selected from a list using a random selection method constitute a random sample. Sometimes, because of issues such as refusal to participate in the study, dropping out and failure

to satisfy the sample inclusion criteria, it is necessary to select replacements for some cases that are unavailable for the study. This can introduce bias into the sample, as the people who refuse may differ consistently from those who accept or volunteer. This impact on sampling validity is sometimes called the volunteer effect.

However, random sampling methods have a number of important advantages over incidental or non-random methods:

- Because the exact sizes of the sample and population are known, it is possible to estimate exactly how representative the sample is: that is, the size of the sampling error. This cannot usually be done with non-random sampling methods.
- Because random samples are usually more representative than non-random samples, the sample size needed for good representation of the population is smaller.

The major disadvantages of random sampling methods are:

- The researcher needs to be able to list every member of the population. Often this is impossible because the full extent of the population is not known. For example, it would be very difficult to sample randomly from the population of Canadians with coronary disease, because no such list exists. Even if it did exist it would be constantly changing.
- Cost. It is usually easier to use conveniently available groups. Random sampling usually involves considerable planning and expense, especially with large populations.

Stratified random sampling

This involves the same approach as quota sampling with set quotas from specific subgroups, except that each quota is filled by randomly sampling from each subgroup, rather than sampling incidentally. For example, if one was drawing a sample stratified with respect to sex, one would prepare a list of all females and all males in the target population and then sample randomly from these lists with the numbers of each group in the sample corresponding to the population proportions. These groups collectively are called the strata.

The advantages of stratified random sampling are:

- All the important groups are proportionally represented.
- The exact representativeness of the sample is known. This has important statistical ramifications.

The disadvantages are:

- A list of all members of the population, their characteristics and the proportions of the important groups within the population need to be known.
- Cost.
- The gain in sample accuracy is usually small in comparison to simple random sampling.

Area sampling

In area sampling, one samples on the basis of location of cases. For example, on the basis of census data, the investigator may select several areas in a city or county with known characteristics, such as high or low unemployment rates. The areas could then be further divided into specific streets and the occupants of, say, every third house contacted for participation in the study. In other words, the locations are randomly selected and then one interviews the occupants of those locations. This can be a very effective, cheap method of sampling in social surveys. It does not require a list of the individual members of the population, merely the location where they live. Recent research has shown that where people live can be an important factor in their health status and their use of health services. The study of the impact of where people live upon health and social issues is sometimes called (geo-) spatial analysis.

Systematic sampling

This involves working through a list of the population and choosing, say, every tenth or twentieth case for inclusion in the sample. It is not a truly random technique but it will usually give a representative sample. It is based on the (usually justified) supposition that cases are not added to the list in a systematic way which coincides with the sampling system. Provided a list of cases is available, systematic sampling is an easy and convenient sampling method. In clinical practice we are using systematic sampling when, for instance, we measure temperature and blood pressure every hour.

Sample size

One of the most poorly understood aspects of sampling is the number of cases that should be included in a study sample. The whole issue of sampling is conceptualized somewhat differently for qualitative and quantitative studies, although the issue of to what extent the results of a study are generalizable is the same whatever the study design.

It is obvious that in one sense the more cases selected the merrier (or the better the sample representativeness), but the costs associated with the sampling and data collection must be weighed against the greater generalizability that is generally associated with larger samples. Also, some studies may involve discomfort, pain, or even danger to patients or laboratory animals. Therefore in this case it is ethically and logistically desirable to ensure that no more than the bare minimum of participants is used to achieve the desired sample accuracy. Health researchers 'walk a tightrope' in deciding the optimum sample sizes for their studies. However, there are some principles available to guide the researcher.

First of all, let us say quite definitely that there is no magic number that we can point to as an 'optimum' sample size. Rather, the optimum sample size depends on the characteristics of an investigation, in the context of which the sample is drawn. In general, the optimum sample size is one which is adequate for making correct generalization from the sample to the target population. Let us discuss these issues by introducing the concept of sampling error.

Sampling error

In the quantitative research framework, sampling error is the discrepancy between the true population parameter and the sample statistic. For example, if I happen to know from census data that the actual average age of males in a district is 35 years and the average age of a sample of males I have surveyed from the district is 30 years, then I have a sampling error of 5 years. However, if we do not know the actual population parameters (which is commonly the case), we can only estimate the probable sampling error.

Sampling error is related to sample size *(n)* by the following relationship:

$$\text{Sampling error} = \frac{1}{\sqrt{n}}$$

The above equation indicates that the greater the sample size, the smaller the probable sampling error.

From this relationship it can be seen that doubling the sample size would only result in a reduction of the error by a factor of the square root of 2 (1.414). Similarly, a nine-fold increase in sample size would result in only a three-fold reduction in the sampling error. Figure 5.2 illustrates this point by showing the graphical relationship between probable sampling error and sample size.

It can be seen from this graph that not much is gained from a sample size of over, say, 300. Yet the cost of the sampling and data collection can be very high with large numbers for relatively little gain in reducing sampling error. In some research situations, even large probable sampling errors have relatively little potential influence on our decisions. In such situations, we can live with a relatively small sample size. In other situations, we need large samples to justify our confidence in the truth of our decisions.

As an illustration, suppose that we are attempting to predict the outcome of an election fought between two political parties: A and B. A representative sample of 100 respondents is polled before the election. Say the outcome is as follows:

Intends to vote for A: 25%.

Intends to vote for B: 75%.

Estimated sampling error: 10%.

In this instance, the estimated sampling error is very small in relation to the size of the effect (i.e. the difference between the percentage of intended votes for the two parties). We can predict confidently, assuming that the respondents were truthful and don't change their minds before the elections, that political party B will romp into government. Increasing sample size, say to 10000, would enormously increase the cost of the survey. The corresponding reduction in sampling error would not justify this cost, as we would still come to the same conclusion. However, say the following sample statistics were obtained in the pre-election poll of 100 respondents:

Intends to vote for A: 48%.

Intends to vote for B: 52%.

Estimated sampling error: 10%.

Now, the same level of estimated sampling error is too large, in relation to the apparent size of the effect, to make a decision concerning which party is likely to win the election. The poll would have to be repeated using a substantially increased sample size to reduce the sampling error.

The above example illustrates the notion that the adequacy of the sample size is affected by the specific situation that we are trying to research. A sample size which is adequate in one situation may be inadequate in another. One benefit of a previous pilot study is that it allows the researcher to estimate the size of the phenomenon under study, and thereby make a more educated guess concerning the sample size required. The concept of statistical 'power' or the ability to detect real effects or differences is discussed later in this text.

Sampling issues in qualitative research

Qualitative research shares with quantitative research a concern with the extent to which findings from one study can be generalized to other settings and people. Therefore the representativeness

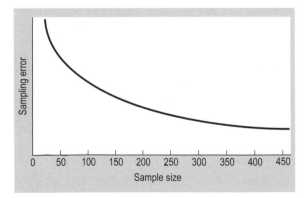

Figure 5.2 • The relationship between sample size and sampling error. The scaling but not the form of the curve will alter with the variability of the data.

of the information obtained from the sample is important in qualitative research. However, there are differences in the way in which a representative sample is conceptualized in qualitative research.

The key difference is the way in which the population is defined. In quantitative research we make the assumption that there is a true knowable state of the population. The true state of the population is represented by an actual parameter, such as '49% of the Australian population are females' or 'the average IQ of Canadian high-school students is 104'. Qualitative research is not concerned with measuring quantities or counting frequencies but with the experiences and meanings of these experiences for individuals and communities. Sampling in qualitative research is referred to as purposive; the researchers deliberately select the participants who are best placed to provide the information for understanding the personal meanings of health-related events. For example, what is it like to survive a heart attack? What does it mean for patients to undergo transplantation surgery? Our sample provides the information which enables us to understand the emotional processes of coping with a heart attack or the psychological demands of being an organ recipient.

Let us consider an example of this approach. Say that you are intending to conduct qualitative research for clarifying issues relevant to the problem of family or 'domestic' violence. The first step would be to clarify the specific aspect of the problem you were studying and define the issues in which you were interested. For example, say that you wanted to collect data concerning the impact of physical violence on the lives of women. A key issue in defining the population is the cultural and historical setting in which it is enmeshed. The moral, legal and health-related problems involved in domestic violence vary across cultures and change with time. In Western societies it is only relatively recently that violence in domestic settings has been recognized as a serious crime and this influences the experiences of the people involved in the events. Therefore, it is essential to carefully define the cultural characteristics of the group being studied and to keep in mind that we must be very cautious in generalizing the findings from one study to other settings and people.

Purposive sampling

Qualitative sampling is designed to be purposive; that is, to select cases for inclusion in the research that are likely to be illustrative of particular issues or circumstances. Patton (1990) has proposed a typology of sampling that is widely used in qualitative research. Table 5.3 shows nine of the commonly used purposive sampling methods. Interested readers can follow up in Rice & Ezzy (1999) for more detailed information.

To illustrate qualitative sampling we have selected four strategies. Considering the example of physical violence against women in domestic settings, what would be the researcher's purpose for selecting the following strategies?

1. *Extreme or deviant case sampling.* We would select respondents who had experienced severe even life-threatening physical violence. Alternatively, we could select women who had experienced minimal violence (such as verbal abuse). Both extremes would illustrate the consequences of violence from the victim's perspective and the understanding of these issues could contribute to developing sensitive and effective interventions.

2. *Maximum variation sampling.* Here we would select across all the categories and severities of domestic violence which have been previously identified. Our purpose here is to identify the common themes emerging from the victims' experiences. This approach would also help to understand how different types of violence might result in varying outcomes from the persons' perspective.

3. *Snowball or chain sampling.* The assumption here is that people sharing similar important experiences might become aware of each other in a community. In particular, key informants who are sympathetic to the researcher's work might be helpful in identifying 'information rich' cases. For example, people who are actively involved in victim support groups would be a good source for further contacts with possible participants. In addition, such key informants can act as 'gatekeepers', protecting participants from unsafe researchers. However, 'snowball' sampling can lead to the biased selection of participants and an inaccurate representation of the issues.

4. *Theory-based sampling.* A researcher might hold the theory that the occurrence and experience of family violence might be shaped by patriarchal traditions. Here the researcher might purposely select couples who have more-or-less equal relationships and couples where there

Table 5.3 Commonly used purposive sampling methods

Sampling method	Brief description of sampling strategy
Extreme or deviant case sampling	The cases in these methods are chosen because of their deviance and the hope that this deviance may illustrate issues about more regular or mainstream cases
Maximum variation sampling	Purposefully picking a wide range of variation on dimensions of interest Documents unique or diverse variations that have emerged in adapting to different conditions Identifies important common patterns that cut across variations
Homogeneous sampling	Focuses, reduces variation, simplifies analysis, facilitates group interviewing
Stratified purposeful sampling	Illustrates characteristics of particular subgroups previously found to be of interest; facilitates comparisons of issues across groups
Snowball or chain sampling	Identifies cases of interest from people who know people who know people who know what cases are information-rich, i.e. good examples for study, good interview participants
Theory-based or operational construct sampling	Finding manifestations of theoretical construct of interest so as to elaborate and examine the construct
Opportunistic sampling	Following new leads during fieldwork, taking advantage of the unexpected, flexibility for discovering new issues
Random purposive sampling	(Still small sample size) Adds credibility to sample when potential purposeful sample is larger than one can handle Reduces judgement within a purposeful category Unlike qualitative research, this strategy is not used for generalizations or representativeness
Convenience sampling	Similarly to quantitative sampling, this strategy saves time, money and effort Poorest rationale; lowest credibility for findings Yields information-poor cases

has been an imbalance of power. The theoretical construct of interest might be 'power' or 'oppression' and this construct might be manifested in the ways in which women experience and interpret violence.

To summarize, we want to make sure the people we are interviewing or the situations we are observing are representative of the targeted issues. We want to gain as complete a picture of the issues from the perspectives of our participants as possible. The usual approach to qualitative sampling is to interview or observe people in situations that fit our criteria until we have reached a point where little or no new observations are being made. This is called saturation.

External validity and sampling

The term external validity refers to the extent to which the results of an investigation can be generalized to other samples or situations. External validity can be classified into two types: population and ecological (Huck et al 1974).

Population validity refers to generalizing the findings from the sample to the population from which it was drawn. We have already examined the importance of having a representative sample in the generalizing of results from a sample to a population. However, an investigator in the health sciences might face another problem: that the accessible population from which the sample was taken might not be the same as the target population; that is, the one of general interest. Let us illustrate this point with an example.

A physiotherapist working in a large private maternity hospital intends to examine the effectiveness of a new antenatal exercise procedure for pregnant women for controlling levels of pain during delivery. A random sample of 50 pregnant women is chosen for the investigation from the population attending the hospital. The sample is then randomly assigned into two groups: one receiving the new antenatal exercise procedure, the other receiving the traditional program. The researcher finds a statistically and clinically significant difference between the two procedures, such that the new program is shown to be effective.

Strictly speaking, these findings can be generalized only to the population of women who attend the hospital. If the target population is *all* women who are having babies, then the generalization will lack external validity, because women attending different hospitals or having children at home had no chance of being included in the study sample. They might have different characteristics, and these different characteristics may interact with the treatment in different ways to that of the sample. For instance, women who chose to deliver at home might respond better than those who chose to go to hospital but we would not know this from this study.

Ecological validity

There is also another facet of external validity: the situation in which an investigation is carried out might not be generalizable to other situations. This is called ecological validity. Consider the following examples:

1. It was shown in a classic study that, for clinical pain (due to disease or injury), morphine is an excellent analgesic. However, in laboratory studies of pain induced by electric shocks, morphine had little effect on participants' reports of pain threshold. Clearly, generalizing from laboratory to clinical settings, or vice versa, has to be done with extreme caution (Beecher 1959).
2. Coronary arteriography involves the insertion of a small-gauge catheter into a coronary artery, and injecting a dye for X-ray visualization. It was initially reported that the mortality rates for this rather dangerous-sounding practice were only 0.1% (1 per 1000) in a first-class medical institution. However, later reports from various other institutions showed mortality rates as high as 8% (80 per 1000) (Taylor 1979). Clearly, the effectiveness of treatments or the usefulness of clinical evaluations can well depend on who implements them.

The above examples illustrate the caution necessary in generalizing findings.

Summary

Appropriate sampling strategies ensure the external validity of studies and their findings. The aim of sampling strategies is to ensure the selection of a sample that is *representative* of the population of objects, persons or events the investigator aims to study. Incidental and quota samples are chosen for convenience, but these sampling strategies do not guarantee a representative sample. Random and stratified random sampling methods ensure that all important groups and characteristics in the population have the best chance to be selected and included in the study sample. Random sampling strategies are the most desirable to obtain a representative sample, although random sampling is not always feasible or desirable in health research. Area sampling and systematic sampling are also strategies that can be used to obtain representative samples.

An adequate sample size reduces the chance of large sampling error. The probable sampling error is inversely proportional to the square root of the sample size. It was argued that optimum sample size is not the maximum number of obtainable participants or a constant number or proportion. Rather, it has to be estimated for a specific investigation on the basis of the parameters of the phenomenon being studied and the study circumstances. Two types of external validity were discussed: population and ecological. External validity is related to inference, which involves using evidence from a limited set of elements to formulate general propositions.

Various approaches to purposive sampling in qualitative research were reviewed and an example of their application to a hypothetical study situation was presented.

Ethics

6

CHAPTER CONTENTS

Introduction 43

Philosophical principles. 43

   A short history of modern health
   research ethics. 44

   Key principles and concepts. 44

Resources 46

   Balancing participants' rights with
   research benefits. 47

   Ethics committees 48

Summary. 48

Introduction

The term ethics is derived from *ethos* referring to the values and customs of a community at a particular point in time. In the present context, ethics are systems of moral principles that guide human action. We are concerned with questions such as 'How should I treat other people?' or 'What research is permissible and how should I conduct it?' Research ethical standards reflect the values of a community regarding what is 'right' or 'wrong'. In health research, where the wellbeing of participants is at stake, ethical considerations play a key role in research planning and implementation.

This chapter deals with the issue of ethics in the context of health research. Research that is conducted within clinics, hospitals, research institutes and universities requires approval from an ethics committee. A research project is deemed 'ethical' if it has been approved by an ethics committee that evaluates the research questions, design and implementation of a proposed study. Sometimes the design of a study may require amendments or be denied approval because of ethical considerations raised by the committee.

In this chapter, we will address the contents of applications and how ethics review processes are conducted. In addition, we will discuss the principles that guide the preparation of submissions and the decisions of ethics committees, and examine the basic ethical principles which govern health research. We will also look at the differences between ethical systems, commonly used ethical principles, ethical dilemmas and the role of ethics committees in determining whether research proposals are accepted or rejected.

Philosophical principles

Ethics is a branch of philosophy concerned with the values and reasoning underlying what constitutes acceptable human conduct. Of course the values that drive ethical considerations are strongly linked to culture. Ethics has a long history with traditions traceable to ideas arising in ancient Greece and Judeo-Christian moral traditions. Four thousand years of debate by philosophers and theologians have ensured many different interpretations (Fara 2009). Two branches of ethics that most directly apply to conducting health research are medical ethics and bioethics. Medical ethics is defined as the moral conduct and principles which govern practices of medical and health professionals. Bioethics refers to the study of social and moral issues raised by developments in biomedicine and the health sciences. The two philosophical frameworks which are most relevant for conducting health care research are *deontology* and *utilitarianism* (Duncan 2010).

Deontology emphasizes that individuals should be treated as an end in themselves, rather than as a means to an end. From this perspective research can only be justified insofar as it benefits the individuals who participate. Some philosophers believe that there are absolute standards of right and wrong which are independent of time and place. Emmanuel Kant promulgated this notion of the 'categorical imperative' which represents right and wrong for all humans. The ancient precept, 'above all, do no harm', can be seen as an *absolute* standard for health practitioners and researchers.

Utilitarianism holds that we should produce the greatest good for the greatest number of people. This is a consequentialist approach to ethics where it is the outcomes of our actions which define our understanding of right and wrong. The benefits of a research project should outweigh potential harm to the research participants. Utilitarianism entails a *relativist* approach to ethics, holding that there are no absolute, universally accepted principles which apply to any given historical or cultural context. Rather, ethics committees need to weigh the risks and benefits for the participants and the community associated with the research proposal.

Philosophical principles are essential; however they do not, in themselves, enable us to determine whether health research can be judged as 'ethical'. Codes of practice are explicit and applicable statements which are directly relevant to conducting ethical research.

A short history of modern health research ethics

The 1964 Declaration of Helsinki by the World Medical Association was a seminal global event in the development of research ethics principles and processes. The Declaration was an elaboration and development of the 1947 Nuremberg Code (World Medical Association 2008). The Code was a response from the judges at the Nuremberg War Crime Trials to the cruel and harmful research projects that had been undertaken in World War II. It specifies basic principles that should govern the conduct of medical research. Most contemporary research ethics codes across the world draw heavily from the Helsinki Declaration and the underpinning Nuremberg Code.

The Declaration has been elaborated a further eight times by the World Medical Association at various meetings since 1964, with the most recent changes being in 2008. The amendments have related to drafting improvements and changes in technology and knowledge. In particular the responsibilities relating to publication and dissemination of research have now been specified.

Although the Declaration is now quite lengthy, it is worthwhile to reproduce the basic principles within the declaration as they provide a clear and definitive guide to the ethics principles that drive ethics processes globally. The language in the guidelines is oriented towards physicians, as it is, after all, a statement made by the World Medical Association, but the content is directly applicable to all research involving humans and it has been used extensively in the design of human research ethics procedures more broadly. The Declaration is the foundation for most ethics statements and procedures throughout the world.

There have been numerous codes of medical ethics published in various countries and professional bodies for guiding health and medical research (Emanuel et al 2000). The Helsinki Declaration has been very influential in the development of ethics codes in different countries. Thus while the codes vary somewhat from country to country they have essentially the same foundation. The Declaration is built upon certain key and basic ethics principles and concepts. These principles and concepts are now discussed.

Key principles and concepts

There are many principles and concepts in ethics processes but some are fundamental. We will now discuss some of the basic ones.

A key ethics principle is that of *informed consent and self-determination, i.e. freedom of choice to participate or not*. That is, the research participants must be fully informed about the purposes of the research, any risks associated with their participation and the uses to which the collected research data will be put. Their participation must be fully voluntary and made with full knowledge of any potential benefits and costs. Special arrangements are implemented where the researchers may have undue influence upon the research participants such as if they are also their patients or have some form of dependent relationship with the researcher.

As discussed later in this chapter, this principle is frequently protected through the use of explanatory statements sometimes called plain language statements. In this statement the researcher explains in plain language to the participants the goals of the research and exactly what is going to happen to them if they agree to participate in the research. The participant's agreement to participate with full information and knowledge about the study is recorded in an informed consent document which they normally sign. In this document they state they have understood the purpose of the study, its risks and the nature of their participation in the research.

Another key ethics principle is *scientific excellence and quality*. Most research ethics committees take the view that the proposed research has to be of high scientific quality and address research questions that have not already been answered. This is safeguarded through the ethics review process where the evaluators consider whether the researchers have the qualifications necessary to conduct the work and whether the scientific rationale for the work is sound. The view is taken that it is unethical to conduct work that is not going to add to the scientific body of knowledge because of its poor quality or a high degree of overlap with existing work. This is a waste of resources and involves participants in unnecessary activities and potential risks.

Another key ethics principle is *minimizing risk and harm to participants*. Of course, most scientific work and indeed all human activities involve some degree of risk and the possibility of harm but this needs to be minimized. The Helsinki Declaration and all ethics processes that derive from it centrally consider the risk of harm to the participant. They seek to see that all risks have been minimized and that the participant is fully aware of such risks before they have agreed to participate. In animal research, discussed later in this chapter, minimization of harm to animal research subjects is also a high priority in ethical review.

A further key ethics principle is that of *confidentiality and right to privacy*. This principle is concerned with ensuring that people's private information is not disclosed as a result of their participation in the study. In most ethics processes this involves quite a lot of attention concerning how people's information is to be obtained, stored, processed and disseminated. So the researcher is often asked detailed questions about how the information is to be obtained and handled and how it is to be retained and ultimately disposed of when the project has been completed. Further detail is required of how the work is to be published and disseminated. Many countries also now have privacy legislation that informs the local ethics procedures because any work within that country needs to comply with the local laws.

The risks of identifying individuals in research are increased in the study of small, specialized sub-populations and in qualitative studies where direct quotation of the words of the research participant may be used in the publications. One of the authors of this text was once asked to participate in a study of staff who had left a university with the assurance that the results would be anonymous. However, he was the only male professor who had left over a five-year period in his faculty. With any basic cross-tabulation of the data based upon appointment level and gender, he would be the only respondent in that category, so the chances of being identified would be very high. In qualitative studies involving the direct reporting of the statements of participants the risk is also increased. People have distinctive manners of expression and experiences such that, while there may be no names mentioned, people who know them may be able to identify the person through their language and the experiences they are describing. We know of numerous examples where research participants have been identified by others when their responses have been directly quoted in research reports and publications with the promised protection of anonymity. So given that most researchers promise to maintain anonymity of their research participants, the possibility of 'outing' through publication must be taken seriously and guarded against.

In this discussion we have used the terms confidentiality and anonymity interchangeably as is now common usage in research discussions. However, they actually mean different things. Anonymity means that the identity of the research participant is not disclosed and in some cases may not even be known to the researchers. Confidentiality, however, means that whatever is being maintained as confidential is not revealed to a third party. While some researchers promise confidentiality of the research findings and the participants, what they often really mean is anonymity. A literal interpretation of confidentiality would mean that they could not publish their research results!

A further key ethics principle is *lack of conflict of interest*. Conflict of interest occurs when an individual or an agency is potentially able to exploit their involvement in research in some way for their own personal or agency benefit. Some commentators argue that all researchers have an intrinsic potential conflict of interest in that they are directly impacted by the findings of their research in some way or another. For example, the outcomes for the researcher may be quite different if they identify that a new therapy is effective versus if it does not work. The positive result may mean more support for their work, professional acclaim, press coverage and so on, but a negative or null result may result in de-funding and little prospect of acclaim or favourable publicity. Similarly, a government agency or institution may have a vested interest in showing that a disease or problem within the community is low or even high to legitimize their existence.

The relationship between researchers and research funding bodies is also an area of potential conflict of interest. This is why many journals and professional and scientific bodies require full disclosure of such arrangements. The researchers are required to disclose their funding sources, memberships and relationships that may impact upon their independence and perceived bias. In ethics review, a high standard is imposed upon researchers. Thus for many the appearance of potential conflict of interest is just as important as whether it is an actual conflict. Some researchers, for example, will not accept funding from tobacco companies, or alcohol or gambling interests or pharmaceutical companies or government because of a perceived conflict of interest for them. There is always the fear that the results obtained in such research may be biased in some way either through direct influence or a desire on the part of the researchers to please the funding agency. To address this issue some of these funding agencies have 'arm's length' funding arrangements where they donate to a third party foundation, but some are intricately involved in the approval and conduct of the research. Although government is generally not categorized with tobacco interests, government officials and ministers still have identifiable conflicts of interest and through 'contract research' can potentially exert considerable influence on the conduct and outcomes of the research they fund.

In some instances the pressure upon researchers to produce exciting and fundable research findings results in misconduct whereby the researcher may cut corners through use of low-cost or non-standard protocols or even directly falsify their research findings. There have been a series of celebrated examples in history and modern day of such lapses. The case of Sir Cyril Burt is one such figure. It is claimed by some that Burt falsified some key data sets for his research (a claim hotly contested to this day). Typing the search terms 'medical research fraud' into any Internet search engine brings up hundreds of reported cases of misconduct and fraud, often involving data falsification. However, it must be remembered that this is a very small proportion of the studies that are conducted. For example, in the UK it is typical to exceed more than two million animal study notifications annually. Interestingly some methodologists claim that poorly conducted research and researcher incompetence, notwithstanding ethics approval, is a much more serious threat to science than outright fraud!

Finally, a key principle in ethics protocols is *independent review*. Researchers and funding bodies are not in a good position to independently evaluate the ethical implications of their own work or the work they may wish to fund. They have an intrinsic conflict of interest. This is why most medical research councils and funding bodies, while enunciating the principles and processes for ethical review, do not directly participate in such review. Of course, the independence and expertise of reviewers is in itself an issue in terms of potential conflicts of interest. Expert reviewers in many fields may have friendships or enmities with the person or research group whose work they may be reviewing. Even if they don't know them some professional jealousies may exist. This is why there are particularly detailed guidelines for reviewers to attempt to address these issues. In small, specialized fields obtaining independent review is particularly problematic because 'everyone knows everyone'. A second option is to use reviewers that do not work in the field but the problem then is that it is easy to obtain reviews that are misinformed about important technical details of the research.

Resources

A fundamental value is that the time and effort of researchers and participants and the resources of the community should not be wasted on a badly planned investigation. Of course, there can never be a guarantee that an investigation will produce clinically useful results. However, some poorly designed projects are doomed to failure even before the data collection begins, and lead to confusion and controversy in the professional literature. Therefore, the appropriate use of high-quality and sound research methods is not only useful for solving problems, but constitutes an ethical necessity. Many ethics committees also vet projects for scientific merit before the project is approved.

Selection of appropriate research strategies can also be influenced by the resources available to investigators. Some projects involving the evaluation of the safety and effectiveness of new drugs, or the identification of risk factors in cardiac disease, have taken tens of millions of dollars to finance. Research planning takes into account economic issues, such as:

1. *Availability of participants.* Here the investigator has to consider if enough people can participate in the project under the required conditions. Attention has to be paid to issues such as the frequency of the disorder in the community, problems in identifying participants and their level of voluntary participation. As discussed in Chapter 5, selection of participants is crucial for the validity of a study.

2. *Availability of equipment.* Some equipment is costly to acquire or to operate (e.g. CT (computed tomography) scanners, biochemical assays, experimental drugs). Research planning should take these expenses into account.

3. *Availability of expertise.* Specialized assessment techniques and the administration of clinical treatments require professional expertise. If these are beyond the investigator's competence or if the experimental design requires an unbiased, 'blind' therapist or assessor (see Ch. 5), there must be means for securing them.

4. *Availability of time.* Research projects have a tendency to take considerably longer than an inexperienced researcher might expect, due to the erratic and at times disastrous workings of Murphy's Law: 'If anything can go wrong, it will'. Equipment breaks down and needs to be repaired, participants 'disappear' and collaborators might not deliver services promised. Research planning should take into account possible problems and how these might affect the time scale of investigations. This is a particularly important issue for postgraduate students.

The availability of resources strongly influences the scope of the research program and also the research strategy selected by the investigator. A research project must be shown to be feasible from a cost viewpoint before it is initiated. It is only after the ethical constraints and economic resources have been evaluated that the researchers' questions can be transformed into clearly defined hypotheses or aims.

It is important when conducting research that the identities of all supporting agencies and individuals are disclosed to the participants in order that their agreement to participate is fully informed.

Balancing participants' rights with research benefits

Who is to benefit from the research? One likes to think that 'humanity', 'the participants' or 'health science' are going to be the beneficiaries of health research. A slightly more cynical analysis points to the investigators as having the most to gain, at least in the short term. After all, given a successful outcome for the research project, they stand to satisfy their curiosity, improve their career prospects or to raise their esteem before colleagues. In practice, benefits accruing to the investigator, the participants and health science have to be carefully weighed in relation to the conduct of any project. The protection of the rights and welfare of the participants is the primary consideration of research ethics.

Sometimes harm may be caused by denying participants access to beneficial treatment as part of a study. This can happen when we use 'no treatment', 'placebo' or 'conventional treatments' as controls. This is particularly a problem when a treatment study begins to demonstrate that one treatment is clearly better than another. Many studies now set predetermined criteria to terminate the study if this occurs to allow those who are not receiving a beneficial treatment to do so. Similarly, the reverse is done when a treatment is shown to be harmful.

Ethical research should ensure that the given research methodology minimizes the intrusiveness, distress and potential harm participants may experience. Distress or harm may be caused by research procedures such as the administration of a new assessment or treatment technique. It may be caused also by the strategy the researcher uses to collect information. For example, the use of existing health care records may be less distressing than reassessing patients/clients for a research study.

A range of methods have been developed to reduce the intrusiveness of research into people's lives. These include researchers working together with people in the community on tasks and projects where the participants take major roles in all the stages of conducting the research. Also there are various 'participant observer' methods available (see Ch. 13), where the researcher can unobtrusively become part of the research setting, while collecting the evidence. These strategies are designed to encourage a partnership between the researcher and the participants in the research. From this perspective, the very idea of 'the research subject' is problematic since it implies that the people who participate in research are passive and have research done to them or on them.

There are two types of methodological problems which make research unethical, independent of the potential benefits the research may produce for the community or the informed consent given by the participants. First, there is not much point in conducting research which cannot answer the question that is being posed because it is methodologically flawed. Such research is a waste of everyone's time, energy and money, all of which could be put to better purposes. In circumstances where participants undergo uncomfortable, painful, distressing, intrusive or risky procedures, methodologically flawed research has costs to the participants with no benefit to the community or the individuals concerned.

Second, sometimes researchers with the best intentions make mistakes in the design of their research, which makes it difficult or impossible to draw conclusions. Mistakes like these can be minimized by an independent review and examination of a research proposal before the research is put into place. Unfortunately, in some circumstances, a limited number of researchers have falsified important aspects of their research for personal benefit.

It is important, therefore, that research is open to scrutiny by independent reviewers while it is being conducted and that research findings are replicated independently by other researchers before they are generally accepted.

Ethics committees

Because of the large administrative burden associated with ethics review and the issue of conflict of interest most health and medical research bodies operate under an institutional review board or institutional research ethics committee arrangement. That is, the process of ethics review is conducted within the research or health institution with a specially constituted group consisting of staff from the institution and external members. Most institutions that grant funds to researchers have requirements for the constitution and operation of the institutional review boards to ensure that the reviews are of high quality and conducted without conflict of interest. Specified members frequently include lawyers, ministers of religion, ethics experts and lay members, so the committees are by no means stacked with fellow researchers or people from the institution. In the event of a conflict of interest, members do not participate in the review in which they have the conflict.

If you are working in a small clinical agency or even in a large clinical agency in a developing country it is possible that you will not have direct access to your own institutional review board. If this is the case and you are conducting some research then you will need to gain access to a properly constituted committee to review your work. This will provide protection to you but also it means that you will be able to publish your work. The ethics review is now required for most credible research journals. That is, you will be asked to provide details of your ethics approval in order to have the work accepted for publication. So if the researcher does not have immediate access to a properly constituted and approved ethics review committee the researcher will need to find one to review their work if they wish to publish it in a reputable journal. Some agencies charge for this service but some do not.

Summary

A responsible investigator is required to take into consideration ethical principles and to plan research projects accordingly so that the probable harm to participants is minimized. Therefore, the health researcher must use considerable ingenuity in designing valid investigations, while maintaining ethical values. One of the roles of ethics committees is to guide investigators on complex issues, and to ensure that research is conducted in accordance with accepted community principles.

This chapter has introduced ethics principles and procedures. A short history of the development of ethics in research has been provided noting the development of the Nuremberg Code from the World War II war crimes trials concerning medical research abuses, and the World Medical Association Helsinki Declaration. The Declaration has been updated to reflect contemporary circumstances from its original to the present day. A discussion of the basic principles underlying contemporary ethics thinking and review has been provided including: informed consent and freedom of choice to participate in the research or not; scientific excellence and quality; minimization of risk and harm to participants; lack of conflict of interest; and independent review. The process of ethics review and the documentation required has been described and some tips for effective ethics submissions have been provided.

Section 3

Research designs

7 Experimental designs and randomized controlled trials 53

8 Surveys and quasi-experimental designs 63

9 Single case (n = 1) designs 71

10 Qualitative research 77

The aim of Section 3 is to examine various research designs and outline their applications for conducting research. As in other areas of creative activities, such as architecture or the fashion industry, the term design refers to explicit plans for completing a particular activity.

The conceptual basis for experimental designs is the need for control as outlined in Chapter 7. In experimental research we manipulate one or more variables (independent variables) while controlling extraneous variables through the use of appropriate control groups. If an experiment is well designed and properly conducted we are in a position to demonstrate the causal effects of independent variables on the outcome or dependent variables. The random assignment of participants to treatment or control groups is a common way to achieve control in applied health sciences research. Randomized controlled trials are experimental designs which are currently the preferred (gold standard) designs for evaluating the efficacy of interventions. In Chapter 7, we will examine how the use of randomized controlled trials enables researchers to control for the biases of both the participants and the observers who evaluate the outcomes thus ensuring the internal validity of trials addressing treatment efficacy.

There are settings where for practical or ethical reasons we cannot randomly assign participants to control or treatment groups. In Chapter 8, we will discuss the use of naturalistic comparisons, correlational designs, quasi-experiments and descriptive surveys. These designs enable us to describe and predict relationships amongst health-related variables such as risk factors influencing health. The accuracy of the information collected using these non-experimental designs depends on the use of appropriate sampling strategies for selecting the participants used for comparisons.

In Chapter 9, we discuss the n = 1 or 'single case' designs for conducting clinical case studies. The advantage is that, in using n = 1 designs, we are able to demonstrate causal effects, while using only a few participants without the need for control groups. The major limitation of the n = 1 design (and other types of clinical case studies) is that the findings may not be validly generalizable to other cases and the population at large.

In Chapter 10, we will describe elementary characteristics of qualitative research designs. The aim of this chapter is to examine the many ways in which qualitative research can be used to understand the experiences and actions of research participants. This data enables us to see health care problems and the outcomes of interventions from the perspective of the patients/participants.

Experimental designs and randomized controlled trials

7

CHAPTER CONTENTS

Introduction 53

The concept of causality 54

Confounding and bias in research studies. . . 54

The use of control groups
in applied health research 55

Assignment of participants into groups 56

    Independent groups 56

    Matched groups 56

Types of experimental designs 56

    Post-test only design 56

    Pre-test/post-test design 57

    Repeated measures 57

    Factorial designs. 57

    Multiple dependent variables 58

Randomized controlled trials 58

Controlled research involving
human participants 60

The external validity of experiments and RCTs 60

Summary. 61

Introduction

There is a fundamental need to identify the causes of illness and disability if we are to deliver effective health care for individuals and the population. It is by understanding these causes that we can formulate and justify our assessments, diagnoses and interventions. Furthermore, we justify interventions in that we can point to the evidence that demonstrates interventions are *causing* the beneficial changes in preventing or managing disease. In health research the concept of internal validity is related to the design of research projects and the extent to which the implementations of these designs enables researchers to unambiguously identify causal relationships between interventions and outcomes.

Experiments are an important form of intervention studies. A well-designed experiment enables researchers to demonstrate how manipulating one set of variables (the *independent* variables) produces systematic changes in another set of variables (the outcome or *dependent* variables). Experimental designs aim to ensure that all variables other than the independent variable(s) are controlled; that is, that there are no uncontrolled extraneous variables or factors that might systematically influence changes in the study's outcome variable(s). Control is most readily exercised in the sheltered environment of research settings such as laboratories and this is one of the reasons why these settings are the preferred habitats of experimental research scientists. However, much of epidemiological and clinical research takes place in field settings (e.g. communities, hospitals and clinics), where the phenomena of human health, illness and treatment are naturally located. Even in these natural settings researchers can nevertheless exercise control over extraneous variables.

In this chapter, we will focus on an experimental design referred to as the *randomized controlled trial* (RCT) which is an experimental research design aimed at assessing the effectiveness of a clinical intervention. Our aim is to show how RCTs are used to demonstrate that an intervention is the cause of a subsequent effect(s). RCTs are considered by many researchers and clinicians to be the premier type of evidence for the effectiveness of clinical interventions.

The specific aims of this chapter are to:

1. Examine the basic structure of experimental research designs and RCTs.
2. Consider threats to the validity of the results obtained from experiments and RCTs.

The concept of causality

The notion of causality has been a difficult and controversial topic for philosophers. As health researchers we need to take a pragmatic approach and look to demonstrate causal relationships. Three simple criteria for demonstrating causal associations are:

1. The cause must precede (occur before) the effect.
2. The cause and effect co-vary. If the cause occurs then so does the effect.
3. If the cause does not occur, then the effect does not occur.

The first criterion is quite simple. For example, if we say that injury to the person's arm is the cause of that person's reported pain, we of course assume that the injury was sustained prior to the onset of the pain. Clearly, if the pain had been already present, the injury would not be seen as the cause of the pain. Second, we assume that there will be 'concomitant variation' between the injury and the pain. The worse the injury, the more severe the pain. As the injury recovers, a decrease in the level of pain can be expected. In general, we are establishing evidence for the existence of a causal relationship between the cause and the effect.

However, observing a relationship between two events is not sufficient to demonstrate causality. For example, night follows day in a predictable, lawful fashion, but we do not say that day causes the night or vice versa. We must attempt to eliminate plausible alternative explanations or hypotheses that offer rival causal explanations for the findings. For example, pain might persist even after the injury has healed. There might be other variables operating which maintain a person's experience of pain.

The problem is that, apart from our intervention, there are likely to be other factors that may be influencing the pain outcome. These influences are called 'confounding extraneous variables' or 'bias' and constitute a potentially serious problem when attempting to interpret the results of a trial.

Confounding and bias in research studies

The research designs that are commonly referred to as 'before–after' designs are often used initially to test the safety and efficacy of novel interventions. The use of the design provides a clear example of how confounding variables can threaten the internal validity (or accuracy) of the study. Confounding variables can result in ambiguity in deciding what has caused any observed changes.

As a hypothetical example, consider the introduction of an exercise program for cardiac patients, which aimed at increasing mobility, and thereby improving health. The patients were also smokers, and were strongly encouraged to give up smoking. The researchers used 'distance walked by patients' (in a specified time period) as an indicator of the effectiveness of the program. Figure 7.1 represents (without showing numbers) the average walking distances before and after the exercise program. There is clearly a difference between before and after (i.e. an improvement from baseline). However, was this improvement caused only by the exercise program, or by confounding extraneous variables, or a combination of both?

Consider the following plausible alternative explanations for the difference shown in Figure 7.1:

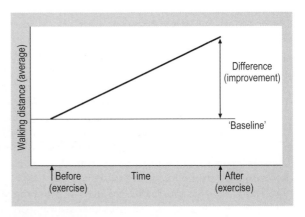

Figure 7.1 • Results for a hypothetical 'before–after' study.

1. The improvement might have been due to natural recovery; the patients' mobility might have improved independently of the exercise program. This is referred to as a threat to internal validity due to *maturation*.

2. The improvement might have been due to other factors, such as the reduction in, or cessation of, smoking among some of the patients, resulting in an average increase in walking distance. Such confounding extraneous variables are referred to as *history*.

3. The improvement might have been due to a placebo effect. Placebo effects (see below) are associated with patient expectations of potential benefits of the intervention. In the example outlined above, the expectations of the patients, rather than the exercise itself, might have been the actual cause of the improvement.

4. An important source of bias is *observer bias* which refers to researchers unknowingly influencing the results of a study by holding expectations regarding the outcome. In the present hypothetical example, the researchers may anticipate that the exercise program will improve mobility.

The above explanations illustrate the influence confounding extraneous variables. That is, each is concerned with factors that are present at the same time as the intervention and which may have produced the observed effect.

Internal validity refers to the ability of a researcher to attribute differences (e.g. Fig. 7.1) to the effect of the independent variable. Maximizing internal validity is important for quantitative research designed to demonstrate causal effects. In order to ensure internal validity, researchers must control for the effects of confounding and bias. Experimental designs are particularly well-suited for controlling for the potential influence of confounding factors. Randomized controlled trials employ experimental designs that are applied for evaluating the efficacy of interventions.

The use of control groups in applied health research

A control group consists of participants that undergo the same conditions as the group receiving the intervention under investigation. For example, in drug trials, control group participants will often receive an injection of saline solution, if the experimental treatment is administered via injection, in order to control for the effects of actual injection. If the medication were administered orally, similar-looking inert tablets would be used for control participants. It has been found that, if people receive any form of 'therapy', improvement may occur even when the 'treatment' or intervention is physiologically and chemically inert. This is referred to as a *placebo effect*. The control group allows the researcher to measure the size of the placebo effect, and to take it into account when interpreting the study results. If we are to include a control group in our intervention studies, it is essential that, at the outset, the experimental and control groups are as similar as possible. We have to take the participants and split them up into the experimental and control groups as equally as possible. This process is called *assignment*. The assignment of participants to their groups by the investigator is an essential feature of an intervention study.

Let us re-examine the investigation outlined in Figure 7.1 in terms of the impact upon internal validity when we use a control group in the study.

1. Assess the walking distances of the patients in a pre-treatment test.

2. Assign participants into experimental or control groups by matching on the basis of pre-test performance, and random assignment within pairs.

3. Administer:
   a. experimental intervention (exercise program, walking, diet and smoking reduction)
   b. control intervention (an alternative activity, walking, diet and smoking reduction).
   The *only* difference between the two groups is that one group receives the exercise program and the other some alternative activity.

4. Test both groups on walking distance, following the treatment.

The results of this fictional study are presented in Figure 7.1.

Let us examine how this new design stands up to threats of internal validity in contrast to the original investigation.

1. *Natural recovery*. Both control and experimental groups had the same time to recover or deteriorate; it is unlikely that this factor explains the difference.

2. *Confounding due to other interventions.* Both groups had walking, smoking decrement and diet. It is unlikely that the difference between the post-test results shown in Figure 7.1 would be due to confounding factors.

3. *Placebo effect.* Given that this is not a double-blind trial, the bias due to expectations remains uncontrolled with this design.

We can see that using a design with a control group resulted in an improvement in the internal validity of the trial. Note that the use of a control group has not removed the effects of placebo. It is still possible, but much less likely, that the differences in the outcomes for the two groups were not a result of the intervention. Nevertheless, the investigator has a much sounder basis for deciding whether or not the exercise program was effective.

It should be noted that there are ways, other than the use of control groups, to minimize the effects of uncontrolled extraneous variables. For example, if 'noise' is a possible extraneous variable in administering a test, we may 'insulate' from it by using a quiet setting. However, if noisy settings are the norm in real life, then, as discussed later, the search for higher internal validity may be at the cost of external validity.

Assignment of participants into groups

Independent groups

The simplest approach is to assign the participants randomly to independent groups. Each intervention group represents a 'level' of the independent variable. Say, for instance, we were interested in the effects of a new drug (we will call this drug A) in helping to relieve the symptoms of depression. We also decide to have a placebo control group, which involves giving patients a capsule identical to A, but not containing the active ingredient.

Given a sample size of 20, we would assign each participant randomly to either the experimental (drug A) or the control (placebo control) group. Random assignment could involve encoding all the 20 names into a computer program and using random numbers to generate two groups of 10. In this case, we would end up with two equivalent groups (see Table 7.1).

Here n_c and n_e refer to the number of participants in each of the groups, given that the total

Table 7.1 Levels of the independent variables

	Control group (placebo)	Experimental group (drug A)
Number of participants	$n_c = 10$	$n_e = 10$

sample size (n) was 20. We can have more than two groups if we want. For example, if we also included another drug 'B', the independent variables would have three levels. We would require a total of 30 participants if the group sizes remained at 10.

Matched groups

Random assignment does not guarantee that the two groups will be equivalent. Rather, the argument is that there is no reason why the groups should be different. While this is true in the long run, with small sample sizes chance differences among the groups may distort the results of an experiment or RCT. Matched assignment of the participants into groups minimizes group differences caused by chance variation.

Using the hypothetical example discussed previously, say that the researcher required that the two groups should be equivalent at the start of the study on the measure of depression used in the experiment. Using a matched-groups design, the participants would be assessed for level of depression before the treatment and paired for scores from highest to lowest. Subsequently, the two participants in each pair would be randomly assigned to either the experimental group or the placebo control group. In this way, it would be likely that the two groups would have similar average pre-test depression scores.

Types of experimental designs

Four types of experimental design will be discussed. These are the post-test only, pre-test/post-test, repeated measures and factorial designs.

Post-test only design

At first it may appear that this would make measurement of change impossible. At an individual level this is certainly true. However, if we assume that the control and experimental groups were initially identical and that no change had occurred in the controls, direct comparison of the post-test scores will indicate the extent of the change. This type of design is fraught with danger in clinical research and should only be used in special circumstances, such as when pre-test measures are impossible or unethical to carry out. The assumptions of initial equivalence and of no change in the control group often may not be supported and, in such cases, interpretation of group differences is difficult and ambiguous. For example, if we conduct a double-blind RCT to determine the efficacy of a drug in treating very severe infections then, if our outcome is proportion of patients surviving, a post-test only design would be appropriate.

Pre-test/post-test design

In this design, measurements of the outcome or dependent variables are taken both before and after intervention. This allows the measurement of actual changes for individual cases. However, the measurement process itself may produce change, thereby introducing difficulties in the clear attribution of change to the intervention on its own. For example, in an experimental study of weight loss, simply administering a questionnaire concerning dietary habits may lead to changes in those habits by encouraging people to scrutinize their own behaviour and hence modify it. Alternatively, in measures of skill, there may be a practice effect such that, without any intervention, the performance on a second test will improve. In order to overcome these difficulties, many researchers turn to the post-test only design.

Repeated measures

In order to economize with the number of participants required in an experimental design, the researchers will sometimes re-use participants in the design. Thus, at different times the participants may receive, say, drug A or drug B. If it were the case that every participant encountered more than one level of the drug variable or factor, then 'drug' would be termed a repeated measures factor. An important consideration is using a 'counterbalanced' design to avoid series effects. For example, half the participants should receive drug A first, and half the participants should receive drug A first, and half

drug B. If all the participants received drug A first and then drug B, the study would not be counterbalanced and we would not be able to determine whether the order of administration of the drugs was important. Time is a common repeated measures factor in many studies. A pre-test/post-test design involves the measurement of the same participants twice. If 'time' is included in the analysis of the study, then this is a repeated measures factor. In statistical analysis, repeated measures factors are treated differently from factors where each level is represented by a separate, independent group. This is true both for matched groups, discussed earlier, as well as for repeated measures, discussed above.

Factorial designs

A researcher will often not be content with the manipulation of one intervention factor or variable in isolation. For example, a clinical psychologist may wish to investigate the effectiveness of both the type of psychological therapy and the use of drug therapy for a group of patients. Let us assume that the psychologist was interested in the effects of therapy versus no psychological treatment, and of drug A versus no treatment. These two variables lead to four possible combinations of treatment (see Table 7.2).

This design enables us to investigate the separate and combined effects of both independent variables upon the outcome measure(s). In other words, we are looking for interactions among the two (or more) factors. If all possible combinations of the values or levels of the independent variables are included in the study, the design is said to be fully crossed. If one or more is left out, it is said to be incomplete. With an incomplete factorial design, there are some difficulties in determining the complete joint and separate effects of the independent variables.

In order that the terminology in experimental designs is clear, it is instructive to consider the way in which research methodologists would typically describe the example design in Table 7.2. This is a study with two independent variables (sometimes called factors): namely, type of psychological therapy and drug treatment. Each independent variable or factor has two levels or values. This would commonly be described as a 2 by 2 design (each factor having two levels). There are four groups (2 × 2) in the design.

Table 7.2 Examples of a factorial design		
	Drug A	**No drug**
Psychological therapy	1	2
No psychological therapy	3	4

If a third level, drug B, was added to the drug factor, then it would become a 2 by 3 design with six groups required. Two groups, drug B with psychological therapy and drug B with no psychological therapy, would be added. It is possible to overdo the number of factors and levels in experimental studies. A 4 × 4 × 4 design would require 64 groups: that is a lot of research participants to find for a study. It is relevant to note that when we evaluate two or more groups over a period of time we are also using a factorial design.

Multiple dependent variables

Just as it is possible to have multiple independent variables in an experimental study, it is also sometimes appropriate to have multiple outcome or dependent measures. For example, in order to assess the effectiveness of an intervention such as icing of an injury, factors such as extent of oedema and area of bruising are both important outcome measures. In this instance, there would be two outcome measures. The use of multiple dependent variables is very common in health research. The outcomes measured are usually evaluated individually, although there are more complex statistical techniques which enable the simultaneous analysis of multiple dependent variables.

Randomized controlled trials

We will now work through each of the steps in conducting an RCT; these steps are summarized in Figure 7.2. The protocol being followed has been developed by the CONSORT Committee, to promote the standardization of RCTs.

1. *Definition of the population.* Researchers define the population to which they wish to generalize. For example, this might be males over 55 years with coronary heart disease or

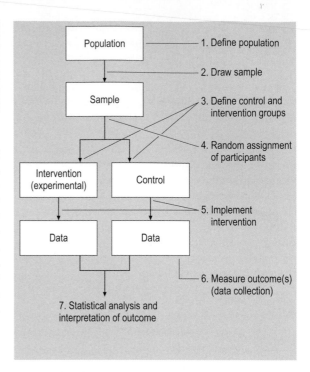

Figure 7.2 • A two independent groups randomized controlled trial.

the local community or a certain type of health care organization.

2. *Selection of the sample.* Using an appropriate sampling method, the study sample is selected from the population. It is desirable that the sample is representative of the population. It is important to note that steps 1 and 2 are common to all research designs (see Ch. 5).

3. *Defining the intervention and control groups.* The simplest RCT design has two groups (see Fig. 7.2): an intervention or experimental group, and a control group. These two groups are sometimes referred to as comprising the two 'arms' of a study. This 'minimalist' design enables the researcher to compare the outcome for the intervention group with the outcome for the control group, and thereby discount the effects of confounding factors. It is possible, of course, to produce far more complex designs, including ones with numerous intervention groups and outcome measures. It is likely that, in the course of searching for research evidence that can be applied to practice, you will encounter more complex designs.

An essential consideration in planning an RCT is the type of control group. There are several possibilities, including:

No intervention/waiting list control group.

Traditional intervention control group.

Placebo control group.

The first of these (no intervention) is the most economical to implement, in the sense that little has to be done to the participants in the control group, beyond making predetermined assessments. The problem is that there is no control for some confounding factors, such as differences in the behaviour of the participants in the two groups. Thus, for example, participants in a no intervention control group may feel neglected and (unbeknown to the researcher) may seek alternative interventions, while remaining in the trial. Finally, no-treatment controls might be unacceptable on ethical grounds (i.e. it is usually unethical to deny treatment if it is available).

When an intervention needs to be provided to all participants, and when there are interventions already available to prevent or to treat a particular health problem, then the traditional or currently available intervention can be provided to the control group. The outcome for the new intervention group is then compared to that for the control group, principally in terms of any superiority of the new intervention.

4. *Assignment procedures.* Random assignment means that each participant has an equal chance of being assigned to any of the groups. In an RCT, one of the groups receives a control intervention with the active component of the intervention missing. For example, in an experimental study of the effectiveness of different types of weight-loss programs, one group might receive an instruction manual, another might receive supervised dietary training and a third group may receive no intervention. The purpose of the randomized assignment procedure is to ensure that the groups are as similar as possible on all the relevant variables. If the groups are substantially different, it will be very difficult to attribute any differences in final outcome to the 'treatments' being administered.

5. *Administration of intervention (treatment).* The researcher then administers the intervention(s) to the various groups participating in the experiment. This is called the independent variable(s). It is important that the intervention is administered in an unbiased way, in order that a fair test of any differences in outcomes may be provided. As will be discussed later, awareness of the expected outcomes on the part of participants may lead to a spurious biasing of the outcomes for those participants. Therefore, the true aims and expectations of the researcher are sometimes concealed from the participants in an attempt to control expectancy effects.

6. *Measurement of outcomes.* The researcher assesses the outcome of the experiment through measurement of the dependent or outcome variable(s). Sometimes, the dependent variable is measured both before and after the experimental intervention (this is called a pre-test/post-test design) and other times only afterwards (this is called a post-test only design).

7. *Statistical analysis and interpretation of the outcomes.* In general, outcome measures index any changes in the health status and functioning of the participants, subsequent to the intervention, and the greater the change, the more effective the intervention is likely to be. Of course, when the intervention is implemented as part of an RCT, the intervention group(s) is always compared with the control group, so it is the difference between the intervention and control groups that represents the true effect of the intervention. Measures of the effect of the intervention are discussed briefly below. The calculation of such measures and procedures for determining if the effect is statistically or practically significant, are discussed in Chapters 20 and 21.

There are a number of ways of designing and implementing RCTs. An important consideration is whether the trial is an explanatory study or a pragmatic study. A pragmatic trial tests the *efficacy* of the intervention in a controlled research setting with selected participants and under ideal conditions. An efficacy study is designed to test whether the intervention works under ideal circumstances.

An effectiveness or pragmatic RCT study tests the *effectiveness* of the intervention in everyday practice. The study includes participants representative of normal patients and with less controlled conditions that more closely reflect everyday clinical practice. Pragmatic or effectiveness RCTs are used in research translation studies to check that interventions that work under highly controlled circumstances will work in normal clinic circumstances.

It is typical to conduct an efficacy study under ideal circumstances before conducting an effectiveness study in an everyday clinical setting.

Controlled research involving human participants

Investigations involving human participants require that researchers should consider both psychological and ethical issues when designing experiments. Human beings respond actively to being studied. When recruited as a research participant, a person might formulate a set of beliefs about the aims of the study and will have expectations about the outcomes. In health research, placebo effects are positive changes in signs and symptoms in people who believe that they are being offered effective treatment by health professionals. These improvements in signs and symptoms are in fact elicited by 'inert' treatments probably mediated by the patients' expectations. Health professionals who hold strong beliefs about the effectiveness of their treatments communicate this attitude to their patients and possibly increase the placebo effects.

Placebo responses as such are not a problem in everyday health care. Skilled therapists utilize this effect to the patients' benefit. Of course, charlatans exploit this phenomenon, masking the poor efficacy of their interventions. In health research, however, we need to demonstrate that an intervention has therapeutic effects greater than a placebo, hence the need for a placebo control group. The ideal standard for an experiment is a *double-blind* design, in which neither the research participants nor the health providers/experimenters know which participants are receiving the active form of the treatment. Placebo controlled double-blind RCTs, with large sample sizes, are the strongest method for controlling confounding extraneous variables, and have a greater degree of internal validity than does any other research design. This is because the only thing that differs between the groups is whether or not they receive the active version of the intervention. Therefore if an effect of the active version of the intervention is demonstrated (i.e. there is a difference between groups that favours the intervention group), then we can have a good deal of certainty in the conclusion that the intervention was the cause of this effect. Placebo controlled double-blind RCTs are therefore sometimes referred to as constituting a 'gold standard for research design'. However,

there are situations where double-blind RCTs are not appropriate. An obvious example is where it is impossible or very difficult to devise and to conceal a placebo intervention. For example, psychologists, speech pathologists and occupational therapists find it difficult to devise behavioural placebo interventions that can be concealed from participants. Also, as stated earlier, placebo controls might be unethical and therefore inappropriate when established treatments are available. Another source of ethical concern has been the use of placebo or 'sham surgery' for implementing double-blind RCTs of the effectiveness of some surgical interventions. It is one thing to administer inert treatments to volunteers, but another thing entirely to cut open people's bodies for the sake of creating a control group. Polgar & Ng (2005) argue that it is unethical to use placebo surgery as a means for creating a control group. Rather, novel surgical procedures are best evaluated using 'traditional intervention' control groups.

It is not always possible, however, to form placebo control groups. In the area of drug research and some other physical treatments it can be possible; but with certain behaviourally based interventions, in areas such as psychotherapy, physiotherapy or occupational therapy, double-blind placebo interventions may be impossible to implement. For instance, how could a physiotherapist offering a complex and intensive exercise program be 'blind' to the treatment program being offered? In these situations researchers employ no treatment or traditional intervention control groups when evaluating the safety and effectiveness of a novel intervention.

Also, there are ethical issues that need to be taken into account when using placebo or non-intervention control groups. Where people are suffering from acute or life-threatening conditions, assignment into a placebo or no-treatment control group could have serious consequences. This is particularly true for illnesses where prolonged participation in a placebo control group could have irreversible consequences for the sufferers. Under such circumstances, placebo or no-treatment controls might well be unethical and the selection of a traditional treatment group would be preferred.

The external validity of experiments and RCTs

As we discussed previously, all health research which relies on drawing representative samples may involve systematic sampling error. Sampling error or selection bias may threaten the external validity of a study, defined as the extent to which we are confident when applying the findings to a specific group or the overall population.

To consider an obvious illustration, say that you are working with a group of adults (65 years or older) with heart disease living in Montreal. You are looking for a diet program which will help to optimize weight. Your literature search identifies a well-designed RCT which clearly indicates that a given diet 'X' has provided large weight losses in overweight children living in Shanghai. Would you adopt diet 'X' for your patients? Before you did, would you carefully consider the differences between your patients and the study sample, including the variables age, health status and environmental and cultural settings?

The highly structured and controlled implementation of RCTs may also influence the extent to which their findings can be applied to everyday health care situations. As an example, consider the use of double-blind RCTs to evaluate the efficacy of cellular therapies for the treatment of Parkinson's disease (see Ch. 6). The double-blind design stipulates that volunteers with Parkinson's disease are assigned to either a sham-operated control group or a treatment group in which the patients were administered human fetal cells to replace the dopaminergic neurones lost through the disease process. Therefore, the concealment of the treatment means that the patient is uncertain whether she or he has actually received new cells or just a sham operation. This uncertainty is quite different to actual cellular therapy where the patient is certain of the intervention and may carry out activities for optimally integrating the new cells into their impaired neural network. That is, the trade-off between ensuring internal validity may compromise the external validity of double-blind RCTs.

Summary

The experimental (RCT) approach to research design involves the active manipulation of the independent variable(s) through the administration of an intervention often with a non-intervention control group and the measurement of outcome through the dependent variable(s). Good experimental design requires careful sampling, assignment and measurement procedures to maximize both internal and external validity.

Common experimental designs include the pre-test/post-test, post-test only, repeated measures and factorial approaches. These designs ensure that investigations can show causal effects. More recent approaches to evidence-based health care have emphasized the importance of employing experimental trials wherever possible.

External validity is concerned with the researcher's ability to generalize her or his findings to other samples and settings, i.e. the generalizability of the study findings. The external validity or generalizability of a study is affected by the sample size, the method of sampling, and the design characteristics and measures used in the study. If we say a study has high external validity, we mean that its findings generalize to other settings and samples outside the study. It does not make sense to talk about the external validity of a particular test.

Internal validity is concerned with the design characteristics of research projects. If a study is internally valid, any effects/changes or lack thereof in the dependent (outcome) variable can be directly attributed to the manipulation of the independent variable. It is important not to confuse the meanings of these terms.

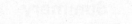

Surveys and quasi-experimental designs

8

CHAPTER CONTENTS

Introduction 63

Non-experimental research designs 63

Surveys 64

Epidemiology 64

Designs for comparing groups 65

   Naturalistic comparison studies 65

   Case-control designs 66

   Correlational designs 66

Quasi-experimental designs 67

   Time-series designs 67

   Multiple-group time-series designs 68

The internal and external validity of naturalistic designs. 69

Summary. 70

Introduction

In the previous chapter, the basic features of the randomized controlled trial were presented. Randomized controlled trials (RCTs) allow the study of causal relationships between variables. Although the RCT is held up by some commentators, such as those using the Cochrane Collaboration framework, as producing the highest level of research evidence, most health sciences research does not use an experimental design. In this chapter we will examine a variety of approaches used for investigation of research questions that do not lend themselves to an experimental approach.

The specific aims of this chapter are to:

1. Examine the uses of naturalistic non-experimental designs.
2. Discuss the use of surveys in health sciences research.
3. Outline the characteristics of designs involving naturalistic comparisons, correlations and quasi-experiments.
4. Identify some of the limitations of these designs.

Non-experimental research designs

If experimental designs are supposed to provide the tightest possible control of extraneous factors, why should we resort to alternative non-experimental research designs? There are a number of reasons why non-experimental research designs ought to be employed instead of experimental designs:

1. Many variables are not amenable to experimental manipulation, i.e. they are unchangeable. For example, if the research question is concerned with sex differences in responses to heart surgery, then sex cannot be manipulated by the researcher. Similarly, if the researcher is interested in age differences, the ages of the participants cannot be altered by the researcher.
2. Often, it is ethically inappropriate to investigate research questions using an experimental design (see Ch. 6). For example, if a researcher wished to perform a study on the effects of smoking upon health, studying this in an intervention

study would require the researcher to allocate participants randomly to the smoking or non-smoking group. Clearly, it is unethical to force some participants to smoke and others not to smoke. In intervention studies using a non-treatment control group, valuable and effective treatment might be withheld from participants. This situation involves serious ethical concerns that might lead to an experiment not being approved by the relevant ethics committee because of potential harm to the participants.

3. Experiments are best used to study simple causal relationships between variables, i.e. does the intervention cause positive therapeutic effects? However, many human diseases and illnesses are not determined by a single cause but rather by a number of causes interacting in a complex fashion. For example, heart disease may be caused by a combination of factors such as smoking, excessive stress, inappropriate diet or genetic factors. To identify such possible causal (or risk) factors, we need to study systems as they function in nature. That is, we should investigate patients in their natural setting, even with the difficulties this entails.

Depending on the nature of the evidence we require, non-experimental designs are appropriate alternatives to experimental designs. In the health sciences, experimental designs are focused on a rather narrow band of research questions that relate to the effectiveness of interventions and the causes of diseases. There are many other interesting research questions that do not relate to intervention effectiveness and, even when the questions do relate to interventions, there are circumstances in which non-experimental methods are more appropriate. Descriptive surveys are non-experimental designs, which provide data essential for progress in the clinical sciences and public health.

Surveys

Surveys are investigations aimed at describing accurately the characteristics of populations for specific variables (see Fig. 8.1). Surveys are commonly used in health research for the following purposes:

1. To establish the attitudes, opinions or beliefs of persons concerning health-related issues. The data collection techniques often include questionnaires or interviews.

2. To study characteristics of populations on health-related variables, such as utilization of health care, blood pressure, emotional problems or drug use patterns.

3. To collect information about the demographic characteristics (age, sex, income, etc.) of populations. A government census can be an important source of knowledge concerning population characteristics.

The statistics obtained from surveys can present us with an overview of the patterns of states of health, illness and the use of health services in a given community. In this way, we can gain insights into issues such as the prevalent causes of death or the health-related requirements of the population. The outcomes of the surveys can be the bases for hypotheses and theories concerning the causes of illness in a community. The area of health science concerned with such matters is called *epidemiology*.

Epidemiology

Epidemiology is the field of study that is concerned with the distribution and determinants of health and illnesses in groups of people. Epidemiology has been defined as the study of determinants of health and illness in a given population. Epidemiological studies may be descriptive, where researchers study the incidence and prevalence of health and illness, or analytical, where researchers aim to identify the multiple and interacting factors that determine health and illness in a specific community. Epidemiological investigations are essential to data collection in public health, as this discipline is concerned with the study of health populations. It differs from much clinical research in that it is oriented to the population or group rather than individual level. Epidemiology goes back to the time of Hippocrates who was concerned with the effects of environments upon the health of populations. The work of John Snow in the 19th century concerning the epidemiology of cholera is also considered to be a major landmark in the development of the discipline. Snow mapped the distribution of cholera cases in London and demonstrated that the water supply to different houses supplied by different water companies was involved with the transmission of the disease. The existence of the cholera organism was inferred from these observational data.

Descriptive epidemiology focuses on specific target populations and compares the occurrence of different health or disease states within these populations. Thus the numbers of cases, new cases and the relative risk of having the target condition are key components of the epidemiological approach. Two key terms in epidemiology are incidence and prevalence. The *incidence* of a disease is the rate at which new cases occur in a specified population during a specified period. The *prevalence* of a disease is the proportion of a specified population that have the target condition at a specified point in time.

These basic definitions are often used to construct indicators of population health that can be compared across different countries. The World Health Organization (WHO) maintains statistics concerning rates such as the birth rate, the infant mortality rate and perinatal mortality rate. The WHO website provides a wealth of comparative epidemiological data (http://www.who.int/en/).

Analytical epidemiology is concerned with how diseases are transmitted or spread within populations. The classic epidemiological approach conceptualizes disease within the framework of host, agent, vector and environment. The host is the human, the agent is the infection or health problem, the vector is the means by which the disease is carried (e.g. in the case of malaria this may be a mosquito) and the environment is the setting or mechanism that promotes the exposure. Disease can be transmitted directly (from person to person) or indirectly (via water, such as was demonstrated in Snow's classic study of London water supplies). Although this framework was developed initially within the context of infectious diseases, it is actually much more broadly applicable. Contemporary epidemiologists also study the prevalence and determinants of non-communicable diseases (e.g. Parkinson's disease) in the population.

The pattern of outbreaks of disease within populations is also an area of interest to epidemiologists. Common patterns of occurrence of diseases include endemic, epidemic and pandemic patterns. A disease is said to be endemic to a particular area if it habitually occurs within the area. An epidemic is the occurrence of a disease that is above and beyond the usually expected rate. We often talk of flu epidemics, meaning an unexpectedly high rate of the occurrence of influenza. A pandemic is a worldwide epidemic. We have become acutely aware of pandemics such as human immunodeficiency virus/acquired immunodeficiency syndrome (HIV/AIDS) and other feared pandemics such as severe acute respiratory syndrome (SARS), and, more recently, avian flu.

Epidemiology uses both experimental and non-experimental designs for collecting evidence. (Interested readers should consult Bonita et al 2006.)

Designs for comparing groups

Naturalistic comparison studies

Essentially, this type of study involves the comparison of naturally occurring groups or populations. For example, a researcher may be interested in the relative performances of males and females on a test of spatial abilities. The researcher might take a sample of each sex studying at a university and then compare the relative performances of the males and females on the test. Alternatively, a researcher might be interested in whether people growing up in different cultures have different pain reactions. Here, the researcher would select a sample of volunteers from the cultural groups of interest and compare their pain responses to standard pain stimuli.

There are extraneous variables which can be controlled in this type of investigation. In these studies, the researcher can control variables such as the ages or educational backgrounds of the participants by selecting similar groups. However, the researchers have not actually changed or manipulated the variables being studied. All that has been done is the measure of differences between naturally occurring groups.

To relate this to our first example, if our researcher determines that there is indeed a statistically significant difference in the performance of males and females on the measure(s) chosen, well and good. If our researcher then claims that biological factors are solely responsible for the differences, this is another matter altogether. This inference is only one of a number of alternative explanations that could be advanced to account for the differences observed. It is possible, for instance, that males and females in a sample have been exposed to different types of toys and games during their development, so that males might perform better or worse on some tasks. In the second example, any significant results in the pain responses might not be due to 'culture', but rather to systematic biological differences among the groups or a complicated interaction between these factors.

The simple fact of the matter is that it is difficult to demonstrate causation in natural comparison studies. However, if consistent evidence emerges from a logical sequence of studies, the investigators will gain crucial information about the differences between groups on clinically relevant measures. Natural comparison studies are vital components of the researcher's methodological tools.

Case-control designs

Researchers using this design select a group of participants or patients who have a specific disease or disability (case) and compare them with a control group. The cases and the controls are compared on previous exposure to defined risk factors, such as pathogens, life events or diseases. The method of data collection is usually *retrospective*. To illustrate the use of case-control designs, let us look at a simple hypothetical example. Say that there is an outbreak of food poisoning in a community with 20 people diagnosed with this condition. These people constitute the 'cases'. The control group would consist of people in the community who are not suffering from food poisoning. The hypothesis driving the investigation is that the outbreak was due to a specific unsafe food which was consumed by the affected individuals.

Data collection would involve interviewing the cases to identify the source of the contamination. Say that 18 out of 20 cases had eaten oysters at 'Oscar's Oyster Bar' in the previous two days. It is also found that only two of the healthy controls had eaten at Oscar's, but had eaten food other than oysters. The analysis of this hypothetical data would clearly indicate the risk factor for the food poisoning outbreak. Following further analyses of Oscar's Oyster Bar and samples from the cases for pathogens (e.g. salmonella), the hypothesis would be confirmed and Oscar would have to rethink his seafood supplier.

This simple example understates the complexity of the multiple and interacting determinants of health outcomes, in particular chronic diseases such as stroke or cancer. However, case-control designs are relatively simple to implement and provide useful evidence which requires further verification.

Correlational designs

The aim of correlational studies in the health sciences is to identify interrelationships among variables. In epidemiology these studies are referred to as 'ecological' designs. Epidemiologists refer to correlational designs as *ecological* designs. As correlational designs, they aim to establish associations between groups or variables, e.g. association between socio-economic class and the incidence of type 2 diabetes. A correlation is a statistic that expresses numerically the strength of association that exists between two or more variables.

Let us look at a simple illustration of correlational or ecological study. Say that clinical observations indicate that people who suffer from coronary heart disease tend to be overweight. Such observations might generate the hypothesis: 'There is a positive correlation between being overweight and the probability of coronary heart disease'. Here, the investigator will need to draw a representative sample of the population of interest (let's say 500 men and 500 women randomly selected from a population of healthy men and women aged 40 living in a specified district). The next step would be to measure the participants' weights and heights. These measures might be monitored over a period of time to check for drastic changes in weight. The second variable would be measured by the criterion of whether or not the participant suffered from heart disease during a specified period (e.g. 10 years), representing the length of the study. The incidence of coronary disease can then be converted into a probability for a particular category of weight (see Table 8.1).

It can be seen from Table 8.1 that the higher an individual scores on one variable (percentage overweight), the higher the scores on the other variable (probability of coronary heart disease). In this way, the fictional data presented in Table 8.1 are consistent with the predictions of the hypothesis stated above.

Two points should be considered at this stage. First, no evidence has been presented that one variable is causally related to another. This type of investigation does not, by itself, allow us to conclude that, for instance, 'being overweight causes coronary heart disease'. There are several alternative hypotheses, such as 'stress causes both being overweight and heart disease', which can also account for the findings. Second, it is clear that, at least for the period of the investigation,

Table 8.1 Fictional data representing the relationship between the variables 'percentage overweight' and 'probability of coronary heart disease' (for a 10-year period)

Percentage overweight	Number of participants	Number suffering coronary heart disease	Probability of coronary heart disease
Underweight or normal	600	30	30/600 = 0.05
10–19% overweight	200	20	20/200 = 0.10
20–29% overweight	100	15	15/100 = 0.15
30–39% overweight	75	20	20/75 = 0.27
40% or more overweight	25	10	10/25 = 0.40

the variable 'percentage overweight' does not account for all of the other variable 'probability of coronary heart disease'. That is, according to the data presented in Table 8.1, there are normal or underweight individuals who suffer from coronary heart disease and very overweight people who do not. Clearly, there must be other variables which influence the incidence of coronary heart disease. There are many other variables such as smoking, blood cholesterol level, personality type, stress and family history of heart disease that also correlate with the probability of coronary heart disease.

Some diseases (e.g. lung cancer and chronic back pain) have complex, interacting causes. Natural comparison, correlational and ecological designs can help us to identify risk factors: that is, factors that might elevate the risk of the onset or progress of these illnesses in individuals and populations.

Quasi-experimental designs

If preventive interventions are to be undertaken to reduce the risk factors associated with a disease, then we require reasonable evidence that these factors are, in fact, causally related to the disease. *Quasi-experimental* and *cohort* designs are often used for this purpose. The term *cohort study* is preferentially used in the domains of epidemiology and public health. These designs can resemble experiments, with the important difference that there is no random assignment into treatment groups. However, the investigator can control the time and place in which a treatment is introduced or withdrawn. One such method is a time-series design. This type of design is used by both clinical

and epidemiological researchers. Usually, these designs are *prospective* in that the participants are assessed at the beginning and then followed and assessed over a period of time.

Time-series designs

Time-series designs involve repeated observations before and after the administration of a treatment or intervention. In this way, changes in the sequence of observations following the introduction of a treatment may represent the effects of the treatment on the observed variable. Let us look at an example illustrating the use of time-series designs in health sciences research.

Returning to the risk factor of 'being overweight' we discussed previously, the following investigation using a time-series design could provide evidence for a causal relationship between this variable and cardiac disease.

1. Select an appropriate population to study.
2. Specify the dependent variable; that is, some clear-cut measure of 'coronary heart disease'. A commonly used measure may be the incidence of the disease. By 'incidence' we mean the number of new cases of the disease reported in relation to the population within a specified period of time (e.g. 50 per 100 000 per year).
3. Introduce an appropriate treatment that reduces the magnitude of the risk factor. In our example, a health promotion package could be introduced, emphasizing exercise and good eating habits. Let us assume that this intervention is adequately financed and a significant proportion of the population adheres to the program.

It could then be hypothesized that introduction of the health promotion package will result in a decrease in the incidence of coronary heart disease in the community.

4. Monitor the dependent variable over a period of time. It is essential to have readings of the variable both before and after the introduction of treatment. In this instance, the incidence of coronary illness would be determined from the medical records of hospitals, clinics and physicians. Public health authorities often gather and make available such statistics.

Epidemiologists are involved in the monitoring and surveillance of the health of human populations to track the occurrence of existing and possibly new health problems. The existence of HIV/AIDS was established very early by epidemiologists at the US Centers for Disease Control using sophisticated monitoring and surveillance systems. At the heart of such systems are sophisticated data-gathering procedures.

While the language and concepts of epidemiology are different from the classical clinical disciplines, the approaches to data collection are quite similar to those disciplines. Epidemiologists rely upon the collection of (especially longitudinal) survey data as the basis for their analyses of the distribution and transmission of diseases, they are involved in the analysis of RCTs and, like clinicians, attempt to build causal and statistical models of disease occurrence.

Figure 8.1 represents two of the many possible empirical outcomes using time-series designs. We will assume that the incidence of the illness was monitored for six years before and after the introduction of the treatment.

There are, of course, other possible outcomes. However, in this case, Figure 8.1A would be consistent with the predictions of our hypothesis, while the outcome shown in Figure 8.1B would be inconsistent with our hypothesis. Discussion of the way in which data generated by time-series designs are analysed is beyond the scope of the present text. Briefly, it involves the analysis of trends (increase or decrease) found in the dependent or outcome variable.

Time-series designs may have problems with internal validity. What assurance have we that the decrease in the incidence of coronary heart disease, shown in Figure 8.1A, was caused by the introduction of the health promotion program? Perhaps

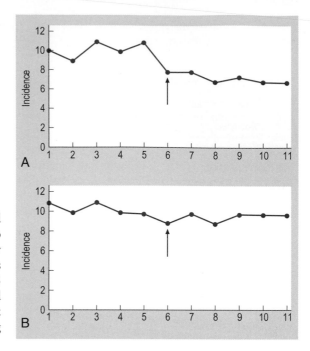

Figure 8.1 • Possible outcomes of time-series designs.

there was another cause, such as the introduction of drugs to control high blood pressure.

Multiple-group time-series designs

The introduction of multiple-group time-series designs involves the comparison of two or more naturally occurring groups or cohorts. Let us examine a simple illustration of such designs by a fictional further investigation of the coronary heart disease problem. Using a multiple-group time-series design, the investigator would select a community which is as similar as possible on demographic variables (socio-economic classes, age, size of the community, etc.) to the community or cohort being studied. In this way we would have:

- *Community A.* Control. Do not introduce health promotion program.
- *Community B.* Introduce health promotion program.

Figure 8.2 shows two of the several possible outcomes for such an investigation. Some researchers would call this type of design a prospective cohort design; prospective refers to the fact that the data

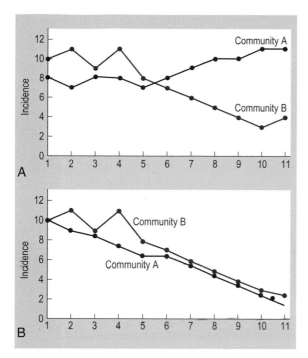

Figure 8.2 • Possible outcomes of multiple-group time-series designs.

The internal and external validity of naturalistic designs

We have noted several types of problems concerning the internal validity of investigations using natural comparison, correlational and time-series designs. These are similar to the problems of internal validity found in experimental RCT investigations. However, because researchers have generally less control over the phenomena being investigated, the use of natural comparison designs makes it more difficult to evaluate causal hypotheses. That is, given uncontrolled extraneous variables, a variety of plausible alternative hypotheses might be offered to account for the findings. Therefore, in areas such as epidemiology, researchers use evidence arising from a variety of investigations using different types of designs to evaluate their theories and models of the causes of human diseases.

When evaluating evidence from natural comparison designs, the external validity of the findings must be considered. In Chapters 3 and 5 we stated that external validity refers to the generalizability of the results of an investigation. Strictly speaking, the results of an investigation should be generalized only to the population from which the sample was selected. For instance, consider the example discussed previously, where a sample of male and female students were compared on a test of spatial ability. Any differences between these two groups can be generalized validly only to the population of students from which the samples were drawn. Investigators sometimes forget this obvious point, and try to make inferences about males and females in general. Such sweeping generalizations are invalid. For instance, other cultures with alternative child-rearing practices might well have males and females with completely different relative spatial abilities. Just because a variable is found to be a risk factor in one community does not guarantee that it will have the same influence on diseases in another community. Clearly, the finding that cigarette smoking is a serious risk factor for coronary heart disease in Western societies does not necessarily mean that cigarette smoking is a risk factor for coronary heart disease among other cultural groups and settings. Given the complex, interacting causes of coronary heart disease, there may be different risk factors in communities which follow different lifestyles or have different physical constitutions. It is not surprising, therefore, that advances

are collected after the commencement of the intervention and cohort refers to the fact that we have multiple intervention/non-intervention groups in the study.

Where the two communities show different trends, the outcome shown in Figure 8.2A is consistent with our previously stated hypothesis. However, in Figure 8.2B there is a trend for decrease in both communities A and B, and therefore the evidence is not consistent with the prediction of the hypothesis.

Even with multiple-group time-series (prospective cohort) designs, some threats to internal validity remain. There are no guarantees that the communities A and B were equivalent on all relevant factors, or that there were no important changes during the study in the communities which might have influenced the incidence of coronary heart disease. The best that researchers can do is to identify and try to estimate the effect of such extraneous factors on the dependent variable. There are problems such as insulating the two groups: when people in community B learn about the program being carried out in community A they, by themselves, might initiate aspects of the program.

in knowledge concerning systematic differences between culturally, racially or sexually different groups have been slow and controversial.

Summary

Descriptive surveys were shown to be important ways of studying the attitudes, behaviours and health problems of a community. Research evidence of this kind can be used to propose theories or test hypotheses of the nature and causes of illness. We examined several types of non-experimental research designs including epidemiological approaches, naturalistic comparisons, correlational and ecological designs, and time-series and prospective cohort designs. It was argued that these designs are appropriate alternatives to experimental designs, especially in field settings. However, as with experimental intervention and RCT designs, investigations using these designs must confront the same problems of internal and external validity.

Single case (*n*=1) designs

CHAPTER CONTENTS

Introduction 71

AB designs. 71

ABAB designs 72

Multiple baseline designs 73

Interpretation of the results
for *n* = 1 designs 74

  Hypothetical example 74

The validity of *n* = 1 designs 75

Summary 75

The aims of this chapter are to:

1. Identify methodological similarities between clinical problem solving and designing $n = 1$ studies.
2. Examine the use and comparative advantages of AB, ABAB and multiple-baseline designs.
3. Comment on the validity of $n = 1$ designs.
4. Demonstrate how the interpretation of single case studies is related to generally applied methodological principles.

Introduction

We have discussed research designs involving the comparison of groups of participants selected from a population. These designs provide evidence concerning the general causes of diseases, or the overall efficacy of interventions. However, before large-scale trials are undertaken, case studies, sometimes referred to as safety and efficacy studies, should be completed. Health professionals often work with individual patients and need to understand the specific causes of their problems and the effectiveness of treatments as applied to them as individuals. $n = 1$ designs illustrate the close relationship between the principles for conducting research and everyday clinical practice.

The purpose of the present chapter is to examine single case $(n = 1)$ designs, as applied by a variety of health professionals in natural clinical settings. You will be able to recognize close similarities between these designs and the quasi-experimental designs discussed in the previous chapter.

AB designs

Let us consider a simple example to illustrate the basic procedures involved in using $n = 1$ designs. Imagine that a patient is admitted to your ward suffering from a condition that involves having a high temperature. Before an appropriate intervention is devised, the patient's temperature is recorded every 15 min, for 2 h. Following this time interval, the patient is given medication to reduce temperature. The question here is: 'How do we show that the medication was effective for reducing the patient's temperature?' Obviously, we need to show that the patient's temperature had fallen following the administration of the medication. Figure 9.1 illustrates a possible outcome.

Let us assume that the drug is known to act quickly, say in 20 min. The evidence shown in Figure 9.1 would be clearly consistent with the hypothesis that the medication caused a decrease in the patient's temperature. Let us generalize this example to $n = 1$ designs used in various settings.

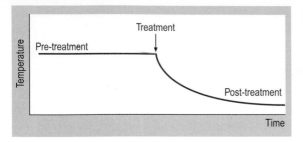

Figure 9.1 • Possible outcome of an AB design.

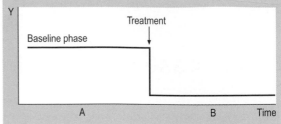

Figure 9.2 • General structure of $n=1$ designs.

Figure 9.2 illustrates the general conventions used in $n = 1$ designs.

1. We can see that the y-axis (Y) represents the outcome or *dependent variable* (DV): observations made of specific physical characteristics or behaviours.
2. The x-axis represents the time over which the observations were carried out.
3. The period A represents the sessions during which no intervention was administered. This is the 'control' level of the *independent variable* (IV). The observations recorded during A form the baseline.
4. Period B represents the sessions during which intervention was administered, i.e. the active stage.
5. The observations taken during A are compared with those taken during B. Systematic changes in the DV between A and B phases (increases or decreases) are assumed to reflect the influence of the intervention.

Therefore, an AB design involves taking observations during phase A, introducing an appropriate intervention, and then taking observations during B. It might have occurred to you that several of the threats to validity can be identified in AB designs. An obvious threat to validity is maturation: that is, recovery or deterioration occurring in the patient that might influence the readings on the outcome variable. Another possible threat is history: that is, influences on the patient other than the actual intervention. In the example we just looked at, one could also argue that perhaps the patient's temperature would have gone down even without the drug, because of the condition improving by itself or the environment of the ward (maturation), or perhaps the ward was air-conditioned and the patient would have cooled down anyway, drugs or not (history).

Next, we look at ABAB designs, which provide stronger control for extraneous variables than AB designs.

ABAB designs

The basic feature of ABAB designs is the alternation of intervention with no-intervention or baseline phases. That is, the researcher introduces the intervention following a baseline or no-intervention phase, then the intervention is withdrawn and then re-introduced later. Observations are recorded during each phase and this approach permits control for the previously discussed threats to validity.

Figure 9.3 illustrates the outcomes for a hypothetical drug study using an ABAB design. When the drug is withdrawn (second A) the patient's temperature returns to previous levels. When the drug is re-introduced (second B), the patient's temperature declines. Clearly, such an outcome is consistent with a causal relationship between the independent variable (intervention) and the outcome or dependent variable (observations of temperature). Figure 9.4 demonstrates the idealized results expected using ABAB designs with a highly effective rapid-onset intervention.

Although the above design is useful for demonstrating causal effects in a single individual, there are situations where it is inappropriate. ABAB designs are not particularly useful when there is a good reason to expect that the effects for an intervention are known to be irreversible following the intervention. For example, if the medication used in the previous example involved antibiotics, then the discontinuation of such drugs after a period might not result in the re-emergence of the symptoms since the antibiotics might well cure the underlying problem. Even when reversal is possible, it might not be ethical. Clearly, if we have succeeded in establishing

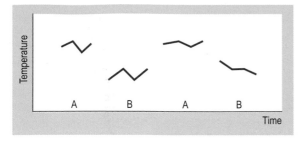

Figure 9.3 • Graph of patient's temperature under different treatment conditions.

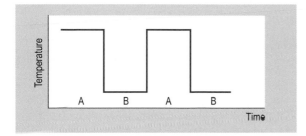

Figure 9.4 • General structure of ABAB designs.

desirable effects in our client during the first B period, we might well be reluctant to reverse this for the sake of demonstrating causal relationships.

Multiple baseline designs

Multiple baseline designs involve the use of concurrent observations to generate two or more baselines. Given two or more baselines, the investigator has the opportunity to introduce intervention affecting only one set of observations, while using the other(s) as a control. We will examine a hypothetical clinical problem to illustrate these designs.

Imagine that we have a brain-damaged client showing aggressive behaviours that disrupt therapy. Therapy is offered in two situations, say occupational therapy (situation 1) and speech therapy (situation 2). A behavioural program is devised, aimed at reducing the frequency of the aggressive outbursts. A multiple baseline design involves the observation of the frequency of the target behaviour in both situations 1 and 2. After establishing a baseline, the intervention is introduced first in one of the situations and then in the other. Evidence demonstrating the effectiveness of the behavioural intervention is shown in Figure 9.5.

The hypothetical data presented in Figure 9.5 indicates that the frequency of the target behaviour

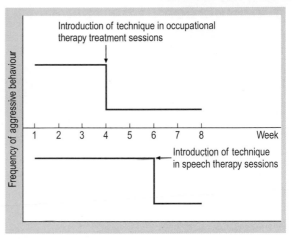

Figure 9.5 • Aggressive behaviour of a brain-damaged patient in two situations.

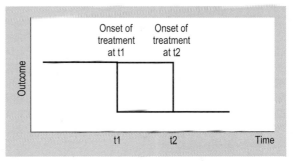

Figure 9.6 • General structure of multiple baseline designs.

(aggression) declined in situation 1 when the intervention was introduced, while it remained stable in situation 2. The subsequent introduction of the intervention in situation 2 resulted in a decrease of the behaviour.

Multiple baseline designs can also be introduced by generating baselines for two or more behaviours, or for two or more individuals. Just as in the example involving the different situations, the interventions would be introduced first for one of the behaviours or individuals, and subsequently for the others. Figure 9.6 illustrates a general example for multiple baseline designs.

Clearly, by introducing the intervention at different times, we are controlling for the effects of extraneous variables that might have influenced our dependent variable. Both ABAB and multiple baseline designs are appropriate for demonstrating the benefits of therapeutic procedures in individual patients.

Interpretation of the results for *n* = 1 designs

The principles for conducting and interpreting health research are also relevant for evaluating the effectiveness of everyday health practices. The need for control and accurate measurement arises when we intend to demonstrate that particular interventions or preventive interventions are causally related to beneficial outcomes.

As we have seen previously we can exercise control by systematically introducing and withdrawing interventions and measuring concomitant changes in the signs and symptoms of a disorder.

Hypothetical example

Let us examine a hypothetical example for illustrating four different methodological principles relevant to the interpretation of *n* = 1 studies. Imagine that you are caring for a young man called John who had suffered a severe fracture of the femur following a motorbike accident. He is gradually recovering with intensive rehabilitation but he is still in severe pain when narcotic analgesics are not provided.

Previous research has shown that transcutaneous electrical nerve stimulation (TENS) is a safe and effective modality for managing acute pain. However, the intervention is not equally effective for all patients so that there are no absolute guarantees that TENS will control pain in this particular patient. Also, even biologically inert pain control techniques can reduce pain through placebo effects. In this case you decide to investigate two clinically relevant research questions:

1. TENS is effective in reducing John's pain.
2. The pain reduction is causally related to the action of TENS.

Having obtained your patient's informed consent you decide to conduct an ABAB, *n* = 1 design for obtaining evidence to answer the above research questions. The variables here can be defined as follows:

1. *IV.* The independent variable is the pain control strategy using the TENS machine. The electrical stimulation produced by the TENS machine can be regulated such that you are in a position to vary the output of the machine. Two settings are selected:
   a. A represents a TENS output which is known to be physiologically *ineffective* for activating

the 'pain-gating' mechanisms (see Section 1). A represents the 'placebo control' level of the IV
   b. B represents a TENS output which is known to be physiologically *effective* in activating 'pain-gating' mechanisms. B represents the 'intervention' level of the IV.

2. *DV.* The outcome or dependent variable is an explicit measure of aspects of the signs and symptoms of the patient's condition. In this case we can select 'pain intensity' as a relevant dependent variable, measured on a 10-point scale (on this scale 0 represents 'no pain at all' and 10 'excruciating pain').

3. *EV.* Extraneous variables are variables other than the IV which can influence the DV and may 'confound' the demonstration of causal effects (see Ch. 7). In the present *n* = 1 study we are controlling for extraneous variables by:
   a. using a placebo control condition
   b. introducing and withdrawing the active intervention over time (ABAB).

The therapeutic effectiveness of the TENS for pain control will be represented by the changes in the pain intensity or the differences between the A and B phases of the intervention. Table 9.1 provides the procedure for conducting the data collection.

The A phase gives us the baseline against which we can compare the effectiveness of the active TENS intervention for reducing pain intensity. The outcome indicates a large and consistent difference between the A and B levels of the independent variable, and the large difference between A and B indicates a clinically useful reduction in the pain intensity experienced by John, your patient. You are now justified in continuing the intervention until he is sufficiently recovered to be pain-free.

We hope you will agree that this was an inspiring little story, the problem with it being that things just do not normally happen this way in the real world. The data we hypothesized above clearly illustrate an ideal, easily interpreted outcome appropriate for educational purposes. However, there may be some factors in the real world that impact upon these idealized findings. These include:

1. *Variability.* The above results are idealized, as opposed to 'variable'; that is to say, appearing to be all over the place. We will look at the concept of variability in Chapters 16 and 17. At this stage it suffices to say that, the more variable the findings, the more difficult it is to identify the trends and differences in results of *n* = 1 studies.

Table 9.1 Data collection procedure for hypothetical example

Time period	Independent variable level	Dependent variable
Week 1	A phase (placebo)	Daily assessment of pain intensity (at 08:00 hours)
Week 2	B phase (treatment)	
Week 3	A phase (placebo)	
Week 4	B phase (treatment)	

2. *Effect size.* The effect size is indicated by the difference between the baseline (A) and the intervention (B) phases. If the effect size is large in relation to the variability of the data, changes in pain intensity will be easy to see. However, if the effect size is small in relation to the variability of the data, then changes in pain intensity will be hard to see. Thus, the ability to detect the effects of interventions is affected by natural variability in the measured variable.

The validity of *n*=1 designs

We examined three (AB, ABAB, multiple baseline) designs in the previous sections. However, more complicated, 'mixed' designs are available for $n = 1$ investigations. The mixed designs include elements of both reversal and multiple baseline strategies. We will not discuss these in detail in this text; interested readers are referred to Morgan & Morgan (2009).

A basic requirement for the valid interpretation of all $n = 1$ designs is the production of a stable baseline. Unless this requirement is met, the interpretation of the results is extremely difficult. In some clinical situations, the production of a stable baseline might be unethical as it could involve withholding treatment. The intervention phase must also be long enough for the effectiveness of the treatment to emerge. Some interventions, such as those involving physical rehabilitation or psychotherapy, might need to be administered for months before their effectiveness, or lack of it, becomes apparent. Clearly, we cannot assume that the baseline and intervention phases are of equal duration.

It is essential that the observations should be valid and reliable. Some observations are straightforward, such as those based on taking temperatures. However, given a more complex variable such as 'aggression' we need to establish with clarity that different observers agree on the type of behaviours we are going to observe; behaviours that might seem 'aggressive' to one observer might not be classified as such by another.

We have already discussed how $n = 1$ designs attempt to control for the influence of extraneous variables. Although the $n = 1$ designs can be conceptually adequate to demonstrate causality, the patients, being in their natural setting, can be influenced by all sorts of uncontrolled events. After all, it is not possible to insulate individuals from their environment. Therefore, sources of invalidity must be evaluated with respect to each $n = 1$ investigation. It must also be remembered that no matter how sophisticated the $n = 1$ design, the observed outcomes for any given case may not generalize to other cases.

Summary

In this chapter, we examined three of the designs (AB, ABAB and multiple baseline) available for studying single individuals in their natural settings. It was argued that ABAB and multiple baseline studies provide a valid means for evaluating the causal effects of variables on therapeutic outcomes. These $n = 1$ designs are particularly useful for establishing the usefulness of interventions for individual patients. Although some limitations and ethical constraints might emerge in conducting $n = 1$ studies, they provide a useful tool for practising health professionals interested in evaluating the effectiveness of their interventions.

Although the statistical analysis of $n = 1$ studies is beyond the scope of this introductory text, it should be noted that graphing our observations, as discussed in this chapter, provides evidence for possible causal relationships. A precondition for interpreting the results of $n = 1$ studies is having an adequate number of stable observations across the various conditions.

The $n = 1$ designs are quite similar to quasi-experimental designs, in that the investigator has control over the type and timing of the interventions. In general, case studies are important adjuncts to conducting large-scale studies with representative samples.

Qualitative research

CHAPTER CONTENTS

Introduction 77

Research problems and questions 77

Approaches to qualitative research 78

What defines qualitative research? 79

An example of qualitative research 80

Summary 81

Introduction

Qualitative (interpretive) research aims to understand people through discovering the meanings of their experiences and actions. Understanding people requires the study of their beliefs, desires and intentions (Minichiello et al 2008). We *infer* what people think and feel by observing and recording what they say and do and take into account the cultural settings in which these actions occur. Qualitative research is well suited for exploring peoples' experiences of health and disease and their views on the benefits of the treatment and care being offered.

The aims of this chapter are to enable you to:

1. Identify the research questions addressed by qualitative research.
2. Describe key approaches to qualitative research.
3. Explain the shared features of qualitative research designs.
4. Explain how qualitative research designs are implemented for producing evidence.

Research problems and questions

When there are significant differences in the cultural backgrounds and experiences of persons, the understanding of personal meanings becomes problematic. There are numerous areas of health care and medicine where the interpretation of personal meanings is essential to ensure effective practices. The following four examples illustrate areas where qualitative field research can make strong contributions for clarifying personal meanings.

1. *Evaluating interventions.* Previously (see Ch. 7), we discussed how randomized controlled trials (RCTs) are used to evaluate the safety and efficacy of interventions. In addition to objective evidence, we should also look at the treatment/intervention experience, including the benefits obtained, from the participants' perspectives.
2. *Understanding cultural differences between health workers and clients.* In countries such as the US, Australia, Canada or the UK we live in multicultural societies. There is persuasive evidence that the way people experience their bodies, or events such as childbirth, pain or illness, depends to a large extent on their cultural backgrounds. When health practitioners misconceive their clients' view concerning their illness or injury, the outcome may be erroneous diagnoses and useless interventions. A particularly important area of qualitative field research is to clarify personal meanings of clients and

therapists with regard to health care problems, in an attempt to improve communications and enhance treatment outcomes.

3. *Evaluating the effects of health care environments.* Health care institutions, such as general and mental hospitals, can be seen as 'subcultures' having strong influences on the lives of both staff and clients. Persons with chronic illnesses and disabilities requiring long-term care might come to view themselves and their life situations from an 'institutionalized' perspective. The development of critical theories in these areas is particularly relevant for understanding the influences of health care environments. Research findings in this area have been applied to devise strategies to empower people such as those with intellectual disabilities to live and participate in the community.

4. *Relating to people with neurological or psychiatric problems.* People diagnosed as suffering from problems such as schizophrenia, intellectual disability or brain disorders may, to some extent, experience themselves and the world in ways different from people living without a mental illness. How such persons experience aspects of their world is by no means obvious, as these clients may demonstrate severe information-processing impairments such as delusions, hallucinations or memory problems, which may make it extremely difficult to establish empathetic relationships. However, in order to ensure that persons with such severe impairments or disabilities are treated appropriately and with understanding, health professionals must learn to see things from their perspectives. Qualitative field research has provided evidence which has helped to clarify the personal perspectives of people with severe disabilities.

The above are examples where qualitative research is appropriate for clarifying personal meanings and enhancing understanding and communication in health care settings. However, personal meanings are relevant to all health care situations, not only in the obvious areas discussed above. The following exemplify questions which are appropriately approached through field research strategies:

- What is it like to have a speech disorder? In what ways does it disrupt the person's life, from their point of view?

- How do caregivers interact with terminally ill patients? How do health professionals experience the death of a patient?

- How do health professionals break the news of unfavourable diagnoses, such as heart disease, to their patients? How are such situations seen from the perspectives of the health professional or the patients?

Approaches to qualitative research

There are several schools of thought that have contributed to the development of qualitative research (see, for example, Denzin & Lincoln 2011). These different traditions influence the way in which individual research projects are designed and analysed. We will outline, very briefly, four of the major approaches to qualitative research.

1. *Phenomenology.* Phenomenology, which is both a system of philosophy and an approach to social science, emphasizes the direct study of personal experience and the understanding of the nature of human consciousness. Research in this area involves 'bracketing' or putting aside the usual preconceptions and prejudices that influence everyday perception so that we can uncover the pure constituents of conscious experience. Within this framework, conscious experience is seen as the basis for personal meaning as we reflect on our experiences in the context of our goals and purposes. An important concept adopted from phenomenology is the notion of 'multiple realities': that is, different people may experience the world in quite diverse ways. This suggests that, in order to understand the meanings of a person's actions, we must become adept, through empathy, at seeing things from their point of view.

2. *Symbolic interactionism.* Symbolic interactionists emphasize that a social situation has meaning only in the way people define and interpret what is happening. That is, people do not react to 'objective' aspects of their environments, but rather their actions are guided by their personal interpretations of the situation. It follows that different people, on the basis of their past experiences and their particular social positions, may come to interpret a specific situation in quite divergent ways, and act in conflicting fashions.

The central issue is how symbols, in particular those of language, express meaning and enable communication and understanding between people.

3. *Ethnomethodology*. Ethnomethodologists study the processes associated with the way in which people perceive, describe and explain the world. Ethnomethodologists argue that the meanings of specific actions and events are not necessarily obvious, but are in fact rather ambiguous and problematic. People select and apply specific rules and principles in order to define and give meaning to situations in which they find themselves and in order to justify their actions in a given situation. Ethnomethodologists assert that we take an enormous amount of cultural context, such as norms and rules, for granted in our everyday communications and social interactions, and we tend to 'bracket' this as obvious or common sense. It must be remembered, however, that when the cultural backgrounds of individuals diverge, the understanding of personal meaning becomes less obvious or common sense.

4. *Grounded theory*. This approach was developed by American sociologists, Glaser and Strauss in the 1960s. Strauss & Corbin (1990, p 23) define a grounded theory as one which is '... discovered, developed and provisionally verified through systematic data collection and analysis of data pertaining to that phenomenon'. The core idea is to begin the research process without holding an explicit theory or hypothesis which is to be tested through the data. Rather, the theory emerges gradually as more data are collected. This method enables health researchers to develop an understanding of how participants actually experience health and illness, rather than 'filtering' these experiences through preconceived theoretical ideas. There are currently several versions of grounded theory applicable to qualitative health research.

Each of the above four traditions leads to somewhat different approaches to the conduct of qualitative research. Qualitative researchers are expected to make explicit which particular tradition was selected to guide their project. At the same time, there are characteristics which are common to quantitative research, as outlined in Chapters 2 and 3.

What defines qualitative research?

Given the different approaches, the question is: What is common among the various interpretive methods? We have already discussed these commonalities in Chapter 2. Qualitative health researchers believe that society exists as a result of meaningful social interaction and that the social actors themselves define it best. Therefore, a qualitative researcher needs to work towards empathy with the research participants through the sensitive collection of data and maintaining that commitment to validity by interpreting their perspectives in a manner which fits with their intended meanings. Qualitative research is a disciplined enquiry examining the personal meanings of individuals' experiences and actions in the context of their social environments. 'Qualitative' refers to the nature of the data or evidence collected. Qualitative data consist of detailed descriptions based on language or pictures recorded by the investigator. By 'disciplined' we mean that the enquiry is guided by explicit methodological principles for defining problems, collecting and analysing the evidence and formulating and evaluating theories.

'Personal meaning' refers to the way in which individuals subjectively perceive and explain their experiences, actions and social environments. Qualitative research provides systematic evidence for gaining insights into other people's view of the world: 'putting ourselves into someone else's shoes'.

The purpose of a research design is to formulate a plan to enable the collection of the data relevant to answering the research question. Regardless of the details, designs for qualitative research projects share the following characteristics:

1. Research questions are about people's experiences, beliefs and the meaning of events from their point of view. Qualitative designs therefore aim to ensure the creation of close, personal contact between the researchers and the participants.

2. Qualitative researchers use inclusive language. For example, where quantitative researchers will refer to 'subjects', qualitative researchers prefer to view the individual as a 'participant' or a 'consumer' of health services.

3. Qualitative designs are associated with purposeful sampling, as discussed in Chapter 5. Designs guide the researcher to look for participants

who will provide data to enable the development of a theory.

4. Implicit in all qualitative research is that the data represents the authentic communications or self-expressions of the participants. Designs must ensure that participants are approached in a way which inspires confidence in the importance of the project and the trustworthiness of the researcher (see Minichiello et al 2008).

5. The research plan must also ensure that persons conducting qualitative data collection (see Ch. 13) are skilled in techniques of effective interpersonal communications. All research traditions (including quantitative) take it as given that human beings respond actively to their environments so that the way in which participants disclose personal meanings and values are sensitive to the settings and interpersonal dynamics. Therefore it is essential that during data collection the researcher 'brackets' their preconceptions and values regarding the phenomenon being studied.

6. A well-formulated design should ensure that the research process is rigorous, conforming to rules of evidence (Dawes et al 2005.) An important consideration is 'bias' where the researchers adopt a preconceived theoretical framework for collecting and interpreting data. Bias has different connotations in qualitative research in comparison to quantitative research. As Dawes et al (2005, p 139) state:

> The whole point of the study is usually to look specifically at the experience of the participant and this process will be influenced by the researcher's perspective. What is key here is that this perspective is clearly recorded.

In other words, we must make explicit the political and personal biases which may colour the evidence. There are a number of strategies referred to as 'participatory action research' where there is an explicit commitment to a particular cause (Kindon et al 2007). For example, a researcher who has had experience of being a refugee may participate in action research aiming to improve the social circumstances of refugees.

An example of qualitative research

The following outline of a qualitative paper illustrates the role of design in the context of the overall research project. We will follow the stages for conducting applied health research as stated in Chapters 2 and 4. The paper authored by Van Lith et al (2011) is titled 'The lived experience of art making as a companion to the mental health recovery process'. This research is an illustration of how qualitative designs are implemented when evaluating therapeutic interventions.

1. *Research problems and questions.* The 'introduction' provides the background to the research in the form of a brief review of studies about the relationship between 'art making' and the process of recovery in 'consumers in mental health psychosocial rehabilitation services' (Van Lith et al 2011, p 652). Recovery is seen as a process of personal growth, a journey through, and '…which one develops purpose beyond the symptoms, disability and stigma of mental illness' (Van Lith et al 2011, p 652). Art making is defined as a variety of creative activities provided to consumers, in particular painting, sculpting and drawing. The research problem is implied by the aims of the study, i.e. the lack of specific information regarding the ways in which consumers benefit from art making. The research question addresses the consumers' experiences of art making and *their* interpretations of the ways in which these experiences contributed to their recovery.

2. *Planning.* The researchers collaborated with '…two of the biggest psychosocial rehabilitation services in Victoria' (Van Lith et al 2011, p 653). Both of these organizations provide extensive services for people recovering from mental health problems. The participants were initially approached by program managers and then selected by the researchers on the bases of their involvement in art-based therapies. Eighteen people volunteered to participate in the study. As the authors indicated, they were using a 'purposive sampling strategy' (Van Lith et al 2011, p 654) as this approach best identified the participants most capable of discussing their experiences of art-based therapies.

3. *Ethical permission* was granted by the various organizations including the university to which the researchers were associated. Consumers were also offered the opportunity to ask questions, assured of anonymity and had the right to withdraw from the study at any stage.

4. *Design.* A qualitative design functions to position researchers in a face-to-face, personal relationship with the participants. An interpretive, phenomenological approach was selected in order to collect and analyse data. This approach enabled the researchers to understand the '… lived experiences of individual consumers during their recovery' (Van Lith et al 2011, p 653).

5. *Data collection.* In-depth interviews were conducted in the setting of the art studio which the participants found comfortable. The researchers reported that each interview, which was tape recorded, was between 45 and 90 min duration. Participants could bring any of their artwork for facilitating the discussion. According to the researchers, '…each interview aimed to encourage an emergence of the participants' narrative about art-making and its relationship to mental health recovery' (Van Lith et al 2011, p 654).

6. *Organization and presentation of data.* The tapes of each interview were transcribed to produce a written record of the discussions between the researchers and the 18 participants. The interpretive phenomenological approach used by the researchers does *not* require using statistical procedures essential for making sense of numerical data characteristic of quantitative research.

7. *Data analysis.* The data analysis involved reading each interview several times and by tabulating key phrases and concepts a number of themes emerged. The authors identified '11 overarching themes' (Van Lith et al 2011, p 654) which represented the experiences of the participants. These themes were linked as closely as possible to the participants' actual words. Further, it was found that the 11 themes could be grouped into three 'meta-themes' which revealed how the art-making process contributed to mental health recovery.

The researchers concluded that art therapy had many benefits for the consumers, including '… insight, self-esteem, and confidence; empowerment; social connectedness and social engagement; context; and moving on' (Van Lith et al 2011, p 657). When evaluating interventions, qualitative researchers focus on the benefits from the perspective of the participants rather than using the objective outcome criteria of quantitative methods. In Chapter 22, we will take a further look at analysing qualitative evidence.

Summary

Qualitative research strategies include data collection that is aimed at understanding persons in their social environments. Rather than generating numerical data supporting or refuting clear-cut hypotheses, interpretive research aims to produce accurate descriptions based on face-to-face knowledge of individuals and social groups in their natural settings. The role of the researcher in this context is crucial and usually involves physical and social closeness between the participant and the researcher (see Ch. 2). In this chapter, we looked at a number of traditions for conducting qualitative research, including phenomenology, symbolic interactionism, ethnomethodology and grounded theory. We will examine how to conduct qualitative data analysis in Chapter 22.

Section 4

Data collection

11 Questionnaires 85

12 Interviewing techniques 91

13 Observation 99

14 Measurement 105

There are numerous methods available for data collection in health research. The appropriate methods are chosen depending on the research aims, design, the ethical considerations and the resources available for the research project.

Questionnaires are commonly used with survey designs. In Chapter 11, we examine a number of ways in which we can construct and validate questionnaires. There are different types of questionnaires, ranging from highly structured, standardized scales to unstructured open-ended formats suitable for qualitative research.

An interview (see Ch. 12) is essentially a conversation between the interviewer and the person being interviewed. As they require the presence of an interviewer, this increases the cost and effort needed to obtain data. The presence of an interviewer may also influence the respondent's answers. Qualitative research studies often employ in-depth interviewing techniques that are preferably carried out in the 'natural' settings (homes, hospital, etc.) in which the respondents are living or receiving treatment.

Observational methods are also commonly used strategies for data collection (see Ch. 13). They may range from highly structured observational protocols, indicating precisely which behaviours or clinical signs should be recorded, to unstructured records of the experiences of participant observers, as used in qualitative research.

Depending on how the data are recorded and analysed, interviews and observations may be used for both quantitative and qualitative research. However, the use of instrumentation and measurement tools to produce numerical data is most appropriate for quantitative research. A variety of standardized measurement instruments are now available for measuring biological and psychological functions (see Ch. 14).

Whatever data collection strategy is being used, we must ensure that it is reliable (replicable) and valid (accurate). Otherwise, as discussed in Chapter 14, the measurement error due to unreliable and invalid data collection strategies may prevent the researchers from achieving their goals.

Questionnaires

11

CHAPTER CONTENTS

Introduction 85

Questionnaire construction 85

Questions and questionnaire formats 86

    Open-ended and closed-response
    question formats 87

    Likert scales and forced-choice response
    formats 88

    The wording and design of questions 88

The overall structure of questionnaires 90

Summary 90

Introduction

Questionnaires and interviews (see Ch. 12) have in common the underlying assumption that some information is most accurately known by the informants themselves. Questionnaires are particularly useful for obtaining evidence for mental states, attitudes and events experienced by the participant such as symptom levels or degrees of satisfaction with treatments and information about the use of health services. This chapter focuses on questionnaires and questionnaire design, since they are frequently used to collect data in health sciences research.

The specific aims of this chapter are to:

1. Introduce basic concepts in questionnaire design.
2. Discuss the construction and administration of questionnaires.

Questionnaire construction

A questionnaire is a set of questions designed with the purpose of seeking specific information from the respondents. Questionnaires are best used with people who are fluent in written and/or spoken communication. The design of the questionnaire is crucial to its success. The process of design and implementation of a questionnaire is usually termed *questionnaire construction*.

Questionnaire construction usually involves the following steps:

1. *The researcher specifies the information that is being sought.* This may involve considerable thinking and discussion. Inspiration for selection of the required information comes from the investigator's research objectives, discussions with others, reading and other sources. At this stage, the document is typically a list of information yet to be translated into specific question form.
2. *Drafting of the questionnaire.* The researcher next takes the list of information he or she wishes to obtain from the respondent and attempts to devise draft questions. As is discussed later in this chapter, the phrasing and design of the questions and the overall design of the questionnaire are important for the validity of the obtained information. If the questionnaire is badly designed, then the responses obtained may not accurately reflect the real situation for the respondents.
3. *Questionnaire pilot.* It is wise to pilot or trial a new questionnaire with a small group of the intended respondents and with clinical or

research colleagues, in order to improve its clarity and remove any problems before the main survey. The pilot respondents may be asked whether the questions were clear.

4. *Redrafting of the questionnaire.* If the pilot phase uncovers problems with the questionnaire, it will need to be redrafted in order to address these problems. If they are of a major nature, it is usual to repeat the pilot phase. If they are minor, the researcher may make the necessary changes and then proceed to administration of the revised questionnaire to the full sample of respondents.

5. *Administration of the questionnaire.* After the questionnaire has been developed, it is administered to the full sample of respondents. The responses are then analysed in terms of the researcher's aims and objectives.

As with all research, the ethics of conducting surveys and designing questionnaires must be considered. For example, respondents should not be misled concerning the true aims of a survey. A blatant example of unethical conduct is if one is asked to respond to a general 'market survey' and then finds a high-pressure salesperson on the doorstep. If the survey is said to be anonymous, then it is questionable practice by the investigator to code the forms secretly so as to identify respondents. The follow-up of non-responders can cause a dilemma; people choosing not to participate in a survey should not be pestered. However, forms are sometimes mislaid or forgotten and it is necessary to follow these up to ensure that a representative sample is obtained.

In clinical research, the ethical issues relating to the possible effect of the contents of the questionnaire on the respondent must be taken into account. As an example, one of the present authors was involved in a survey aimed at establishing levels of knowledge of Huntington's disease and certain attitudes of people at risk for the condition. Before the survey was undertaken, a pilot study was carried out to establish whether or not the questions were upsetting to the participants. The actual participants were randomly selected from a 'pedigree chart'. However, the questionnaires could not be sent out before it was clearly established that each of the prospective participants already knew that they were at risk of developing the condition. It would have been appalling if people learned from receiving this questionnaire that they were at risk of a severe genetic disorder.

Questions and questionnaire formats

Questions and questionnaires come in a variety of formats. The researcher must decide which format is the most appropriate for the purpose of the study. Let us first consider the issue of the questionnaire format.

In some instances, researchers will not prepare a formal ('structured') questionnaire to be filled in by the respondent, but will design a general interview schedule to guide the interviewer who asks the questions of the participant. (Interviews are discussed in more detail in Chapter 12.) There are costs and benefits in both approaches, as shown in Table 11.1.

The interviewer-administered question schedule approach requires expert interviewers to administer the questions and this is expensive and time-consuming. Further, interviewer bias has been shown to influence responses, as some respondents may modify their responses to fit in with what they perceive to be the opinions of the interviewer. It is important to note that the structure and content of a questionnaire convey a lot of information about the researcher's agenda to the respondent. The respondent generally has little opportunity to

Table 11.1 Costs and benefits of interviews and questionnaires

	Costs	Benefits
Interview schedule administered by interviewer	Expensive to administer; requires expert help Responses much more susceptible to interviewer bias	Lower rejection rate More detailed responses can be elicited Greater control over filling out of response form
Self-administered questionnaire	Higher rejection rate Difficult to elicit detailed responses Less control over how response form is filled out	Cheap to administer Less susceptible to interviewer bias Can be administered by mail

influence the agenda in the case of structured questionnaires. A questionnaire is not really a conversation or dialogue but is essentially a monologue from the researcher to which the potential respondent may or may not respond.

However, the self-administered questionnaire approach is relatively cheap, is less susceptible to interviewer bias and can be administered by post (although it must be said that mail surveys traditionally have low return rates). Thus the disadvantages of this approach include higher rejection or refusal rates and much less control over how the response forms are filled out. Quality control of responses is certainly a problem with some questionnaires returned by mail. Frequently questionnaires that have been returned may need to be rejected because they are only part completed or they are poorly completed. Anyone involved in self-administered questionnaire analysis will attest to the sometimes remarkable talents of respondents in returning incomplete questionnaire response forms.

Having decided whether the questionnaire will be self-administered or administered by interviewers, the researcher must then decide upon the format for the individual questions.

Open-ended and closed-response question formats

There are two major question formats: the open-ended and the closed-response types. The distinction between the two is best illustrated by example (see Table 11.2).

In Table 11.2 the first question is an open-ended question whereas the second question is a closed-response question. In an open-ended question, there is no predetermined response schedule into which the respondent must fit a response. In a closed-response question, the respondent is supplied with a predetermined list of response options. The advantages and disadvantages of both question types are represented in Table 11.3.

Although open-ended questions elicit more detailed responses, there are some possible disadvantages associated with this type of question. The responses generated by such questions require a very large amount of effort to encode for data analysis and, when they are coded, tend to give rise to categorical scales. Categorical measures are at the low end of the types of measurement scales that may be used in health research. These scales

Table 11.2 Open-ended and closed-response formats

Open-ended	Q1. How do you feel about the standard of the treatment you received while you were a patient at this hospital?		
Closed-response	Q2. How would you rate the standard of the treatment you received while you were a patient at this hospital? (circle one number)	Excellent	1
		Good	2
		Moderately good	3
		Fair	4
		Poor	5

Table 11.3 Costs and benefits of open-ended and closed-response formats

	Costs	Benefits
Open-ended	Less structured Responses difficult to encode and analyse using powerful statistical methods Greater time taken by respondent to answer Respondent may find writing an essay more difficult than circling a number	More detailed answers elicited
Closed-response	Less 'depth' in answers May frustrate respondents	Tightly structured Responses easily encoded and analysed Less time taken to collect responses

Table 11.4 Questionnaire

Why did you choose XYZ Insurance to insure your car?	Newspaper advertisement TV advertisement Personal recommendation Previous insurance with us

necessitate the use of less powerful statistical methods. Further, some respondents may take a long time to answer this type of question. Or if they do not want to invest the effort, there is a greater chance of refusal to complete some questions. It is easier for the respondent to 'tick and flick'.

Of course, to a researcher employing a qualitative orientation, these 'disadvantages' may not be seen as such. The opportunity to study respondents' interpretations expressed in their own words might lead a qualitative researcher to advocate extensive use of open-ended questions. However, in this situation it is more likely that interview techniques rather than a written questionnaire would be employed. Questionnaires, particularly of the self-administered variety, are generally used for convenience and speed, not for depth of analysis.

It is important that the lists of options for closed-response questions are carefully designed by the questionnaire designer. It is very easy to bias responses by restricting the range of answers in this type of question.

This brings to mind a short questionnaire distributed by an insurance company to one of the authors (see Table 11.4). Two features are remarkable about this question. First, it does not allow for any answers other than the ones listed. Second, the range of available answers is very limited. What we wanted to say was that the insurers were cheap and reliable, i.e. were likely to pay up in the event of a claim. Clearly, the survey designer was a marketing person who had not satisfactorily trialled the questions with a non-marketing audience. While the designers may well have obtained the answers they wanted, the answers may not have been the ones the respondents wished to give. In the health sciences, there are often large differences in the ways in which health professionals and consumers approach the same problems. In questionnaire design, it is vital that the researchers do not impose their own conceptualizations of the situations under investigation to the extent that validity is compromised.

A further example of this danger is provided by the results of a survey conducted at a major teaching children's hospital in Australia. The survey was designed to study why many parents chose to stay with their children in the hospital, in order to plan better facilities and services. One of the questions asked of the respondents was 'Why did your child come to hospital today?' The investigators deliberately chose an open-ended response format for this question in order to tap into the parents' interpretations of the situation in their own words. What a treasure trove of answers! The answers provided considerable insight into the issues of importance to the parents, most of which we could not have predicted. Thus, the ways in which the questions are asked and the answers sought can have a major impact on the value of the information collected.

Likert scales and forced-choice response formats

In attitudinal questions, two possible response formats may be chosen: the traditional five- or seven-point Likert-type format (e.g. strongly agree, agree, neutral, disagree, strongly disagree), or the four-point forced-choice format (e.g. strongly agree, agree, disagree, strongly disagree). These are best illustrated by examples, as shown in Table 11.5. The first example is a conventional five-point Likert-type scale. The second is a four-point forced-choice type. The advantages and disadvantages are summarized in Table 11.6.

The forced-choice format does not allow respondents to give a 'middle of the road' or undecided answer. This is to guard against respondents using an *acquiescent response mode*. Acquiescent response mode refers to the phenomenon that occurs when respondents give middle responses all the time perhaps because of laziness or a wish to conceal their true opinions. *Extreme response mode* occurs when a respondent never selects an intermediate point on the rating scale. For example, if the respondent always chooses 'strongly agree' as their answer to all questions then one needs to be a little wary about the accuracy of these answers.

The wording and design of questions

The construction of good questions is an art, and a time-consuming art at that. In order to obtain valid

Table 11.5 Likert and forced-choice response formats

Likert-type	Q1. My medical practitioner always explains the chosen treatment to me (circle one number)	Strongly agree	1
		Agree	2
		Undecided	3
		Disagree	4
		Strongly disagree	5
Forced-choice	Q2. My medical practitioner always explains the chosen treatment to me (circle one number)	Strongly agree	1
		Agree	2
		Disagree	3
		Strongly disagree	4

Table 11.6 Advantages and disadvantages of response formats

Response format	Advantages	Disadvantages
Likert-type	Allows middle 'undecided' response	Acquiescent response mode
Forced-choice	Respondent forced to give either a positive or a negative response	'Undecided' response not allowed

and reliable responses one needs well-worded questions. There are a number of pitfalls to be avoided. Some of the following are the common mistakes made in constructing questions:

1. *Double-barrelled questions.* This is where two questions are included in one: for example, 'Do you like maths or science?' These questions should be separated so that it is perfectly clear to the respondent (and the researcher) which component of the question is being answered.

2. *Ambiguous questions.* It is important to avoid vacuous words and terms that may mean different things to different people. For example, 'old people' may mean everyone above 30 years old to a teenager, but everyone above 60 to a 50-year-old.

3. *Level of wording.* It is important to tailor the level of wording of questions to accord with the intended respondents. Jargon is to be avoided, and it should be established in the pilot study that the respondents will understand the concepts. For instance, asking

questions about 'Trisomy 21' might be inappropriate, whereas 'Down syndrome' could be intelligible. Using double negatives should be avoided. In general, questions should be simple and concise.

4. *Bias and leading questions.* The wording of the question should not lead the respondent to feel committed to respond in a certain way. For example, the question 'How often do you go to church?' may lead respondents to respond in a way that is not entirely truthful if they in fact never go to church. Not only can the wording of a question be leading but the response format may also be leading. For example, if a 'never' response was excluded from the available answers to the above question, the respondent would be led to respond in an inaccurate way. Bias might also arise from possible carry-over effects from answering a pattern of questions. For example, a questionnaire on health workers' attitudes to abortion might include the question 'Do you value human life?' followed by 'Do you think unborn babies should be murdered in their mothers' wombs?' In this case, the respondent is being led both by the context in which the second question is asked and the bias involved in the emotional wording of the questions. Surely one would have to be a monster to answer yes to the second question, given the way it was asked.

Finally, it should be kept in mind that even a good questionnaire might be invalidly completed. For example, a survey on 'attitudes to migration' might be answered less than honestly by respondents who may not want to reveal their negative attitudes to the researcher if the researcher is obviously of immigrant background.

The overall structure of questionnaires

Questionnaires may be structured in different ways, but typically the following components are included.

1. *Introductory statement.* The introductory statement describes the purpose of the questionnaire, the information sought and how it is to be used. It also introduces the researchers and explains whether the information is confidential and/or anonymous.

2. *Demographic questions.* It is usual to collect information about respondents, including details such as age, sex, education history and so on. It is best to position these questions first as they are easily answered and serve as a 'warm-up' to what follows.

3. *Factual questions.* It is generally easier for respondents to answer direct factual questions, for example 'Do you have a driver's licence?' than to answer opinion questions. Often, this type of question is also positioned early on in the questionnaire to serve as a warm-up.

4. *Opinion questions.* Questions that require reflection on the part of the respondent are usually positioned after the demographic and factual questions.

5. *Closing statements and return instructions.* The closing statements in a questionnaire usually thank respondents for their participation, invite respondents to take up any issues they feel have not been satisfactorily addressed in the questionnaire and provide information on how to return the questionnaire.

It is best to avoid complicated structures involving, for example, many conditional questions such as 'If you answered yes to Question 6 and no to Question 9, please answer Question 10'. Conditional questions usually confuse respondents and ought be avoided where possible.

Summary

Questionnaires are frequently used for data collection in health sciences research. This chapter has reviewed the principles of questionnaire design, including issues arising from the selection of appropriate questions and response formats.

Interviewing techniques

12

CHAPTER CONTENTS

Introduction 91

Interviewing models. 91

Methods of conducting interviews 92

The interview process. 93

Methods of recording interview information . . 94

    Advantages and disadvantages
of interview-recording methods 94

    Focus groups 95

The analysis of interview data 96

    Quantitative analysis of interview transcripts 97

    Qualitative analysis of interview transcripts . 97

    Coding and thematic analysis 97

Summary. 97

The aims of this chapter are to:

1. Distinguish between structured and unstructured interviews.
2. Outline commonly used strategies for conducting interviews.
3. Compare and contrast quantitative and qualitative strategies for conducting interviews.

Interviewing models

Many researchers distinguish between structured and unstructured interviews. Sometimes the terms 'formal' and 'informal' or 'guided' and 'open-ended' are also used (see, for example, Morse & Field 2003).

Denzin & Lincoln (2011) distinguished between three forms of interviews: (i) the schedule standardized interview in which the wording and order of all questions are exactly the same for every respondent; (ii) the non-schedule standardized interview where certain types of information are desired from all respondents but the particular phrasing of questions and their order are redefined; and (iii) the non-standardized interview in which no prescribed set of questions is employed.

If one defines an interview as a conversation, then a schedule-standardized interview is a very rigid form of conversation, almost like a play with a fixed script. In its most structured form, a structured interview may involve the reading of a prepared questionnaire to respondents and then filling in an answer form or response sheet for them on the basis of their answers. The questions are provided in a systematic order, with minimal or no

Introduction

A very commonly used method of data collection in the health sciences is interviewing. An interview can be thought of as a dialogue or conversation between the interviewer and the research participant with the purpose of eliciting information from the participant. Interviews are a key tool for the clinician and the health researcher as a means of collecting information about the opinions and experiences of patients and research participants. Interviews vary substantially in their structure, content and the way in which they are conducted. This chapter is concerned with the design and conduct of interviews and the analysis of interview data.

deviation from the prepared script. In a structured interview, the role of the interviewer is to ask the questions and the role of the respondent is to provide the answers with minimal extraneous information. Conversely, an unstructured interview may involve the interviewer in asking no direct questions, but simply prompting respondents to reflect on their current interests and concerns. Clearly, between these extremes lie a variety of different types of interview strategies and degrees of structure. The three different approaches to conducting interviews can be seen as being on a continuum: (i) structured, (ii) semi-structured, and (iii) unstructured. Semi-structured and unstructured interviews may include in-depth approaches designed to elicit more detailed and personal information from participants (Minichiello et al 2008). The extent of 'structure' or 'formality' is determined by a number of factors, including the following:

1. *Whether there is a fixed set of questions or schedule.* In a structured interview, the interviewer has a pre-planned set of questions or schedule. These questions may or may not be presented in a fixed order. In an unstructured interview, there may be particular 'themes' to be explored without a specific order required or specific question wordings.

2. *The way in which the information is recorded.* There are a number of ways in which interview information may be recorded. Structured interviews tend to employ pre-planned answer sheets or response schedules. Unstructured interviews have less expectations and restrictions on the answer formats of the respondents. The interviewer may record the interview or take free-form notes.

3. *The types of questions.* Structured interviews tend to employ more closed-response questions in which the valid answers have been pre-planned, rather than open-ended questions. With open-ended questions the respondents

provide their answers in their own words, whereas closed-response questions involve a choice of answers provided by the interviewer.

4. *The extent of control by the interviewer.* In a structured interview, the interviewer explicitly guides or directs the conversation (e.g. 'Mr. Smith, let's discuss how your family feels about your problem') rather than the respondent setting the agenda. In an unstructured interview, the respondent may assume a more active role in the conversation.

Quantitative researchers often favour highly structured, standardized interviews, while qualitative researchers often prefer semi-structured or unstructured approaches. This is consistent with the way data is analysed and interpreted under the two methods (see Ch. 2). It is useful to consider some of the advantages and disadvantages of the different types of interview approaches. These are summarized in Table 12.1.

The appropriateness of the different interview approaches is determined by the objectives of the researcher. If the researcher simply wishes to collect some basic symptom data, an unstructured interview would be inefficient. However, if the researcher wishes to study people's conceptualization and interpretation of their illness, an unstructured interview may be quite suitable. Some clinical interviews, such as history taking, are highly structured whereas other clinical interviews, such as those involving management of a long-term problem, may be less so.

Methods of conducting interviews

Since an interview is a conversation, there are several possible ways of conducting it. The interview may be conducted in person ('face to face') or by remote means such as by telephone or by using a

Table 12.1 Advantages and disadvantages of structured and unstructured interviews

	Advantages	Disadvantages
Structured interviews	May be less time-consuming The same information is collected for all respondents	Responses may not be recorded in the respondents' own words
Unstructured interviews	Responses may be recorded in the 'own words' of the respondents, hence less bias through interpretation The respondent has some input into the research agenda	May be time-consuming Not all the same information is collected for all respondents

system such as Skype™. There are a number of advantages associated with face-to-face interviews. (These are also discussed in Chapter 9.) Face-to-face interviews permit the non-verbal reactions of the respondent to be observed and perhaps the development of a closer rapport arising from the more 'natural' setting. Interviewers may use their observations of non-verbal cues to supplement the verbal information being provided and use their own non-verbal cues in a similar fashion. This is a particularly important consideration for qualitative researchers. However, the face-to-face interview may require a substantial amount of participant travel time and hence higher costs than for a telephone interview. With certain interview objectives, however, telephone interviews may not be suitable. If the interviewer and his or her credentials are not well known to the interviewee, it is unlikely that participants in a telephone interview would provide valid and reliable information about personal topics. Some people find disclosure of sensitive information to be easier by telephone or by the use of anonymous self-completion questionnaires. The face-to-face interview may be too confrontational or embarrassing for them. Tools such as Skype™ provide an interesting combination of the two methods if the video-cam is enabled.

The interview process

1. *Selection of the types of participants to be interviewed.* One of the interviewer's first tasks is to select the types of participants to be interviewed. In quantitative research, strategies such as random sampling are used to ensure a representative sample (see Ch. 6). As qualitative researchers, the interviewer selects those who are most likely to provide the required insights into the situation or issue under study, i.e. the 'key informants'.

2. *Recruitment of research participants.* The interviewer must then enlist the participation of the research participants. Typically, the interviewer will contact the prospective participant, explain the purposes of the interview and make a number of assurances. These assurances may include protection of privacy, the ability to vet materials based on the interview and the extent of time involvement of the research participant. Often, the interviewer might write to participants first and then contact them via telephone in order

to arrange the interview to be less 'confronting' (see Ch. 6).

3. *The interview.* The process of the interview varies substantially according to the methodology to be employed by the interviewer. The process of a structured interview is quite different from that of an unstructured interview. However, some basic goals are shared. The desirability of eliciting the participant's views rather than reflecting those of the interviewer (i.e. maximization of validity) is paramount. To achieve this, interviewers need to be sensitive, non-evaluative, alert and skilled at delivering and sequencing their questions. In in-depth interviewing, multiple interviews may be required. In this type of approach, the emphasis is on depth of analysis with a smaller number of interviewees rather than the breadth of coverage of interviewees offered by a sample survey. Substantial practice and good interpersonal skills are required to achieve competence in interviewing. Both video and audio recording of interviews have one large advantage over other methods of recording interview information. This is that the interviewer's interpretation of the interviewee's answers is open to independent scrutiny, because the primary research materials are available for study by others (with appropriate ethical clearance).

4. *Use of response schedules/answer checklists.* When conducting an interview, the interviewer may record the information provided by the interviewee on a pre-designed response schedule/answer checklist. For example, the schedule may contain information such as the sex and age of respondents and areas for recording their answers to particular questions. Typically, the response sheet is completed during the interview, although it can be completed at some time following the interview. Immediate recording is probably more valid and reliable although, once again, the mere presence of a recording device may be of concern to the respondent. Unless the response sheet is well designed, there is a major problem of handling novel or unexpected turns in the interview. The interviewer is interpreting, on the fly, the answers and information provided by the interviewee. If those do not conform to the assumptions designed into the response sheet, these interpretations may not be satisfactory or well considered. Telephone interviews may involve the use of computer

assistance where the interviewer is prompted by, and records the responses on, a computerized schedule.

5. *Free-form (unstructured) notes.* This method of recording involves interviewers making free-form notes to record information they believe to be salient, either during or following the interview. This method of recording is used extensively by clinicians in case notes. There are a number of advantages and problems with such recording; these result from the process whereby the interview is distilled into the notes. This process involves substantial judgement and interpretation on the part of the interviewer. Such distillations result in highly refined (or biased) and reduced data, the validity of which, at least in terms of the interview, is inaccessible to scrutiny. Further, free-form note-taking may not result in the recording of the same type of data across interviewees. Often, when case audits from records are being performed, it is not possible to derive the required data from clinical notes because of this problem. For the participant, it can be a bit off putting, watching the interviewer write down all the answers. So, although a recorder may be initially intrusive, it is far less intrusive than watching the interviewer write down everything during the interview.

6. *Follow-up.* Having completed the interviews, the interviewer may wish to follow up the participants. Some interviewers undertake to give the respondents copies of their transcribed interview and may offer the right of vetting the materials included in the transcript.

Methods of recording interview information

Interviewers may use a number of different means of recording interview information, ranging from written summary notes of the interview to an actual video or audio recording of the live interview. These recording methods have a number of advantages and disadvantages, as discussed below.

1. *Video recording.* Video technology has reduced in cost and improved to such an extent that high-quality video recordings of interviews are well within the budgets of many organizations and individuals. Video recordings provide a wealth of information about the interview. It is possible to observe non-verbal communication channels as well as to construct audio transcripts of the interaction between the participants. However, some interviewees find the presence of the camera to be threatening. This may have a number of effects: one may be to refuse to participate, another may be to alter the normal flow of the interview. Some respondents may be unwilling to commit personal information and/or controversial views to tape, if they believe there is a risk that the interviewer might disclose the interview to others. Interviewees would find it difficult to deny their views when they have been videotaped expressing them. This is why the police in some countries videotape their interviews with suspects.

2. *Audio taping.* Many interviewers use audio recording of interviews in order to be able to prepare transcripts for later study. Many of the same issues that pertain to video recording are also relevant to audio recording. The use of audio recording may result in greater refusal rates and the 'sanitization' of the views expressed by participants for fear of reprisals arising from disclosure of the interview to others. However, audio recording is often considered to be less intrusive by the participant than video recording. Qualitative research methodologists have developed systematic methods in note-taking and coding of interview information. For a more detailed treatment of these issues, the reader is referred to Minichiello et al (2008).

Advantages and disadvantages of interview-recording methods

The advantages and disadvantages of the various recording methods are summarized in Table 12.2. Thus, video recording is intrusive, requires substantial post-interview analysis and may result in less disclosure, yet provides very rich information that can be independently analysed. The use of a recording method such as a response sheet requires great trust in the judgement and recording abilities of the interviewer. There is a potential for bias arising from the interviewer 'adjusting' the information provided by the interviewee to fit the recording

Table 12.2 Advantages and disadvantages of different ways of recording interview information

	Advantages	Disadvantages
Video recording	Full transcripts of interview possible Non-verbal data available Accessible to independent analysis	Intrusive Less disclosure Necessity for substantial, and costly, post-interview analysis Potentially greater rates of refusal to participate
Audio recording	Full transcripts of interview possible Accessible to independent analysis	Intrusive (but probably less than video) Reduced disclosure Necessity for substantial, and costly, post-interview analysis Potentially greater rates of refusal to participate
Response sheets	Same data recorded for all interviews Little post-interview analysis required, reducing costs	Unexpected answers may not be well handled Interviewers may bias data in their recording Inaccessible to independent analysis
Unstructured notes	Cheap and simple	Interviewers may bias data in their recording Some data may be omitted Inaccessible to independent analysis Necessity for some post-interview analysis

method and/or expectations of the interviewer. Further, there is no opportunity for re-analysis.

So which information-recording method for interviews is the most appropriate? The appropriateness of the method of recording interview information is determined by the needs of the person using the information. For example, if the information user simply wants some basic data such as the age, sex and symptom profile of a patient, it would be absurd to use video recording. This would be very time-consuming. Each tape would have to be made, and then viewed again for analysis. In this instance, a simple response sheet or checklist would suffice. However, if the interviewer was interested in exploring reactions of interviewees to the death of a close relative, perhaps the use of audio or video recording would provide a richness of data suitable for that interest.

Focus groups

Focus groups are a form of group interviewing and can enhance data collection by providing information that may not have been made available through individual interviews. Focus groups were developed by market researchers as an efficient way of gaining commercially important information about consumer preferences. This use is not altogether different from the use of focus groups in health

care research. For instance, one might conduct a focus group with people who experience a chronic illness such as epilepsy in order to learn more about the personal experiences of the socio-economic impact of illness and managing seizures.

Focus groups usually involve a small group of approximately six to ten people in a face-to-face setting who engage in a series of discussions. Focus groups can involve one session, though are typically run over a number of sessions where the researcher conducts the sessions in the role of moderator or facilitator of the discussions. A focus group operates as a discussion rather than a group interview primarily because it relies heavily on participant interaction; there is an underlying assumption that interaction between participants will encourage them to clarify their points of view.

The role of the facilitator is essential to an effective focus group; they must be skilled at controlling the flow or discussion in a manner which enables participants to contribute as much as possible and yet ensure that the direction of the discussion remains within the parameters of the research question. As with any data collection method, focus groups are not without bias and the researcher must remain mindful of any distortions or prejudices arising from group discussions.

Focus groups have a number of advantages. They allow for maximum data collection (versus individual interviews) in one setting. In terms of sampling issues, they can encourage participation from those who are reluctant to be interviewed on their own or who feel that they have little or nothing to contribute. They do not discriminate against those who are illiterate since ideas may be verbally expressed and can therefore be useful in cross-cultural research.

The disadvantages of using focus groups include group dynamics or group culture which may silence some individuals. This may make it difficult to research highly sensitive topics and 'group think' may become a problem. Another issue which is not often discussed is the difficulty in transcribing a multitude of voices which are often talking over one another or interrupting. This can increase the cost of focus group interviewing.

Nevertheless, focus groups have proved to be a very useful data collection strategy because they have assisted in the successful assessment of health education programs, providing insight into people's attitudes towards specific public health issues.

The analysis of interview data

The manner in which interview data may be analysed is determined in part by how the data have been recorded and, in part, by the theoretical orientation of the researcher. In the previous discussion, we have seen that these formats include videotapes, audiotapes, completed response sheets and free-form summary interviewer notes.

The basis for many analyses of interview data is the interview transcript. The transcript of an interview is a verbatim written version of the conversation that took place between the participants. To provide an example, an excerpt from an interview transcript produced by Janet Doyle at La Trobe University follows (Doyle & Thomas 2000). The transcript is of an interview between a clinician and a client, concerning the client's hearing loss.

Clinician: Okay. So what are you noticing with your hearing?
Client: Well, in a crowded area I can't, you know, understand the other people.
Clinician: Right, sound's a bit jumbled up.
Client: And when I am in the next room I can't even hear the phone.
Clinician: Right.
Client: I am not bad, it is like I am not that bad but still at times.

Clinician: Right.
Client: There is a lot of times I can't hear it.
Clinician: If people speak directly to you like this you are fairly good?
Client: Yes I am alright.
Clinician: But in a group have a bit of trouble?
Client: Have trouble.
Clinician: Right, does one ear seem better than the other ear?
Client: Yes, this one seems better than this.
Clinician: Right.
Clinician: How long have you been noticing your difficulty?
Client: Oh, about 12 to 18 months I suppose.
Clinician: Just gradual was it?
Client: Yes.
Clinician: Okay. Do you get any ringing or buzzing in your ears?
Client: Oh, now and again, very seldom though.
Clinician: It doesn't bother you?
Client: No.
Clinician: Okay. Have you had medical trouble with your ears like infection or anything?
Client: No, no.
Clinician: Do you know of any family history of hearing loss?
Client: No, only the older brother, he has got a hearing aid.
Clinician: Right.
Client: That's all.
Clinician: Have you been exposed to excessive noise?
Client: Yes.
Clinician: …machinery or?
Client: Yeah. I worked down the car plant, you know, with the heavy machinery.
Clinician: The assembly line?
Client: Right.
Clinician: Were you doing that sort of work for a long time?
Client: Oh yes, 30 years.
Clinician: Yeah, that's a fair…
Client: I wasn't on the line all the time but.
Clinician: Right.

And so the interview continued.

Let us now consider some of the analysis options under the quantitative and qualitative headings.

Quantitative analysis of interview transcripts

A number of quantitative analysis possibilities are presented with interview transcripts. For example, the researcher might count the number of words spoken by each participant to obtain a quantitative measure of their relative contribution to the conversational process. Another possibility would be to count the number of questions asked by the clinician. These quantitative measures could then be used to test various hypotheses. Analyses of interview transcripts similar to the example shown above, in the study from which it was taken, have demonstrated substantial sex differences between the number of questions asked by male and female clients. It seems that the male clients asked many more questions than the females. Thus, the quantitative researcher might use interview transcripts to count and analyse certain features of the transcripts.

Qualitative analysis of Interview transcripts

Under the qualitative heading there is a broad variety of approaches to the collection and analysis of interview data. Such approaches may, however, be broadly categorized as *descriptive* or *theoretical*.

A descriptive qualitative study is often termed ethnography. They are often written from the perspective of the participant(s) in the first person. The purpose of the ethnography is to provide a detailed description of a particular set of circumstances and to encourage readers to make their own interpretations. To make such interpretations, it is essential to consider and theorize the social and cultural contexts in which the evidence was produced.

Ethnographic studies are primarily used in health and anthropology and can help researchers to understand and address health/social problems from a specific cultural perspective. Some researchers spend decades living in or involved with a particular ethnic community in order to understand and research what issues are considered important to them.

Most qualitative studies, however, are theoretical in nature. That is, they attempt to develop theories and concepts and, often, to verify these concepts and theories. A key approach to theoretical qualitative research is provided by Glaser & Strauss'

grounded theory (Liamputtong 2009). There two methods for the development of grounded theory: the constant comparative method in which the researcher codes and analyses data to develop concepts, and the theoretical sampling method in which cases are selected purposively to refine the 'theory' previously developed. In contrast, however, some qualitative researchers prefer to collect a substantial amount of data before attempting to formulate their theories.

Coding and thematic analysis

Coding is used to organize data collected in an interview and, for that matter, in other types of documents such as field notes. Different qualitative researchers advocate different approaches to coding but it typically involves the following steps. The researchers closely study their materials, in this case the interview transcripts, and develop a close familiarity with the material. During this process, all the concepts, themes and ideas are noted to form major categories. For example, in interviews of nursing home residents, some themes that arise might include personal safety, autonomy and decision making, personal hygiene and so on. Often, the researcher will then attach a number or label to each category and record their positions in the transcript. Coding is an iterative process, with the researcher coding and recoding, as the scheme develops. Some computer programs are now available to assist with the coding analysis of machine-readable transcripts and these ease some of the clerical burden, although most qualitative researchers still employ manual coding methods. The researchers, having developed the codes and coded the transcripts, then attempt to interpret their meanings in the context in which they appeared. The reporting of this process typically involves 'thick' or detailed description of the categories and their context, with liberal use of examples from the original transcripts. The process of analysis of qualitative research materials is examined in more detail later in this book (see Ch. 22).

Summary

Interviews may be defined as a conversation between interviewers and interviewees with the purpose of eliciting information. Structured interviews generally involve a fixed set of questions or schedule, the use of pre-planned response sheets, a greater proportion of closed-response questions and direction from the interviewer. Unstructured interviews tend not to have these attributes, with less structure and control. Interviews may be conducted face to face or by telephone and both these methods have certain advantages and disadvantages. The focus group is a valuable alternative to the individual interview. Interview data may be recorded in a number of different ways, but the transcript is often used. Transcripts may be analysed using quantitative or qualitative techniques.

Observation

13

CHAPTER CONTENTS

Introduction 99

Overview of different approaches to
observation 99

   Who is to make the observations?. 99

   Settings in which observation is conducted 100

   Issues in the use of unaided observation
   or the use of instrumentation 101

Observer roles. 101

Observation in qualitative research. 102

Observation in quantitative research 104

Summary. 104

Introduction

Observation is a common method for data collection in both health research and clinical practice. Observation involves the direct perception and recording of the phenomena under study. The advantage of observational data collection over questionnaires and interviews in research is that the researcher is in a position directly to see and hear what people actually do, rather than relying on the participants' interpretations and perceptions of their actions.

   The aims of this chapter are to:

1. Outline different approaches to conducting observations and examine their relative advantages.
2. Discuss the different roles observers may adopt.
3. Examine observation in the context of qualitative and quantitative approaches.

Overview of different approaches to observation

Depending on the phenomenon being studied and the research questions being asked, several different observational approaches might be employed in the data collection. Each of these approaches has associated advantages and disadvantages. The basic issues are:

- Who is to make the observations.
- The settings in which the observations are made.
- The use of instrumentation.

Who is to make the observations?

When research involves the observation of people, self-observation becomes feasible and, at times, desirable. As an example, consider the study of pain. Here the patients themselves are uniquely positioned to provide subjective evidence concerning the intensity and location of pain over a period of time. Figure 13.1 shows a typical chart for guiding self-recorded pain observations in chronic pain patients, which is used in both research and clinical assessment.

   The self-observations of the patients provide data for understanding how patients' pain experiences change over time, events correlating with the onset and offset of the pain and also evidence for evaluating the relative effectiveness of pain management strategies. Given that the experience of pain may be expressed in the sufferer's overt behaviour, we may observe such pain-related behaviours when assessing pain. For instance, in a study involving comparison of pain behaviours of surgical patients with different cultural backgrounds, independent observers recorded pain-related behaviours in patients at agreed time intervals during physiotherapy treatments. Figure 13.2 is based on whether the observers recorded a yes or no for each category for each time interval in which the behaviours were sampled.

There are probable relative advantages and disadvantages to using self-observation or outside observers, as shown in Table 13.1.

	On average, what was your level of pain during today										
Monday	0 1 2 3 4 5 6 7 8 9 10 no pain very intense										
Tuesday	0 1 2 3 4 5 6 7 8 9 10 no pain very intense										
Wednesday	0 1 2 3 4 5 6 7 8 9 10 no pain very intense										

Figure 13.1 • Typical chart for self-recorded pain observations.

Behaviours	Time		
	t1	t2	t3
Verbal complaint			
Vocalization			
Protective response			

Figure 13.2 • Observation guide for recording pain behaviours.

Settings in which observation is conducted

Some disciplines, such as astronomy or geography, focus on phenomena which are best studied as they occur, in their natural settings. Other disciplines, such as anatomy or chemistry, are more likely to be studied in a laboratory. In the broad range of health sciences research, phenomena are studied in either laboratory or natural settings, and observational data collection may be appropriate in both of these settings.

The general advantage of laboratory environments is that we can impose a considerable degree of control over extraneous factors that may systematically influence (and perhaps bias) our observations. In addition, equipment for facilitating or recording observations is more readily available. For example, in the 1960s, researchers began a series of studies to examine the physiology of the human sexual response. The controlled laboratory setting and the use of appropriate instrumentation enabled these researchers to observe and accurately record poorly understood aspects of human sexual functioning. This work was thought to be fundamental for developing clinically useful interventions aimed at helping people with sexual dysfunction, although it must be noted that this work has been controversial.

The disadvantage with laboratory settings is that the phenomenon being observed may change when it is being observed in an artificial setting. This is particularly true for human behaviour, where the social contexts are important determinants of the behaviours and experiences. Indeed, the discipline of social psychology is devoted to the study of these effects. In other words, laboratory research sometimes has problematic ecological validity in that the findings discovered in this context may

Table 13.1 Advantages and disadvantages of using self-observation or outside observers		
	Advantages	**Disadvantages**
Self-observation	Greater access to participative experience (introspection) Less intrusive Less expensive	Greater bias Less likely to record accurately Less likely to carry out observation as agreed
Outside observer	Greater objectivity Less bias More likely to record accurately More likely to carry out observations as agreed	Cannot directly access participant's perceptions More intrusive More expensive and time-consuming

not generalize well to other 'real world' contexts such as in the clinic or the community. Table 13.2 summarizes some of the relative advantages and disadvantages of laboratory and natural settings for making observations.

Issues in the use of unaided observation or the use of instrumentation

The accurate observation of a variety of phenomena is possible through the unaided senses; for example, observing aspects of human behaviour or clinical symptoms such as abnormal postures, discoloration of the skin, or abnormalities in patients' eye movements. Other phenomena may be inaccessible to unaided observation such as, for example, very small objects and events, where we might need to use a microscope for accurate observations. Some events are also extremely complex and occur relatively quickly in relation to the abilities of the observer. An example of this is human locomotion where recording the event using a device such as a video camera greatly enhances the accuracy of the observation such as in a gait analysis laboratory. A key factor in the advancement of science and clinical practice has been the development of sophisticated instrumentation to enable better observation of clinical phenomena.

There are, however, certain disadvantages associated with using instrumentation. These issues are discussed later in this book, when we review instrumentation and measurement. In other words, observation and measurement are closely interrelated (see Ch. 12). We can note here, however, that the use of instruments may distort the event being observed; for example, the preparation of tissue for electron microscopy changes to some extent the internal organelles of a cell being observed. These effects are very well known and documented. It requires considerable expertise to use more complex instruments, and a strong theoretical background to separate the artefacts from useful data and interpret the observations. Human research participants also react to being observed. The more intrusive the observer is with equipment and instruments, the more likely that the participants' behaviour will change.

The use and relative advantages and disadvantages of recording techniques were discussed in the context of interviewing techniques earlier in the book (see Ch. 12). Table 13.3 represents the relative advantages and disadvantages of using instruments for aiding observations.

Observer roles

Whether or not instrumentation is used, observation involves a person perceiving and recording an event. There are various positions observers may take in relation to observing human behaviour in

Table 13.2 Advantages and disadvantages of laboratory and natural settings for making observations

	Advantages	Disadvantages
Laboratory setting	Better control over extraneous variables Observation aids and recording equipment available	Distortion of phenomena in artificial environments Problematic ecological validity
Natural setting	Increased ecological validity Observation of phenomena as they occur naturally	Little control over extraneous variables Observation aids and recording equipment may be more difficult to use

Table 13.3 The advantages and disadvantages of using instruments for aiding observations

	Advantages	Disadvantages
Unaided observations	Less disruptive Best suited for observing human behaviour Relatively simple and inexpensive	Insufficient for observing some phenomena Insufficient accuracy and detail
Instrumentation	Access to events outside unaided human senses Increased accuracy and detail	May distort phenomena May be complex and expensive to use

health care settings. The fundamental issue is the extent to which the observer becomes involved or participates in the events being observed. There are generally considered to be four main roles that an observer may take. These are: complete participant, participant as observer, observer as participant and complete observer. These are discussed below.

The *complete participant* assumes the role of participant in the setting under investigation and does not normally disclose his or her intent to the other participants. Thus, the researcher actively participates in the setting without the knowledge or consent of the other participants. The purpose behind this approach is to minimize any changes in behaviour of the other participants as a result of their being observed. It can, however, border on the edge of unethical practice and must be used with caution. An example of the use of the complete participant method is provided by Rosenhan's (1975) classic study of 'pseudo-patients' in psychiatric hospitals. Here, the observers posed as (and were admitted as) psychiatric patients in order to study the experiences of psychiatric patients. The pseudo-patients were not recognized as impostors by the staff or the institutions. In this way, they could make and record observations about the interpersonal interactions between the staff and patients. However, in order to be admitted, the observers deliberately misled the staff, who were in fact under study.

The *participant as observer* participates fully in the situation under study, but discloses his or her identity and purpose to the other participants. Examples of this can be seen in anthropological studies, where the observer attempts to participate as an active member of a cultural group.

The *observer as participant* makes no pretence of participation but interacts with the other participants. When using this method in a health setting, the observer obtains permission to record events and observe patients, while interacting with the staff and the patients. An example of this method is provided by a study performed by a PhD student with a nursing background, supervised by one of the authors. The student's objective was to investigate how psychiatric nurses working in the community make decisions to act in a crisis situation with a disturbed person. He accompanied the nurses on their crisis visits. While travelling to the crisis scene, he interviewed the nurses about their expectations. He observed the crisis scene and its participants and, immediately following its conclusion, interviewed the nurses about it.

The *complete observer* does not interact with the other participants at all and, as with complete participation, does not disclose his or her identity or purpose. As an example, one might investigate therapist–patient interactions by observing from behind a one-way mirror. It is a bit like how zoologists may use a 'hide' in a natural setting to observe the animals they are studying. Observers can, if they wish, use a structured schedule for making the observations.

The level of participation chosen involves a tension between the requirements of objective and independent analysis, and the proximity from which the social and clinical phenomena can be studied. Clearly, the participation of the observer introduces changes in the phenomenon under study. It is a question of whether these changes are so large as to negate the benefits obtained by closer observation afforded by actual participation. This question has generated much discussion in the social, behavioural and clinical sciences.

Observation in qualitative research

Observation data collection in the context of qualitative field research requires providing authentic pictures and reports of individuals functioning in their natural environments. There are four principles that are important for conducting field research (Daly et al 1997):

1. The investigator should establish proximity with the participants in both a physical and a social sense. It is desirable that this involvement should be long-term, both to enable understanding and to reduce the participants' reactivity to the presence of the investigator.

2. The report should be truthful. The reporter should not allow ideological biases to distort or censor their observations or deliberately lie to place their participants in a good or bad light.

3. The data should contain a large amount of pure description of action, people, activities and the like. The reality of the place should be conveyed through representation of its mundane aspects in a straightforward manner.

4. The data should contain direct quotations from the participants. Note-taking, audio and video recordings are appropriate for conveying the

actual situation. The obtrusiveness of the data collection methods is a major factor. It would not do to assume the role of a complete participant and turn up with a movie camera, while denying any other motives.

When observing persons in the context of qualitative research, investigators should focus on the following shown in these classic studies:

1. *Acts and activities.* These are actions constituting brief or major involvements of an individual:

> All pseudo-patients took extensive notes publicly. Under ordinary circumstances, such behaviour would have raised questions in the minds of observers, as, in fact, it did among patients. Indeed, it seemed so certain that the notes would elicit suspicion that elaborate precautions were taken to remove them from the ward each day. But the precautions proved needless. The closest any staff member came to questioning these notes occurred when one pseudo-patient asked his physician what kind of medication he was receiving and began to write down the response. 'You needn't write it', he was told gently. 'If you have trouble remembering, just ask me again.'
>
> Rosenhan (1975)

2. *Meanings.* These are verbal productions directly defining or explaining the participant's activities: holding her breath, standing still, sniffing and coughing were all means of countering what she felt as her mother's impingements.

> Mary: I used to hold my breath because my mother used to go on so quick and (pause).
> Interviewer: Moving you mean?
> Mary: Yes.
> Interviewer: You mean your mother was moving about the house quickly?
> Mary: Yes and everything.
> Interviewer: And what did you do?
> Mary: Sort of stand like that.
> Interviewer: Can you demonstrate to me – sitting in a chair?
> Mary: Yes. I just sort of (shows what she did).
> Interviewer: With your elbows?
>
> Laing & Esterson (1970)

3. *Participation.* This describes the participants' involvement in a particular social setting:

> The pseudo-patient behaved afterward as he normally behaved. The pseudo-patient spoke to patients and staff as he might ordinarily. Because there is uncommonly little to do on a psychiatric ward, he attempted to engage others in conversation. When asked by staff how he was feeling, he indicated that he was fine, that he no longer experienced symptoms. He responded to instructions from attendants, to calls for medication (which was not swallowed), and to dining-hall instructions. Beyond such activities as were available to him on the admissions ward, he spent his time writing down his observations about the ward, its patients, and the staff. Initially these notes were written secretly, but as it soon became clear that no one much cared, they were subsequently written on standard tablets of paper in such public places as the day-room. No secret was made of these activities.
>
> Rosenhan (1975)

4. *Relationships.* These are descriptions of the nature of the interrelationships among several people:

> Her absence of social life, her withdrawal, appears to be an unwitting invention of her parents that never seems to have been called into question.
> Ruth: Well the places I like to go to my parents don't like me to go to.
> Mother: Such as?
> Ruth: Eddie's club.
> Mother: Oh, goodness. You don't really –
> Father: ?
> Ruth: I do.
> Interviewer: What is 'Eddie's'?
> Mother: It's a drinking club. She doesn't really drink. It's just that she likes to meet different types.
> Interviewer: She sounds as though the people that she does want to go out with are people she feels you disapprove of.
> Mother: Possibly.
> Father: Yes.
> Mother: Possibly.

Her parents' attitude to the life Ruth actually leads involves both the negation of its existence and the perception of mad or bad behaviour on Ruth's part. Thus, she is said to drink excessively, while, simultaneously, she is said not to drink at all.

Laing & Esterson (1970)

5. *Settings.* These are descriptions of the entire setting for the investigation:

> A stranger entering an ICU is at once bombarded with a massive array of sensory stimuli, some emotionally neutral but many highly charged. Initially, the

greatest impact comes from the intricate machinery, with its flashing lights, buzzing and beeping monitors, gurgling suction pumps, and whooshing respirators. Simultaneously, one sees many people rushing around busily performing lifesaving tasks. The atmosphere is not unlike that of the tension-charged strategic bunker. With time, habituation occurs, but the ever-continuing stimuli decrease the overload threshold and contribute to stress at times of crisis.

As the newness and strangeness of the unit wears off, one increasingly becomes aware of a host of perceptions with specific stressful emotional significance. Desperately ill, sick, and injured human beings are hooked up to that machinery. And, in addition to mechanical stimuli, one can discern moaning, crying, screaming and the last gasps of life. Sights of blood, vomitus and excreta, exposed genitalia, mutilated wasting bodies, and unconscious and helpless people assault the sensibilities. Unceasingly, the ICU nurse must face these affect-laden stimuli with all the distress and conflict that they engender.

Hay & Oken (1977)

Observations of the above classes of behaviours and settings will provide a report representing individuals' experiences and their interactions in a natural setting.

Observation in quantitative research

Research involving human participants may be conducted using either qualitative or quantitative approaches. The following are common features of observations in the context of quantitative research.

1. *Observer roles.* In quantitative research, the observer attempts to be as objective and detached as possible. Therefore, the observer as participant or the complete observer roles are most suited for quantitative approaches.

2. *Definition of relevant variables.* Considerable effort is made in quantitative research to specify precisely what aspect of an object, event or human behaviour the investigator intends to study and observe. In studies where several observers are involved in data collection it is appropriate to discuss and demonstrate that there is a substantial degree of agreement among the observers. The above issues will be discussed in more detail in the context of operational definitions, validity and reliability in the next chapter.

3. *Observation and structure.* For quantitative studies, we prefer the maximum level of control and structure. We have examined this point earlier in Chapter 5 when we discussed the concept of ecological validity. The degree of structure for observation may be further increased by using explicit, previously prepared observation guides or protocols. This is quite similar to how degrees of 'structure' or 'formality' are determined in the context of interview techniques, as outlined in the previous chapters. An excellent example of quantitative observational research is Piaget's work on cognitive development which proposed that an individual's level of moral reasoning is contingent on their level of cognitive development (Gerrig et al 2009).

We have examined two different types of observation guides (shown in Figs 13.1 and 13.2). If they are to be useful for conducting observational data collection, considerable effort must be made in the design of such guides and in establishing their reliability and validity, as we shall see in the next chapter.

The advantages of an observation guide are that the recording of the observations is made simple, and the data are easily summarized and evaluated using descriptive and inferential statistics, as discussed in later chapters of this book. The disadvantage of highly structured observations (as with interview and questionnaire techniques) is that the spontaneity and uniqueness of certain events may be lost, to the extent that only predetermined categories are recorded.

Summary

Data collection based on observation is appropriate for a wide range of research designs, ranging from laboratory-based experiments to qualitative field research. A basic issue is the extent to which a structure is imposed on the observer. Highly structured observational frameworks are most suited for quantitative research while more loosely structured participant observation is better suited for qualitative research. In general, when making observations involving human participants, researchers attempt to minimize participant reactivity and enhance the accuracy of recording the evidence. When appropriate, instrumentation may be used to enhance or record observations. It is worth noting that data collection using questionnaires, interviews and observations may well be used in combination in both research and clinical case work.

Measurement

CHAPTER CONTENTS

Introduction 105

Operational definitions and measurement . . .105

Objective and subjective measures 106

Desirable properties of measurement tools and
procedures. 106

    Reliability. 107

    Validity 108

Standardized measures and tests 109

What makes a good test?. 110

Measurement scale types. 110

    1. Nominal scales 110

    2. Ordinal scales. 111

    3. Interval scales. 111

    4. Ratio scales. 111

Levels of measurement 112

Summary. .112

Introduction

The term *measurement* refers to the procedure of attributing qualities or quantities to specific characteristics of objects, persons or events. For example, how tall you are is an attribute which is measured by a score on the variable 'height'. Accurate and standardized procedures are available such as a ruler to produce the score (e.g. 175 cm) which is your height.

Measurement is a key process in health research as well as in clinical practice. The same issues are important in both settings. If the measurement procedure used in a study or diagnostic procedure is inadequate, its usefulness will be limited. Similarly, in clinical practice, the validity of diagnostic and treatment decisions can be compromised by inadequate measurement processes and tools. The development of accurate instruments or tools is one of the foundations of scientific and clinical advances.

The aims of this chapter are to:

1. Discuss key issues in measurement procedures.
2. Describe good practice in measurement in both research and applied health promotion settings.
3. Compare and evaluate the use of four different types of measurement scales.

Operational definitions and measurement

Sometimes researchers start their projects with rather vague views of how to measure theoretical constructs/key factors in their study. For instance, if researchers are interested in collecting data on 'levels of pain' experienced by patients, then they must convert this general idea about pain to a tightly defined statement of how exactly this is to be measured. Depending on their theoretical interpretation of the concept of 'pain', and the practical requirements of the investigation, one of the many possible approaches to measurement of pain will then be selected.

The process of converting theoretical ideas to a precise statement of how variables are to be measured is called *operationalization*. It is important that researchers give exact details of how the measurements were taken in order that others may judge their adequacy and appropriateness and be in a position to repeat the procedures in a new study. Data collection is a very important stage of the research process. A quantitative study that is adequate in terms of design, sampling methods and sample size may nevertheless have limited value due to the use of inadequate measurement techniques. Let us now discuss operationalization.

The *operational definition* of a construct or associated variables is a statement of how the researcher conducting a particular study chooses to measure the variables being investigated. It should be unambiguous and reproducible by other researchers.

At the outset, let us note that in most circumstances there is no single best way of taking measurements. If a researcher claimed that her therapeutic techniques significantly increased 'motor control' in her sample of patients, the obvious question that arises is 'What was meant by 'motor control' and how is it measured?' If our researcher replied that she was interested in motor control as measured by the Plunkett Motor Dexterity Task scores, she has, in fact, supplied her operational definition. Another researcher may challenge the adequacy of this definition and substitute their own, stating that patients' self-ratings of control on a ten-point scale is a more appropriate definition.

A good operational definition will contain enough information to enable another researcher or clinician to replicate the measurement techniques used in the original study. Similarly, a good operational definition of a clinically relevant variable will enable a fellow professional to replicate the original diagnostic or assessment procedures. An operational definition can be an unambiguous description, a photograph or diagram, or the specification of a brand name of a standard measuring tool. In describing the procedure for quantitative research, we must include operational definitions of the measurement instrument and how they are used, so that readers are quite clear as to what has been done to collect the data.

Objective and subjective measures

A distinction is commonly drawn between objective and subjective measures, often with overtones of suspicion of poor quality directed towards so-called 'subjective' measures. Let us make a much less value-laden distinction and define them as follows: objective measurements involve the measurement of physical quantities and qualities using measurement equipment; subjective measures involve ratings or judgements by humans of quantities and qualities. In general, subjective measures are observations (see Ch. 13) of values measured on nominal or ordinal scales, while objective measures are used to produce scores on interval or ratio scales. We will discuss levels of measurement at the end of this chapter.

One should not confuse the distinction between objective and subjective measures as corresponding to good quality or bad quality measurement techniques. Equipment might be improperly calibrated, complicated to use, or become damaged during an investigation. For instance, a researcher might have an absolutely terrible set of scales that gives results far at variance with the true weights of people. With the sophistication and complexity of much current measurement equipment, it is often difficult to calibrate equipment accurately without a complex calibration procedure. *Just because a tool is involved in measurement does not mean that the results will be accurate.* Furthermore, many quantities and qualities associated with persons and clinical phenomena are difficult to measure objectively, such as the personal attractiveness of individuals, or aspects of patient–therapist relationships, or the intelligence of a person. Ultimately, the issue is whether the best reliable and accurate data has been produced to answer the research and/or clinical question.

Desirable properties of measurement tools and procedures

Measurement tools and procedures ought to yield scores or values that are reproducible, accurate, applicable to the measurement task in hand and which are practical or easy to use. These properties are often given the technical terms of reliability, validity, applicability and practicability. These properties will be reviewed in detail in the following sections. Measurement theory and method are applied to the development of measurement tools that maximize these properties.

Before these specific test properties are reviewed, it is useful to review some basic concepts in test theory. In any measurement, we have three related concepts: the observed value or test score, the true value or test score and measurement error. Thus if I could be weighed on a completely accurate set of weighing scales, my true score might be 110 kg. However, the scales that I use in my bathroom might give me a reading of 100 kg. The difference between the observed score and my true score is the measurement error. This relationship can be expressed in the form of an equation such that:

$$\text{Observed value} = \text{true value} \pm \text{error}$$

Measurement tools are designed with a view to minimizing measurement error so that the observed value we obtain from our assessment process is close to the true or real value.

Reliability

Reliability is the property of reproducibility and consistency of the results of a measurement procedure. There are several different ways in which reliability can be assessed. These include test–retest reliability, inter-observer reliability and internal consistency. Let us examine each.

Test–retest reliability

A common way to assess test reliability is to administer the same measurement procedure twice to the same participants. The results obtained from the first test are then correlated with the second test. Reliability is generally measured by a correlation coefficient that may vary from -1 to $+1$ in value. A test–retest reliability of $+0.8$ or above is considered to be sound. When the measurement process involves clinical ratings, e.g. a clinician's rating of the dependency level of a cerebrovascular accident patient, test–retest reliability is sometimes termed *intra-observer* reliability, i.e. the same observer rates the same patients twice and the results are correlated.

Inter-observer (inter-rater) reliability

A common issue in clinical assessment is the extent to which clinicians agree with each other in their assessments of patients. The extent of agreement is generally determined by having two or more clinicians independently assess the same patients and then comparing the results using correlations. If the agreement (correlation) is high then we have high inter-observer or inter-rater reliability.

Table 14.1 Inter-observer reliability

	Low reliability		High reliability	
Participants	A	B	A	B
1	4	3	4	4
2	2	5	2	3
3	3	4	4	5
4	1	4	2	2
5	3	1	1	1
6	4	4	5	5

Table 14.1 illustrates examples of both high and low inter-observer reliability on ratings of patients on a five-point scale. Let's imagine that this scale measures the level of patient dependency and need for nursing support. As we mentioned earlier, the degree of reliability is quantitatively expressed by correlation coefficients. However, by inspection you can see that in Table 14.1 there is a high degree of disagreement in the two observers' ratings in the 'Low reliability' column. In this instance the clinical ratings would be unreliable, and inappropriate to use in the research project. However, the outcome shown in the 'High reliability' column in Table 14.1 shows a high level of agreement.

Internal consistency

Measurement tools will often consist of multiple items. For example, a test of your knowledge of research methods might include 50 items or questions. Similarly, a checklist designed to measure activities of daily living might have 20 items. The internal consistency of a test is the extent to which the results on the different items correlate with each other. If they tend to be highly correlated with each other, then the test is said to be internally consistent. Internal consistency is also measured by a form of correlation coefficient known as Cronbach alpha; an alpha of above 0.8 is considered to be a desirable property for a test.

Thus, the reliability or reproducibility of an assessment or test can be determined in several different ways including the test–retest, intra-rater, inter-rater and internal consistency methods.

Table 14.2 Predictive validity

Participants	Low predictive validity		High predictive validity	
	Score on X	Score on Y	Score on X	Score on Y
1	4	3	3	3
2	4	8	4	3
3	5	2	5	5
4	5	7	5	5
5	6	4	6	6
6	8	5	8	7

Validity

Validity is concerned with accuracy of the test procedure. Just because one keeps getting the same result upon repeated administrations, or agreement among independent observers, doesn't mean that the results are accurate. If I jump on the bathroom scales and get a result of 40 kg and then jump off the scales and then get back on and it is still reading 40 kg, this reading is certainly reliable, but obviously it is an error (for readers who do not know us, 40 kg as an observed score for our weight entails major measurement error!). Thus the adequate reproducibility or reliability of a test or assessment process is essential, but we also need the results to be accurate or valid.

Types of test validity

As with reliability, test validity may be assessed in a number of different ways. These include content validity, sensitivity and specificity, and predictive validity.

Content or face validity

In many contexts it is difficult to find external measures to correlate with the measure to be validated. For example, an examination in a particular academic subject may be the sole measure of the student's performance available to determine grades. How can it be determined whether the tests administered will be valid or not? One way is to write down all the material covered in the subject and then make sure that there is adequate sampling from the overall content of the material delivered in the subject. If this criterion is satisfied it can be said

that the test has content or face validity. You may have had an experience where you felt that a subject assessment task had low content validity in that it did not reflect the material presented in the subject.

Predictive validity

Predictive validity is concerned with the ability of a test to predict values of it or other tests in the future. Some tests are designed to assist with prognostic decisions, i.e. what is going to happen in the future; for these tests high predictive validity is an important quality.

Let us examine an example of predictive validity. Say a researcher devised a screening rating scale, X, for selecting patients to participate in a rehabilitation program. The effectiveness of the rehabilitation program is assessed with rating scale Y. Say that each rating scale involves assigning scores of 1–10 to the patients' performance. Table 14.2 illustrates two outcomes: low predictive validity and high predictive validity.

Construct validity

Although the calculation of correlation coefficients is needed to examine quantitatively the predictive validity of test X, it can be seen in Table 14.2 that in the 'Low predictive validity' column, the scores on X are not clearly related to the level of scores on Y. On the other hand, in the 'High predictive validity' column, scores on the two variables correspond quite closely. Within the limits of the fact that only six participants were involved in this hypothetical study, it is clear that only the results in the 'High predictive validity' column are consistent with rating scale X being useful for predicting the outcome of the rehabilitation program, as measured on scale Y.

Table 14.3 Possible outcomes of test results

	Real situation	
Test result	**Disease present**	**Disease not present**
Disease present	True positive	False positive
Disease not present	False negative	True negative

At this point we should again refer to the concepts of internal and external validity. The concepts of predictive and content validity apply to the specific tests and measures a researcher or clinician uses. Internal and external validity refer to characteristics of the total research project or program. Test validity should not be confused with other forms of research design validity such as internal and external validity (see Ch. 5).

Sensitivity and specificity

The concepts of sensitivity and specificity are most commonly applied to screening tests, where the purpose of the test is to determine whether the patient has a particular problem or illness. There are four possible outcomes for a test result, as shown in Table 14.3.

Sensitivity refers to the proportion of people who test as positive who really have the disease (i.e. the proportion of true positives out of all positives). Specificity refers to the proportion of individuals who test as negative who really do not have the disease (i.e. the proportion of true negatives out of all negative test results). If a diagnostic test has a sensitivity of 1.0 and specificity of 1.0 it is a perfectly accurate or valid test. Most clinical or screening tests are not perfect and some have unknown or quite low sensitivity and specificity.

A case study in clinical test validity

The early detection of breast cancer in women has been recognized as an important public health initiative in many countries. Common ways of detecting suspicious lumps include breast self-examination and mammography, an X-ray of the breasts. Mammography is a common screening procedure and some countries such as Australia have funded large-scale programs to promote it.

However, commendable as these initiatives may be, there are some doubts about the validity of mammography as a diagnostic tool. Walker & Langlands (1986), in an early evaluation, studied the mammography results of 218 women, who, through the use of a diagnostic biopsy, were known to have breast cancer. Of the 218 women with cancer, 95 (43.6%) had recorded a (false) negative mammography test result. Of these patients, 47 had delayed further investigation and treatment for almost a year, no doubt relieved and reassured by their 'favourable' test results. The delays in treatment, given what we know about the relationship between early intervention and improved prognosis, in all likelihood seriously compromised the health and ultimate survival of these women. In this instance, the accuracy (or lack of it) of the test results has very important consequences for the people concerned. Test quality is of profound importance in research and clinical practice, as demonstrated by this example. In the last 25 years, research has been completed to improve the accuracy of screening tests. Recently, Evans (2012) estimated that improved screening techniques have helped in the early detection of breast cancer and, combined with advances in chemotherapy, have contributed to the survival of thousands of women.

Standardized measures and tests

Because reliability and validity of measures are so important, many researchers have devoted considerable time and energy to the development of measuring instruments and procedures that have known levels of reliability and validity.

The development of measurement standards for physical dimensions such as weight, length and time has been fundamental for the growth of science. That is, we have standards for comparing our measurements of a variable and we can meaningfully communicate our findings to colleagues living anywhere in the world. There are a variety of clinical measures (e.g. the Apgar tests for evaluating the viability of neonates) that represent internationally recognized standards for communicating information about attributes of persons or disease entities.

Furthermore, there are standards relevant to populations, in terms of which assessments of individuals become meaningful. For instance, there are standards for the stages of development of infants: levels of physical, emotional, intellectual and social development occurring as a function of age.

Some tests have been trialled on large samples, and reliability and validity levels recorded. Tests that have been trialled in this way are known as standardized measures or tests. A large variety is available, particularly in the clinical and social areas. Many US firms and cooperatives market standardized tests for health researchers and practitioners. However, many researchers use tests and measures that have not been standardized, and do not report levels of reliability in their literature. This is of particular concern in studies where subjective measures with incomplete operational definitions are employed.

What makes a good test?

Considerable effort has been devoted to developing, standardizing and evaluating novel instruments and measurement procedures. Based on our discussion, the following criteria are relevant for identifying what constitutes 'good' measurement in health research and practice.

1. *Theoretical framework.* As there are complex and abstract concepts in the health sciences, researchers need to have a clear theoretical framework in the context of which the measurement procedure is defined and evaluated.

2. *The measurement process should lead to reliable outcomes.* This means that the results should be consistent and there should be substantial agreement between researchers or clinicians using a measurement procedure. It follows that if a measuring instrument or a procedure produces unreliable results, then its usefulness is questionable.

3. *The measurement procedure should be valid.* This means that we are measuring the targeted, rather than another, construct or variable. Also, the results should be accurate as determined by the criteria for validity discussed in this chapter.

4. *The instrument should be accessible.* This implies that the cost and level of expertise required to use the instrument should not be prohibitive. Of course, there are different criteria for accessibility depending on the questions being investigated or the level of resources available to the researcher or practitioner. For example, PET (positron emission tomography) scans are a very expensive and specialized procedure involving

the use of radio-isotopes. However, the cost and level of expertise required are justifiable in terms of the data produced or the needs of the patients for accurate diagnoses.

5. *The measurement procedure should be acceptable to research participants or patients.* It is important to explain, as an ethical requirement, the measurement process and any possible associated risks or burdens (see Ch. 6). The procedure should be as convenient and safe as possible for research participants.

Measurement scale types

Measurement can produce different types of numbers, in the sense that some numbers are assigned different meanings and implications from others. For instance, when we speak of Ward 1 and Ward 2, we are using numbers in a different sense from when we speak of infant A being 1 month old, and infant B being 2 months old. In the first instance, we used numbers for naming; in the second instance the numbers indicate quantities. There are four scale types, distinguished by the types of numbers produced by the measurement of a specific variable.

1. Nominal scales

The 'lowest' level of the measurement scale types is the nominal scale, where the measurement of a variable involves the naming or categorization of possible values of the variable. The measurements produced are 'qualitative' in the sense that the categories are merely different from each other. If numbers are assigned to the categories they are merely labels and do not represent real quantities; for example, Ward 1 and Ward 2 might be renamed St. Agatha's Ward and St. Martha's Ward without conveying any less information. Table 14.4 shows some other examples of nominal scaling.

The only mathematical relationship pertinent to nominal scales is equivalence or non-equivalence; i.e. $A = B$ or $A \neq B$. A specific value of a variable either falls into a specific category, or it does not. Thus, there is no logical relationship between the numerical value assigned to its category and its size, quantity or frequency of occurrence. The arbitrary values of a nominal scale can be changed without any loss of information.

Table 14.4 Some examples of nominal scaling

Variable	Possible values
Patient's admission number	3085001, 3085002
Sex	Male, female
Religion	Catholic, Protestant, Jewish, Muslim, Hindu
Psychiatric diagnosis	Manic depressive, schizophrenic, neurotic
Blood type	A, B, AB, O
Cause of death	Cardiac failure, neoplasm, trauma

Table 14.5 Some examples of ordinal scales

Variable	Possible values
Severity of condition	Mild = 1, moderate = 2, severe = 3, critical = 4
Patients' satisfaction with treatment	Satisfied = 1, undecided = 2, dissatisfied = 3
Age group	Baby, infant, child, adult, geriatric
Cooperativeness with nurse or patients in a ward	(In decreasing order) Mrs Smith, Mr Jones, Ms Krax

2. Ordinal scales

The next level of measurement involves rank ordering values of a variable. For example, 1st, 2nd or 3rd in a foot race are values on an ordinal scale. The numbers assigned on an ordinal scale signify order or rank.

With ordinal scales, statements about ranks can be made. Where A and B are values of the variable, we can say A > B or B > A. For instance, we can say Mrs Smith is more cooperative than Mr Jones (A > B), or Mr Jones is more cooperative than Ms Krax (B > C). We cannot, however, make any statements about the relative sizes of these differences. Examples of ordinal scales are shown in Table 14.5.

3. Interval scales

Examples of interval scales are shown in Table 14.6. For these scales, there is no absolute zero point; rather, an arbitrary zero point is assigned. For instance, 0°C does not represent the point at which there is no heat, but the freezing point of water. An IQ of zero would not mean no intelligence at all, but a serious intellectual or perceptual problem in using the materials of the test.

The use of an interval scale enables identification of equal intervals between any two values of measurements: we can say A − B = B − C. For example, if A, B and C are taken as IQ scores, and A = 150, B = 100 and C = 50, then it is true that A − B = B − C. However, we cannot say that A = 3C (that A is three times more intelligent than C).

Table 14.6 Some examples of interval scales

Variable	Possible values
Heat (celsius or fahrenheit)	−10°C, +20°C, +5°C, +10°F
Intelligence (IQ)	45, 100, 185

Table 14.7 Variables measured on ratio scales

Variable	Possible values
Weight	10 kg, 20 kg, 100 kg
Height	50 cm, 150 cm, 200 cm
Blood pressure	110 mmHg, 120 mmHg, 160 mmHg
Heart beat	10 per min, 30 per min, 50 per min
Rate of firing of a neurone	10 per millisec, 20 per millisec, 30 per millisec
Protein per blood volume	2 mg/mL, 5 mg/mL, 10 mg/mL
Vocabulary	100 words, 1000 words, 30 000 words

4. Ratio scales

Ratio scales have what is called a meaningful or non-arbitrary zero point. For example, in the kelvin temperature scale, 0°K (or absolute zero) represents an absence of heat, in that the molecules have stopped vibrating completely; whereas 0°C is simply the freezing point of water. The centigrade or celsius zero is an arbitrary one tied to the freezing point of a particular compound. Thus °K is a ratio scale and °C is an interval scale. Examples of variables measured on ratio scales are shown in Table 14.7.

Table 14.8 Characteristics of levels of measurement

Characteristic	Level of measurement			
	Nominal	**Ordinal**	**Interval**	**Ratio**
Distinctiveness	•	•	•	•
Ordering in magnitude		•	•	•
Equal intervals			•	•
Absolute zero				•

Distinctiveness: different numbers assigned to different values of property.
Ordering in magnitude: larger values represent more of the property.
Equal intervals: same distance between points on a scale.
Absolute zero: zero value represents absence of property.

Levels of measurement

Table 14.8 compares the characteristics of different scales or levels of measurement.

Interval and ratio scales represent quantitative measurements. A ratio scale is the 'highest' scale of measurement, in the sense that it involves all the characteristics of the other scales, as well as having an absolute zero. A measurement on a higher level can be transformed into one on a lower level in this framework, but not vice versa, because the higher scale measurement contains more information and the values can be put to more use by permitting more mathematical operations than those on a lower level.

Also, a given variable might be measured on one of several types of scales, depending on the needs of the investigator. Consider, for instance, the variable 'height'. This variable could be measured on any of the four scales, as follows:

1. *Ratio scale.* The height of individuals above the ground, e.g. 180 cm.
2. *Interval scale.* The height of individuals above an *arbitrary* surface, e.g. 100 cm above the surface of a bench.
3. *Ordinal scale.* The comparative heights of individuals, e.g. rank-ordered from tallest to shortest.
4. *Nominal scale.* Categorizing individuals, e.g. 'normal' or 'abnormal'.

The different types of measurement scales are important when considering statistical analysis of data. Statistics are numbers with special properties from data. The type of measurement scale determines the type of statistic that is appropriate for its analysis. This issue is taken up later in this book.

Summary

This section defines good measurement practice and its importance in research and clinical practice.

In good measurement practice we need to define concepts operationally, so that other investigators can also carry out or assess the measurement procedure. We also need to establish the reliability and validity of our measurements. A high degree of reliability and validity is necessary for minimizing measurement error. We have noted that measures involving the exercise of human judgement (i.e. 'subjective' measures) are not necessarily unreliable or invalid.

Four different scale types were discussed: nominal, ordinal, interval, and ratio. These scales have different characteristics, particularly in relation to the permissible mathematical operations. In subsequent sections, we shall see that the scale type involved in our measurements determines the descriptive and inferential statistics appropriate for describing and analysing the data.

Section 5

Descriptive statistics

15 Organization and presentation of data 115
16 Measures of central tendency and variability 125
17 Standard scores and normal distributions 133
18 Correlation 139

Data produced in quantitative research is analysed by applying statistics. Depending on the complexity of the research design and the amount of data collected, we will have generated or collected a set of scores called raw data. Section 5 is concerned with descriptive statistics, which represent the mathematical conventions for organizing and summarizing the raw data.

In Chapter 15 we outline techniques used for tabulating and graphing data. These techniques enable us to visualize trends and identify differences across levels of the independent variables. When the data have been appropriately organized we may calculate statistics, such as the percentages and proportions of scores found in the groups being studied.

Another important use for descriptive statistics is to 'crunch' or condense data into typical values for representing scores. The statistics are discussed in Chapter 16 and include 'measures of central tendency' (mode, median and mean) and also measures of variability (range, semi-interquartile range and standard deviation). Using these statistics enables us to condense the raw data and to convey to the reader information about the research findings.

Statistics such as the mean and the standard deviation can also be applied to calculating standard scores. Standard scores are used to establish the position of a particular score relative to a population. In Chapter 17 we examine how the standardized normal distribution can be used to calculate the position of any specific score within a population and how to interpret the clinical implications of these scores.

In Chapter 18 we examine another important class of statistics called correlation coefficients. Correlation coefficients are used to express the degree and direction of association between two or more variables. For example, we could use correlation coefficients to demonstrate if there is an association between the variables 'level of exercise' and 'body weight'. The closer the calculated correlation coefficient is to 1.0 (the maximum value), the more precisely we may predict from one variable to the other. Although correlation coefficients are extremely important for showing how different variables are associated, they do not necessarily indicate causal relationships between the variables. Showing causal effects requires appropriate research designs, as we suggested in Chapter 7.

Organization and presentation of data

15

CHAPTER CONTENTS

Introduction 115

The organization and presentation of nominal
or ordinal data. 115

   Organization of discrete data 116

   Graphing discrete data. 116

Organization and presentation of interval
or ratio data 118

   Grouped frequency distributions 118

   Graphing frequency distributions 118

Descriptive statistics for discontinuous data .120

   Ratios 120

   Proportions. 121

   Percentages 121

   Rates. 121

   Odds 122

Summary. 123

It can be difficult to make sense of raw data when they consist of a large number of measurements. Before we can interpret or communicate the information provided by a research project, the raw data must be organized and presented in a clear and intelligible fashion. We do this using descriptive statistics. In this chapter we will outline methods used in descriptive statistics for the organization, tabulation and graphic presentation of data. We will also examine the use of some simple statistics directly derived from the tabulation of the data.

The aims of this chapter are to:

1. Outline methods for organizing and representing data in the form of frequency distributions, tables or graphs.
2. Demonstrate how the measurement scale used for data collection influences the organization and presentation of the evidence.
3. Discuss the calculation and use of some simple descriptive statistics for discontinuous data, including percentages, ratios and rates.

Introduction

The summary and interpretation of data from quantitative research entail the use of *statistics*. A statistic is a number that is obtained by the mathematical manipulation of the data. We use descriptive statistics to describe data and inferential statistics to analyse research observations and measurements.

In previous chapters we examined how interviews, observations and measurement are used to produce data in clinical investigations or research.

The organization and presentation of nominal or ordinal data

A primary consideration in selecting appropriate statistics is the question of whether the data are discrete or continuous. Scaled data are necessarily discrete, so that the organization of the data involves counting the number (frequency) of cases falling into each category of measurement.

Let us examine two hypothetical examples as an illustration.

Organization of discrete data

Example 1: nominal (categorical) data

We are interested in the sex of patients (these are nominal or categorical data) undergoing gall bladder surgery (cholecystectomy) at a public hospital over a period of one year. The raw data indicating the sex (M or F) of the patients is simply read off the patients' records, as follows:

F, M, M, F, F, F, M, F, M, F, M, F, F, F, F, F, F, F, F, F, M, F, F, F, M, M, F, M, F, M

Grouping the above nominal data involves counting the number of cases (or measurements) falling into each category. The total is M = 10 and F = 20. The data can be presented in tabular form. Table 15.1 shows the following conventions in tabulating data:

1. Tables must be clearly and fully labelled – both the table as a whole and the categories – so that readers can interpret unambiguously what they are observing.
2. f represents frequency of cases or measurements falling into a given category.
3. n represents the total number of cases or measurements in a sample.
4. N represents the number of cases in a population. (See Section 3 for the difference between samples and populations.)

Example 2: ordinal data

Ordinal data are presented by counting the number of cases (frequency) of each ordered rank making up the scale.

An investigator intends to evaluate the effectiveness of a new analgesic versus placebo treatment.

A post-test only control group design is used: the experimental group receives the analgesic and the control group receives the placebo. Twenty patients are randomly assigned into each of the two groups. Pain intensity is assessed by the patients' pain reports five hours after minor surgery, on the following scale:

5 = Excruciating pain.
4 = Severe pain.
3 = Moderate pain.
2 = Mild pain.
1 = No pain.

The raw data are:

Experimental group: 3, 4, 5, 3, 3, 3, 4, 2, 1, 3, 2, 1, 3, 4, 5, 2, 3, 3, 3, 3
Control group: 5, 4, 4, 4, 5, 3, 4, 3, 2, 4, 4, 2, 4, 5, 3, 4, 4, 4, 5, 5

After tallying the results, the above data can be presented as a frequency distribution, as shown in Table 15.2. This demonstrates that, when the data have been tabulated, we can see the outcome of the investigation. Here, the pain reported by the experimental group is less than that of the control group. Organizing the data is the first step in producing evidence for testing the hypothesis that the new analgesic is more effective than placebo.

Graphing discrete data

Once a frequency distribution of the raw data has been tabulated, a variety of techniques is available for the graphical presentation of a given set of measurements. Frequency distributions of qualitative data

Table 15.1 Frequency distribution of gender of patients undergoing cholecystectomy at a hospital over a period of 1 year

Gender	f
Male (M)	10
Female (F)	20
	$n = 30$

Table 15.2 Reported pain intensity of patients following placebo and analgesic treatments

Pain intensity	Experimental group (analgesic) f	Control group (placebo) f
1	2	0
2	3	2
3	10	3
4	3	10
5	2	5
	$n = 20$	$n = 20$

are often plotted as bar graphs (also termed 'column' graphs), or shown pictorially as pie diagrams.

A bar graph involves plotting the frequency of each category and drawing a bar, the height of which represents the frequency of a given category. Figure 15.1 graphs the data given in Table 15.1.

Figure 15.1 demonstrates conventions in plotting bar graphs:

1. The y-axis, also called the ordinate, is used to plot frequencies.
2. The x-axis, also called the abscissa, is used to indicate the categories.
3. The bars do not touch each other, reflecting the discontinuity of the measurement categories.

It should be noted that care must be exercised in interpreting graphs, as the axes may be translated or compressed causing a false visual impression of the data. Make sure that you inspect the values along the axes, so that you are not misled. It is also acceptable to calculate the percentage of scores falling into each category and to display the percentages instead of frequencies.

It can be seen in Figure 15.2 that, by presenting the data for the experimental and control groups on the same graph, the reader gains a visual impression of the possible effectiveness of the analgesic treatment in contrast to that of the control intervention or treatment. Nominal data can also be meaningfully presented as a pie chart, where the percentage of each category is converted into a proportional part of a circle or 'pie'. For example, in a given hospital we have the hypothetical spending patterns shown in Table 15.3.

Figure 15.3 represents a pie chart of the information. In constructing Figure 15.3, we converted the numbers into percentages and then into degrees (out of a total of 100% = 360°), i.e. each 1% of the total is represented by 3.6° in the circle.

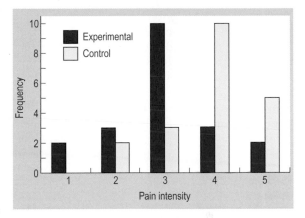

Figure 15.2 • Bar (column) graph of patients' pain intensity.

Table 15.3 Hypothetical spending patterns

Item	Cost ($)	Percentage of total
Wages and salaries	1 500 000	50.00
Medical supplies	500 000	16.67
Food and provisions	500 000	16.67
Administrative costs	500 000	16.67
Total	**3 000 000**	**100.01**

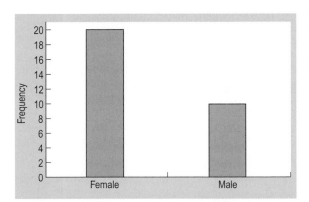

Figure 15.1 • Bar (column) graph of patients undergoing cholecystectomy.

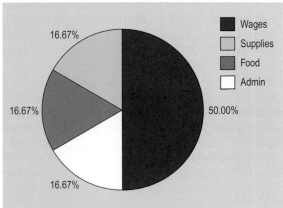

Figure 15.3 • Pie diagram of a hospital's spending pattern.

Organization and presentation of interval or ratio data

Previously we have noted that interval and ratio scales of measurement produce real numbers that can be processed according to the standard rules of arithmetic. Interval and ratio measurements typically produce continuous data (e.g. weight, length, time, IQ), implying that increasingly accurate values of the variable are possible to obtain, depending on the precision of the measurement process. For example, the weight of a neonate could be measured as 4, 4.2, 4.18 or 4.183 kg.

Grouped frequency distributions

When the continuous data are made up of a large number of varied measurements, it is useful to present the data as grouped frequency distributions. When drawing up a grouped frequency distribution, the following conventions should be taken into account:

1. The table of grouped frequency distributions should have no more than nine groups of values, otherwise it is too difficult to inspect. However, if too few groups are used, the meaning of the data is obscured, as varied measurements are combined into too few equivalent categories.
2. There should be equally sized class intervals, the *width* of which is represented by i.
3. Individual scores within a given class interval 'lose' their precise identity. The midpoint of each class interval is taken to represent the class interval.

Example

On admission to hospital, patients are routinely weighed. You are asked to summarize the weights of 50 male patients who were admitted in your ward over a period of time. The weights (raw data) are as follows (to nearest kg):

75, 67, 76, 71, 73, 86, 72, 77, 80, 75, 80, 96, 93, 75, 73, 83, 81, 82, 73, 92, 81, 87, 76, 84, 78, 79, 99, 100, 88, 77, 71, 76, 75, 83, 66, 79, 95, 85, 77, 87, 90, 73, 72, 68, 84, 69, 78, 77, 84, 94

The steps in constructing a grouped frequency distribution are:

1. Organize the data into an ordered array, and find the frequency of each score (see Table 15.4).
2. Find the range of scores. The range is the difference between the highest and lowest score plus 1. We add 1 to include the real limits for continuous data. In this case the range is $100 - 66 + 1 = 35$.
3. Decide on the width (i) of the class intervals; i can be approximated by dividing the range by the number of groups or class intervals. In this instance, if we decide on seven classes, i will be $35 \div 7 = 5.0$. When i is a decimal, it should be rounded up to the nearest whole number: here, $i = 5$. As stated earlier, the number of class intervals is arbitrary and will be chosen by the researcher, depending on the properties of the data. By convention, more than nine class intervals are rarely employed.
4. The next step is to determine the lowest class interval, and then list the limits of each class interval. Clearly, the lowest class interval must include the lowest score in the distribution.
5. Then, the frequency of scores is determined from each class interval and tabulated, as in Table 15.5.

It is easier to understand the data by inspecting Table 15.5 than by looking at the raw data. However, some precision in the data has been lost as somewhat different scores have been assigned into the same class intervals.

Graphing frequency distributions

The two common types of graphs used to graph frequency distribution of quantitative data are histograms and frequency polygons.

Histograms

A histogram resembles a bar graph but the bars are drawn to touch each other. The fact that the bars touch each other reflects the underlying continuity of the data. The height of the bars along the y-axis represents the frequency of each score or class interval plotted along the x-axis. With grouped data, the midpoint of each class interval becomes the midpoint of each bar, and the width of the bar corresponds to the real limits of each class interval.

Table 15.4 Ordered array of data

Score	f	Score	f	Score	f	Score	f
100	1	91	0	82	1	73	4
99	1	90	1	81	2	72	2
98	0	89	0	80	2	71	2
97	0	88	1	79	2	70	0
96	1	87	2	78	2	69	1
95	1	86	1	77	4	68	1
94	1	85	1	76	3	67	1
93	1	84	3	75	4	66	1
92	1	83	2	74	0		

Table 15.5 Grouped frequency distribution of patients' weight in a given ward

Class Interval	f
66–70	4
71–75	12
76–80	13
81–85	9
86–90	5
91–95	4
96–100	3
	n = 50

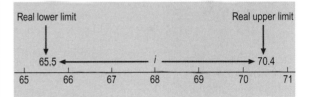

Figure 15.4 • Real limits of a class interval.

For example, consider the lowest class interval, 66–70, in Table 15.5. Because the data are continuous, the real upper and lower limits of the class interval are 65.5 and 70.4 (Fig. 15.4). Although all the weights are given as whole numbers of kilograms, these will in most cases be the result of rounding off by the nursing staff to the nearest whole number. Thus, someone who actually weighed 70.2 kg would have been recorded as weighing 70 kg and would fall into the 66–70 class. As Figure 15.4 shows, $i = 5$, and the midpoint of the class interval is 68.

Frequency polygons

Any data that can be represented by a histogram can also be graphed as a frequency polygon. For this type of graph, a point is plotted over the midpoint of each class interval, at a height representing the frequency of the scores. Figure 15.5 represents a histogram and a frequency polygon for the data in Table 15.5.

Frequency polygons allow the reader to interpolate, that is, to estimate the frequency of values in between those actually measured or graphed. Of course, interpolation cannot be done for discrete data (e.g. Fig. 15.1), as values between categories have no meaning. When a frequency polygon is plotted, it can take on a variety of shapes. The shapes which are of particular importance for frequency polygons are shown in Figure 15.6.

Figure 15.6A represents a bell-shaped, normal distribution. It is symmetrical in the sense that one-half is the mirror image of the other. The curve indicates that most of the scores fall in the middle, with relatively few scores towards either 'tail'. Figure 15.6B represents a negatively skewed distribution, with most of the scores being high and spreading out toward the lower end of the distribution. Figure 15.6C represents a positively skewed distribution, with most of the scores being low, but

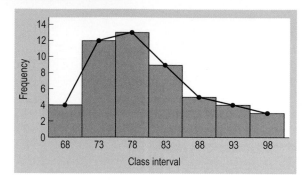

Figure 15.5 • Combined histogram and frequency polygon for the same data (see Table 15.5).

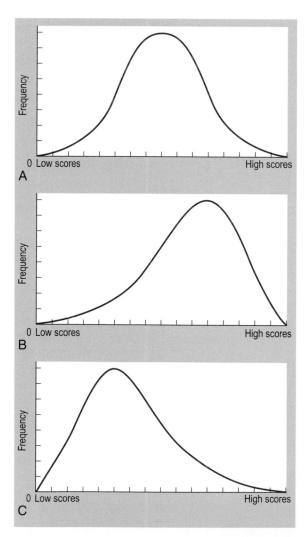

Figure 15.6 • Shapes of frequency polygons: (A) normal distribution; (B) negative skewing; (C) positive skewing.

with some scores spreading out towards the upper end of the distribution.

An easy way to remember the direction of the skew is to consider the region where the 'tail' or portion of the graph with lower frequencies falls. For example, if the tail is located at the low score end of the x-axis, the graph is negatively skewed. The significance of the skew or a symmetrical, normal distribution will be discussed in subsequent sections.

Descriptive statistics for discontinuous data

Once the data have been summarized in frequency distribution, it is often useful to make comparisons concerning the relative frequencies of scores falling into specific categories. As stated earlier, a statistic is a number generated by computations based on the raw data. The calculation of statistics is essential for 'crunching' the raw data into single numbers that represent the characteristics of the full data set. The following statistics are useful for understanding comparative trends in the data, and can be used for measurements on any scale: nominal, ordinal, interval or ratio.

Ratios

Ratios are statistics which express the relative frequency of one set of frequencies, A, in relation to another, B. The formula for ratios is:

$$\text{Ratio} = \frac{A}{B}$$

Therefore, the ratio of males to females for the data presented in Table 15.1 is:

$$\text{Ratio (males to females)} = \frac{10}{20} = 0.5$$

or

$$\text{Ratio (females to males)} = \frac{20}{10} = 2.0$$

Ratios are useful in the health sciences when we are interested in the distribution of illnesses or symptoms or the categories of participants requiring or benefiting from treatment. The ratio calculated above tells us about the relative frequency of gall bladder surgery for males and females.

Proportions

Proportions are statistics which are calculated by putting the frequency of one category over that of the total number in the sample or the population:

$$\text{Proportion of A} = \frac{A}{A+B}$$

Therefore, the proportion of males in the sample represented in Table 15.1 is:

$$\text{Proportion of males} = \frac{f(\text{males})}{n} = \frac{10}{30} = 0.33$$

Percentages

Proportions can be transformed into percentages, by multiplying by 100. Of course, this is how we obtained the values of the y-axis for Figure 15.2. To illustrate, patients scoring 5 (excruciating pain) in the control group:

$$\% \text{ scoring } 5 = \frac{5}{20} \times 100 = 25\%$$

The values of the pie chart (see Fig. 15.3) also involved such calculations.

Rates

When summarizing the results of epidemiological investigations it is often useful to use this statistic to represent the level at which a disorder is present in a given population. The two rates which are commonly used in the health sciences are:

1. *Incidence rate*, which represents the number of new cases of a disorder reported within a time period:

$$\text{Incidence rate} = \frac{\text{number of new cases of a disorder}}{\text{total population at risk of the disorder}} \times \text{base}$$

2. *Prevalence rate*, which represents the total number of cases suffering from a disorder:

$$\text{Prevalence rate} = \frac{\text{number of existing cases of a disorder}}{\text{total population at risk of the disorder}} \times \text{base}$$

Let us illustrate the above equation by applying it to hypothetical data. Let us consider the condition herpes, a nasty little condition associated with the virus herpes simplex that attacks various parts (lips, etc.) of the body. Assume that an epidemiologist is interested in the spread of the condition in a given community.

1. Assume that all the population above the age of 15 years ($N = 1\,000\,000$) is at risk of herpes.
2. In 2005, 5000 new cases were reported.
3. In 2005, there was a total (old and new active cases) of 15\,000 known cases.

Here, substituting into the equation:

$$\text{Incidence rate for herpes} = \frac{5000}{1\,000\,000} \times \text{base}$$
$$= 0.005 \times \text{base}$$

The statistic 0.005 is not seen as the best way to represent a rate.

Often, epidemiologists select a base to make the statistic more understandable. The base represents a number for transforming the rate. The base selected depends on the magnitude of the rate; conventionally a multiple of 10, such as 1000, 10\,000 or 100\,000 is selected. In this instance we select 1000 as the base. Therefore, substituting into the equation, we obtain:

Incidence rate for herpes simplex
$$= \frac{0.005 \times 1000}{1} = 5 \text{ per } 1000$$

Prevalence rate for herpes simplex
$$= \frac{15\,000}{1\,000\,000} \times \frac{1000}{1} = 15 \text{ per } 1000$$

The above statistics can be graphed. For example, we may wish to represent pictorially the incidence of herpes simplex in the community over a period of five years. The (fictitious) evidence is shown in Table 15.6.

Table 15.6 Incidence of herpes

Year	Incidence of herpes (per 1000)
1982	8
1983	15
1984	17
1985	16
1986	10

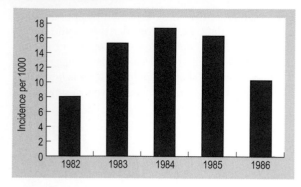

Table 15.7 Frequency data from a hypothetical RCT of an exercise program

Group	No diabetes	Diabetes	Total
Intervention (exercise)	80 a	20 b	100
Control	60 c	40 d	100
Total	140	60	200

Figure 15.7 • Incidence rate of genital herpes 1982–1986.

The graph of the time-series for the incidence over time (Fig. 15.7) gives us a visual impression of the changing incidence rate of the problem in question.

Odds

Odds refer to a ratio of the number of cases favouring an event to the number of non-events. For example, the odds of throwing a six with a dice are:

Odds = number of events favouring

'1'/number of non-events '2, 3, 4, 5, 6'

$$= \frac{1}{5}$$

$$= 0.2$$

In other words, the odds of throwing a six are 1 in 5 or 0.2. As you probably know, gamblers are very expert in using odds. These statistics are also important in health research as illustrated by the following example.

One way of assessing the effect of an intervention is to count up the number of people who have, or who develop, a disease or health condition that the intervention aimed at remediating. As a comparison, we also count the number of people who do not have or do not develop this disease or health condition. When there are two groups, this procedure produces dichotomous outcomes. The data for dichotomous outcomes can be summarized (see Table 15.7). Say that 200 obese, but otherwise healthy 55–65-year-old males are randomly assigned to two equally sized groups: the participants in the intervention group

receive a carefully targeted exercise program, while participants in the control group, maintain their usual lifestyle. The outcome measure is diagnosis of diabetes (yes or no) at the end of the trial. The hypothesis being tested is: the odds of being diagnosed with diabetes in the intervention group will be reduced in comparison to the control group. The hypothetical findings are shown below.

A number of values can be calculated from the data, shown in Table 15.7, and these can be used to test the hypothesis regarding the benefits of the exercise program.

The proportion of people in each group who do not develop diabetes, is calculated as follows:

Intervention group:

$$\text{Proportion} = \frac{a}{a+b} = \frac{80}{100} = 0.8$$

Control group:

$$\text{Proportion} = \frac{c}{c+d} = \frac{60}{100} = 0.6$$

The proportion of people without diabetes is higher in the intervention group than in the control group.

Intervention group:

$$0.8 \times 100 = 80\%$$

Control group:

$$0.6 \times 100 = 60\%$$

The hypothetical results indicate that 80% of participants in the intervention group did not develop diabetes, in comparison to 60% of participants in the control group. This outcome would support the efficacy of the exercise program.

The odds for each group, of experiencing the adverse event, is calculated as follows.

Intervention group:

$$\text{Odds} = \frac{a}{b} = \frac{80}{20} = 4.0$$

Control group:

$$\text{Odds} = \frac{c}{d} = \frac{60}{40} = 1.5$$

The odds of not developing diabetes in the intervention group are better than the odds for the control group. This is not the complete story; in Chapter 21 we will look at how these results are used for determining the efficacy of the intervention. To do this, we will use a statistic referred to as the odds ratio. To illustrate the concept of an odds ratio (OR) for the present example:

$$\text{OR} = \frac{\text{odds intervention group}}{\text{odds control group}} = \frac{4}{1.5} = 2.7$$

In other words, participants had 2.7 times the odds of not developing diabetes if they had followed the exercise program.

Summary

We outlined several techniques for organizing, tabulating and graphically presenting both discontinuous (nominal, ordinal) and continuous (interval, ratio) data. It was shown that raw data can be organized and tabulated as a frequency distribution, by counting the number of cases falling into specific categories or class intervals. Data composed of a large number of highly varied measurements were shown to be best presented by grouping the scores into class intervals.

Several techniques of graphing data were discussed: bar graphs and pie charts for discontinuous data, and histograms and frequency polygons for continuous data. The possible shapes of frequency polygons were also examined. It was shown that discrete data grouped in frequency distributions can be represented as ratios, proportions, percentages, rates and odds. In the next chapter, we will examine further techniques of 'crunching' or condensing data by using appropriate descriptive statistics suitable for continuous data.

Measures of central tendency and variability

16

CHAPTER CONTENTS

Introduction 125

Measures of central tendency 125

   The mode 125

   The median 125

   The mean 126

Comparison of the mode, median and mean .127

Measures of variability 128

   The range 128

   The average deviation 128

   The variance 129

   The standard deviation. 129

   The semi-interquartile range 130

Summary. 130

Introduction

In the previous chapter we examined how raw data can be organized and represented by the use of statistics in order that they may be easily communicated and understood. The two statistics that are necessary for representing a frequency distribution of data are measures of central tendency and variability.

Measures of central tendency are statistics or numbers expressing the most typical or representative scores in a data distribution. *Measures of variability* are statistics representing the extent to which scores are dispersed (or spread out) numerically. The overall aim of this chapter is to examine the use of several types of measures of central tendency and variability commonly used in the health

sciences. As quantitative evidence arising from investigations is presented in terms of these statistics, it is essential to understand these concepts.

The aims of this chapter are to:

1. Discuss the selection and use of measures of central tendency.
2. Discuss the selection and use of measures of variability.
3. Outline the relationship between the skew of frequency distributions and the selection of appropriate descriptive statistics.

Measures of central tendency

The mode

When the data are nominal (i.e. categories), the appropriate measure of central tendency is the mode. The mode is the most frequently occurring score or category in a distribution. Therefore, for the data shown in Table 16.1 the mode is the 'females' category. The mode can be obtained by inspection of grouped data (with the largest group being the mode). As we shall see later, the mode can also be calculated for continuous data as well as discrete data.

The median

With ordinal, interval or ratio scaled data, central tendency can also be represented by the median. The median (Mdn) is the score that divides the distribution into half: half of the scores fall under

Table 16.1 Table of sample data

Score	Real class interval	f	cum f
1	0.5–1.4	2	2
2	1.5–2.4	5	7
3	2.5–3.4	4	11*
4	3.5–4.4	3	14
5	4.5–5.4	3	17
		n = 17	

*Class interval containing median.

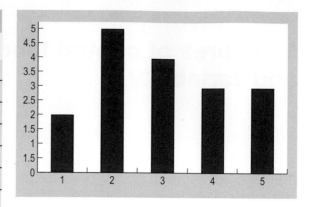

Figure 16.1 • Distribution of pain scores.

the median, and half above the median. That is, if scores are arranged in an ordered array from say highest to lowest or vice versa, the median would be the middle score. With a large number of cases and scores, it may not be feasible to locate the middle score simply by inspection. To calculate which is the middle score, we can use the formula $(n + 1)/2$, where n is the total number of cases in a sample. This formula gives us the number of the middle score. We can then count that number from either end of an ordered array.

In general, if n (i.e. the number of cases) is odd, the median is the middle score; if n is even, then the median falls between the two centre scores. The formula $(n + 1)/2$ is again used to tell us which score in an ordered array will be the median. For example:

5, 8, 9, 10, 28. Mdn = 9 (n is odd)
6, 17, 19, 20, 21, 27. Mdn = 19.5 (n is even)

For a grouped frequency distribution, the calculation of the median is a little more complicated. If we assume that the variable is continuous (e.g. time, height, weight or level of pain), we can use a formula for calculating the median. This formula (explained in detail below) can be applied to ordinal data, provided that the variable being measured has an underlying continuity. For example, in a study of the measurement of pain reports we obtain the following data, where $n = 17$:

1, 1, 2, 2, 2, 2, 2, 3, 3, 3, 3, 4, 4, 4, 5, 5, 5

These data can be represented by a bar graph (Fig. 16.1).

Here we can obtain the mode simply by inspection. The mode = 2 (the most frequent score). For the median, we need the ninth score, as this will divide the distribution into two equal halves (see Table 16.1). By inspection, we can see that the median will fall into category 3. Assuming underlying continuity of the variable and applying the previously discussed formula, we have:

$$Mdn = X_L + i \left[\frac{(n/2) - cum\ f_L}{f_i} \right]$$

where X_L = real lower limit of the class interval containing the median, i = width of the class interval, n = number of cases, cum f_L = cumulative frequency at the real lower limit of the interval and f_i = frequency of cases in the interval containing the median. Substituting into the above equation:

$$Mdn = 2.5 + 1 \left[\frac{(17/2) - 7}{4} \right]$$

$$= 2.5 + 1 \left[\frac{1.5}{4} \right]$$

$$= 2.875$$

The mean

The mean, $\overline{X}$ or μ, is defined as the sum of all the scores divided by the number of scores. The mean is, in fact, the arithmetic average for a distribution. The mean is calculated by the following equations:

$$\overline{X} = \frac{\Sigma x}{n} \text{ (for a sample)}$$

$$\mu = \frac{\Sigma x}{N} \text{ (for a population)}$$

where Σx = the sum of the scores, $\overline{X}$ = the mean of a sample, μ = the mean of a population, x = the values of the variable, that is the different elements in a sample or population, and n or N = the number of scores in a sample or population.

The formula simply summarizes the following 'advice':

> To calculate the average or mean of a set of scores ($\overline{X}$), add together all the scores (Σx) and divide by the number of cases (n).

Therefore, given the following sample scores:

2, 3, 5, 6, 7

To calculate the mean:

When n or N is very large, the average is calculated with the formula above but usually with the assistance of computers.

Comparison of the mode, median and mean

The mode can be used as a measure of central tendency for any level of scaling. However, since it only takes into account the most frequent scores, it is not generally a satisfactory way of presenting central tendency because it does not take into account scores from the whole of the distribution. For example, consider two sets of scores, A and B, shown in Table 16.2. It can be seen, either by inspection or by sketching a graph, that the two distributions A and B are quite different, yet the modes are the same, i.e. 1.

The median divides distributions into two equal halves, and is appropriate for ordinal, interval or ratio data. For interval or ratio data, however, the mean is the most appropriate measure of central tendency. The reason for this is that, in calculating this statistic, we take into account all the values in the study sample. In this way, it gives the best representation of the average score. Clearly, it is inappropriate to use the mean with nominal data, as the concept of 'average' does not apply to discrete categories. For example, what would be the average of 10 males and 20 females?

There is some justification for using the median as a measure of central tendency when the variable being measured is continuous. However this is controversial, and the mean should be preferred. Alternatively, when a distribution is highly skewed, the median might be more appropriate than the mean for representing the 'typical' score. Consider the distribution:

2, 2, 2, 5, 7, 8, 9
mode = 2

Table 16.2 Example data sets

A		B	
x	*f*	*x*	*f*
1	16	1	8
2	1	2	7
3	1	3	6
4	7	4	4
	$n = 25$		$n = 25$

median = 5
$\overline{X}$ = 5

Let us change the 9 to 44:

2, 2, 2, 5, 7, 8, 44
mode = 2
median = 5
$\overline{X}$ = 10

Clearly, the median and the mode are less sensitive to extreme scores, while the mean is pulled towards extreme scores. This might be a disadvantage. For example, there are seven people working in a small factory, with the following incomes per week:

$100, $200, $200, $300, $400, $400, $1900
median = $300
$\overline{X}$ = $500

The distribution of wages is highly skewed by the high income of the owner of the factory ($1900). The mean, $500, is higher than six of the seven scores; it is in no way typical of the distribution. In cases like this the median is more representative of the distribution.

Figure 16.2 illustrates the relationships between the skew of frequency distributions and the three measures of central tendency discussed in this chapter. We should remember that the mode will always be at the highest point, the median will divide the area under the curve into halves, and the mean is the average of all the scores in the distribution. Also, the greater the skew in distribution, the more the measures of central tendency are likely to differ.

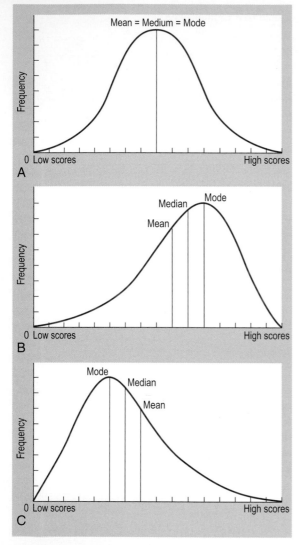

Figure 16.2 ● Measures of central tendency in (A) normal distribution, (B) negative skewing, (C) positive skewing.

Measures of variability

We have seen that a single statistic can be used to describe the central tendency of a frequency distribution. This information is insufficient to characterize a distribution; we also need a measure of how much the scores are dispersed or spread out. The variability of discrete data is of little relevance, as the degree of variability will be limited by the number of categories defined by the investigator at the beginning of measurement.

Consider the following two hypothetical distributions representing the IQs of two groups of intellectually disabled children:

Group A: 45, 50, 55, 60, 60, 70, 80
Group B: 57, 58, 59, 60, 61, 62, 63

It is evident that, although $\overline{X}_A = \overline{X}_B = 60$, the variability of the scores of group A is greater than that of group B. Insofar as IQ is related to the activities appropriate for these children, group A will provide a greater challenge to the therapist working with the children.

The three statistics commonly used to indicate the numerical value of variability are the *range*, the *variance* and the *standard deviation*.

The range

The range is the difference between the highest and lowest scores in a distribution. As we mentioned, given the IQ data above, the ranges are:

Group A: $80 - 45 + 1 = 36$
Group B: $63 - 57 + 1 = 7$

Although the range is easy to calculate, it is dependent only on the two extreme scores. In this way, we are not representing the typical variability of the scores. That is, the range might be distorted by a small number of atypical scores or 'outliers'. Consider, for instance, the differences in the range for the data given. The earlier example of the distribution of wages shows that just one outlying score in a distribution has an enormous impact on the range ($1900 - $100 = $1800). Obviously, some measure of average variability would be a preferable index of variability.

The average deviation

A convenient measure of variability might be average deviation about the mean. Consider group B shown previously. Here $\overline{X} = 60$. To calculate the average variability about the mean, we subtract the mean from each score, sum the individual deviations, and divide by n, the number of measurements (see Table 16.3). Therefore:

$$\Sigma (x - \overline{X}) = (-3) + (-2) + (-1) + (0) + (1) + (2) + (3) = 0$$

This is a general result; the sum of the average deviations about the mean is always zero. You can demonstrate this for the average deviation of group A.

Table 16.3 Average variability about mean for group B	
x	x − X̄
57	−3
58	−2
59	−1
60	0
61	+1
62	+2
63	+3

Table 16.4 Calculation of variance		
x	x − X̄	$(x - \bar{X})^2$
57	−3	9
58	−2	4
59	−1	1
60	0	0
61	+1	1
62	+2	4
63	+3	9
$\bar{X} = 60$		$\Sigma(x - \bar{X})^2 = 28$

The problem can be solved by squaring the deviations, as the square of negative numbers is always positive. This statistic is called the sums of squares (SS) and is always a positive number. This leads to a new statistic called the variance.

The variance

The variance (σ^2 or s^2) is defined as the sum of the squared deviations about the mean divided by the number of cases:

$$\sigma^2 = \frac{\sum (x - \mu)^2}{N} \quad \text{(for a population)}$$

$$s^2 = \frac{\sum \left(x - \bar{X}\right)^2}{n - 1} \quad \text{(for a sample)}$$

Divide by $n - 1$ when calculating the variance for a sample, when we use s^2 as an estimate of population variance. Dividing by n results in an estimate which is too small, given that a degree of freedom has been lost calculating $\bar{X}$.

For the IQ example shown above, the variance is calculated as shown in Table 16.4.

Substituting into the formula:

$$\sigma^2 = \frac{\sum \left(x - \bar{X}\right)^2}{n - 1} = \frac{28}{6} = 4.67$$

The problem with this measure of variability is that the deviations were squared. In this sense, we are overstating the spread of the scores. In taking the square root of the variance, we arrive at the most commonly used measure of variability for continuous data: the standard deviation.

The standard deviation

The standard deviation (σ or s) is defined as the square root of the variance:

$$\sigma = \sqrt{\sigma^2} = \frac{\sqrt{\sum (x - \mu)^2}}{N}$$

$$s = \sqrt{s^2} = \frac{\sqrt{\sum \left(x - \bar{X}\right)^2}}{n - 1}$$

Therefore, the standard deviation for group B is:

$$s = \sqrt{s^2} = \sqrt{4.67} = 2.16$$

The size of the standard deviation reflects the spread or dispersion of the frequency distribution representative of the data. Clearly, the larger σ or s, the relatively more spread out the scores are in a distribution. Calculation of the variance or the standard deviation is extremely tedious for large n using the method shown above. Statistics texts provide a variety of calculation formulae to derive these statistics. However, the accessibility of statistical packages for analysing data (see Ch. 20) in research and administration makes it superfluous to discuss these calculation formulae in detail as almost all data are analysed using statistical packages.

The semi-interquartile range

We have seen previously that, if we are summarizing ordinal data, or interval or ratio data that is highly skewed, then the median is the appropriate measure of central tendency. The statistic called interquartile and semi-interquartile range is used as the measure of dispersion when the median is the appropriate measure of central tendency for a distribution. The interquartile range is the distance between the scores representing the 25th (Q1) and 75th (Q3) percentile ranks in a distribution.

It is appropriate to define what we mean by percentiles (sometimes called centiles). The percentile or centile rank of a given score specifies the percentage of scores in a distribution falling up to and including the score. As an illustration, consider Figure 16.3, in which:

- 25% of cases or scores fall up to and including Q1.
- 50% of cases or scores fall up to and including the median.
- 75% of cases or scores fall up to and including Q3.
- 25% of cases or scores fall above Q3.

The distances A and B represent the distances between the median and Q1 and Q3. When a distribution is symmetrical or normal, the distances A and B will be equal. However, when a distribution is skewed, the two distances will be quite different. The semi-interquartile range (sometimes called the quartile deviation) is half of the distance between the scores representing the 25th (Q1) and 75th (Q3) percentile ranks in a distribution. Let us look

at an example. If we have a sample where $n = 16$ and the values of the variable are:

1, 5, 7, 7, 8, 9, 9, 10, 11, 12, 13, 15, 19, 20, 20, 20

clearly, a frequency distribution of these data is not even close to normal as the distribution is not symmetrical and the mode is at the maximum value. Therefore, the median is selected as the appropriate measure for central tendency, and we should use the interquartile range as the measure of dispersion.

Looking at the data, we find:

1 5 7 7 * 8 9 9 10 † 11 12 13 15 ‡ 19 20 20 20

where * denotes the 25th centile, † denotes the 50th centile and ‡ denotes the 75th centile.

The score that cuts off the first 25% of scores (25th centile) is the first quartile (Q1). Since we have $n = 16$, Q1 will cut off the first four scores (25% of 16 is 4). Thus:

$$Q1 = \frac{7+8}{2} = 7.5$$

The third quartile (Q3) is the score which cuts off 75% of the scores. As $n = 16$, Q3 will cut off 12 scores (75% of 16 is 12).

$$Q3 = \frac{15+19}{2} = 17$$

Therefore, the semi-interquartile range is:

$$\frac{Q3 - Q1}{2} = \frac{17.0 - 7.5}{2} = 4.75$$

The larger the semi-interquartile range, the more the scores are spread out about the median.

Summary

In this chapter, we discussed two essential statistics for representing frequency distributions: measures of central tendency and variability. The measures of central tendency outlined were the mode and median for discrete data, and the mean for continuous data. Measures of variability were shown to be the range, average deviation, variance and standard deviation. These statistics are appropriate for crunching the data together to the point that the distribution of raw data can be meaningfully represented by only two statistics. That is, the raw data representing the outcome

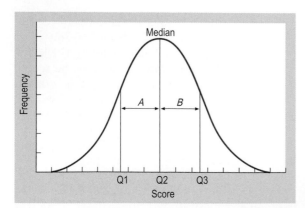

Figure 16.3 • Interquartile ranges.

of investigations or clinical measurements are expressed in this manner. We have seen that the mean and the standard deviation are most appropriate for interval or ratio data. The median and semi-interquartile range are used when the data are measured on an ordinal scale, or when interval or ratio data are found to have a highly skewed distribution. The mode represents the most frequent scores. The contents of the chapter focused on the use and meaning of these concepts, rather than stressing calculations involved. These calculations are obtained by using statistical software packages. In Chapter 17, we discuss the application of the mean and standard deviation for relating specific scores to an overall distribution.

Standard scores and normal distributions

17

CHAPTER CONTENTS

Introduction 133

Standard scores (z scores) 133

Normal distributions. 134

　The standard normal curve 135

Calculations of areas under the normal curve .135

　Critical values 136

Standard normal curves for the comparison of distributions 136

Summary. 138

Introduction

In this chapter we will discuss standard distributions. Standard scores represent the position of a score or measurement in relation to an overall set of scores. Standard distributions are also useful for comparing scores from different sets of measurements. Standard scores are used in both clinical practice and research in the health sciences. In clinical practice the score of a patient is often compared with a known distribution to interpret the score. Measurements such as blood pressure or cholesterol levels are compared with a distribution to interpret the patient's result.

The aims of this chapter are to:

1. Define 'standard' scores.
2. Describe the characteristics of normal and standard normal curves.
3. Show how standard normal curves can be used for calculating percentile ranks.

4. Show how standard normal curves can be used to compare scores from different distributions.

Standard scores (z scores)

Consider this example: infant A walked unaided at the age of 40 weeks, while infant B is 65 weeks old but still cannot walk. What sense can we make of these measurements? Could infant B need further clinical investigation in case he has some neurological abnormality? The fact that infant B is unable to walk at the age of 65 weeks is not very informative in the absence of additional information about how this compares with norms for other children. However, say that it is known that the distribution of walking ages is such that $\mu = 50$ weeks and $\sigma = 5$. Assuming that the frequency distribution is normal, the frequency polygon representing the population would look something like that shown in Figure 17.1.

In this instance, infant B's score is clearly above the mean. In fact, by inspection, we can see the infant's score at this point of time was three standard deviations above ($+3$) the mean ($65 = 50 + (3 \times 5)$). In contrast, infant A began walking earlier than the mean, his score of 40 being two standard deviations below (-2) the mean. In general, any 'raw' score in a frequency distribution can be described in terms of its distance from the mean. The process of transforming a score into a measurement based on its distance from the mean in standard deviations is called *standardizing* the score. Such 'transformed' scores are called *z* scores or standard scores.

A *z* score represents how many standard deviations a given raw score is above or below the mean.

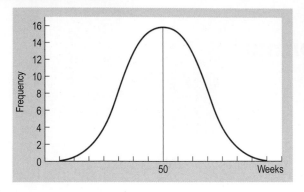

Figure 17.1 • Age at which children walk unaided.

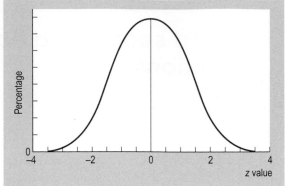

Figure 17.2 • Standard normal distribution.

The equation for transforming specific raw scores into z scores is given as:

$$z = \frac{x - \mu}{\sigma} \text{ (for a population)}$$

$$z = \frac{x - \overline{X}}{s} \text{ (for a sample)}$$

For the above equation, x is the raw score, $\overline{X}$ or μ is the mean of the distribution from which the score was drawn and s or σ is the standard deviation of the distribution. That is, when we know the mean and standard deviation of a distribution, we can transform any raw score into a z score. Conversely, when the z score is known, we can use the above equations to calculate the corresponding raw scores.

In the above example, the z scores corresponding to the infants' raw scores are:

$$\text{Infant A: } z = \frac{x - \mu}{\sigma}$$

$$= \frac{40 - 50}{5}$$

$$= -2$$

$$\text{Infant B: } z = \frac{x - \mu}{\sigma}$$

$$= \frac{65 - 50}{5}$$

$$= -3$$

These calculations support our previous observations that A's score was two standard deviations below the mean and B's score was three standard deviations above the mean. In other words, A walked very early and B was a very late starter. The particular value of standardizing scores for understanding clinical or research evidence will be discussed in the context of the concepts of normal and standard normal distributions.

Normal distributions

Many variables measured in the biological, behavioural and clinical sciences are approximately 'normally' distributed, i.e. they have a characteristic 'bell-shaped' curve. What is meant by a normal distribution is illustrated by the normal curve (see Fig. 17.2), which is a frequency polygon representing the theoretical distribution of population scores. We assume here that the variable x has been measured on an interval or ratio scale and that it is a continuous variable such as weight, height or blood pressure.

The normal curve has the following characteristics:

1. It is symmetrical about the mean, so that equal numbers of cases fall above and below the mean (mean = median = mode).
2. Relatively few cases fall into the high or low values of x. Most of the cases fall close to the mean. (For the theoretical normal distribution, the arms of the curve do not intersect with the x-axis, allowing for a few extreme scores.)
3. The precise equation for the normal curve was discovered by the mathematician Gauss, so that it is sometimes referred to as a Gaussian curve.

We need not worry about the actual formula for the normal curve. Rather, the point is that, given that the functional relationship between f and x is known, integral calculus can be used to calculate areas under the curve for any value of x. All normal curves have the same general mathematical form; whether we are graphing IQ or weight, the same bell shape will appear. The only differences between the curves are the mean value and the amount of variation. This is why the mean and the standard deviation provide us with important information about any particular normal distribution. Note that it is unlikely that any real data are exactly normally distributed. Rather, the normal distribution is a mathematical model that is useful for representing real distributions.

The standard normal curve

If we transform the raw scores of a variable into z scores and then plot the frequency polygon for the distribution, we will have a standard curve. If the original distribution was normal, then the frequency polygon will be a standard normal curve. Standard normal curves are identical regardless of the nature of the original variables.

By transforming raw scores into z scores we are adjusting for differences in means and standard deviations, which are the only things that distinguish between non-standardized normal curves.

The standard normal curve has the following additional properties:

1. The mean is always 0 (zero). For the previous example, the z score corresponding to $\mu = 50$ (as in the 'infants' walking age' example) is:

$$z = \frac{50 - 50}{5} = 0$$

2. The mean = median = mode, as the curve is symmetrical.

3. The standard deviation of z scores is always 1 (one). For instance, the z score for 55 (which is one standard deviation above the mean) is:

$$z = \frac{55 - 50}{5} = 1$$

4. It is assumed that the *total area under the curve adds up to 1.00*. Since the normal curve is symmetrical, 0.5 of the area falls above $z = 0$ and 0.5 falls below $z = 0$. This is another way of saying that 50% of the total cases fall below the mean, and 50% of the cases fall above the mean (which is equal to the median).

5. More generally, we can use appropriate *statistical tables* to estimate the area under the standard normal curve for any given z scores. These areas are available in table form (see Appendix A) so that for any value of z we can read off the corresponding area.

6. The area under the curve between any two points is directly proportional to the percentage

of cases falling above, below or between those two points. We can use the standard normal curve to calculate the percentage of scores falling between any specified two scores.

In the next section, we will examine the use of the table of areas under the standard normal curve to understand the meaning of measurements in relation to distributions.

Calculations of areas under the normal curve

We have already examined the concept of percentile or centile ranks. The normal curve is useful for evaluating the percentile rank of scores in normal distributions. Appendix A gives the proportion of areas under the standard normal curve which lies:

- between the mean and a given z score
- beyond the z score.

Since normal distributions are symmetrical, the same proportions are also true for the area between the mean and any negative z score. Only the positive values are given in Appendix A.

Let us see how we can use this information to estimate the percentile ranks of the two infants' walking ages. We have shown previously in our hypothetical example that, for infant A, $z = -2$. Let us now turn to Appendix A. In going down the column of z scores, we find that the area corresponding to $z = 2.00$ is 0.4772 (between) and 0.0228 (beyond).

We know that the area A1 under the curve in Figure 17.3 must be:

$$\text{Shaded portion} = 0.5000 - 0.4772$$
$$= 0.0228 \text{ (as half the scores fall under the mean)}$$

This proportion can be expressed as a percentage, so that 2.28% of the cases in the distribution fall below $z = -2$. We have defined percentile rank for a score as the percentage of cases in a distribution falling up to and including a specific score. Therefore, the percentile rank for infant A's walking is 2.28%. Of all children, only 2.28% learn to walk as early as or earlier than infant A. Clearly, he is doing well.

What then is the percentile rank for infant B's performance? As you remember, $z = +3$. Looking up the area corresponding to $z = 3.00$ in Appendix A we find the area (A1 in Fig. 17.4) is equal to 0.4987. Therefore, the proportion of scores falling up to and including $z = +3$ is $0.5 + 0.4987 = 0.9987$.

135

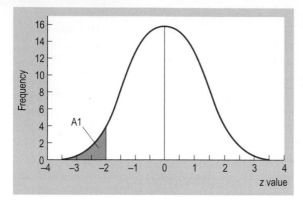

Figure 17.3 • Area (A1) corresponding to $z = -2$.

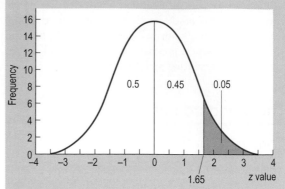

Figure 17.5 • Determining z score of 95th percentile.

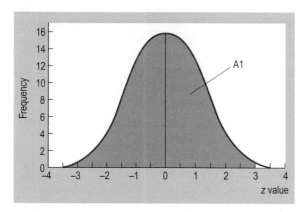

Figure 17.4 • Area (A1) corresponding to $z = +3$.

Expressing this finding as a percentage, we find that 99.87% of children learn to walk by the age of 65 weeks. As we said earlier, infant B is still not walking. Perhaps further clinical tests are indicated, although we should keep in mind that an unusual or extreme score is not necessarily indicative of pathological states.

Critical values

We can work the other way by determining the raw scores corresponding to areas under the normal curve in Appendix A. For example, say that the slowest 5% of infants (i.e. the 5% with the highest age first walked scores) are offered some special exercises in learning to walk. What would be the age at which the exercises should be offered, should the child not be walking? The key here is to determine the score that corresponds to the

slowest 5% (5th percentile) of the distribution. This can be represented as shown in Figure 17.5.

From Figure 17.5 we can see that we need to discover the z score that corresponds to an area of 0.45 above the mean. By consulting the normal distribution table (see Appendix A), it can be seen that the corresponding z score is $z = 1.65$. This is a critical value for the statistic in defining an area.

Given the z score, we can calculate the corresponding raw score from the formula:

$$z = \frac{x - \mu}{\sigma}$$

$$\text{Therefore } 1.65 = \frac{x - 50}{5}$$

$$x = (5 \times 1.65) + 50$$

$$= 58.25$$

That is, if the slowest 5% are thought to be in need of help, then children somewhat over 58 weeks old and still not walking would be recommended for the remedial exercises. Of course, we can use the tables for reading off the z scores corresponding to any specified area or percentage. It must be emphasized that if a distribution is *not* approximately normal, e.g. markedly skewed or bimodal, then the above critical values do not apply. It is always appropriate to check if a distribution is approximately normal or not before conducting statistical analysis. Most statistical software packages have this as an inbuilt feature.

Standard normal curves for the comparison of distributions

One of the uses of standard distributions is that we can compare scores from entirely different distributions. For example, if a student scored 63 on test A,

Table 17.1 Scores for example in text

Raw scores	z scores	Percentile ranks
x = 63	−0.25	40.1
x = 52	+1.50	93.3

Table 17.2 Blood cholesterol

	Mean blood cholesterol (mg/mL)	Standard deviation
Meat eaters	0.6	0.15
Vegetarians	0.4	0.1

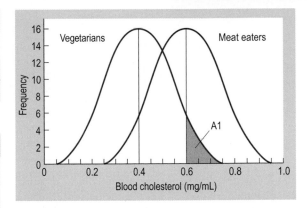

Figure 17.6 • Area A1 corresponds to the percentage of vegetarians with blood cholesterol higher than 0.6 mg/mL.

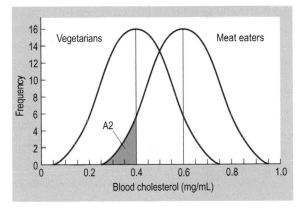

Figure 17.7 • Area A2 corresponds to the percentage of meat eaters with lower blood cholesterol than the mean for vegetarians.

and 52 on test B, on which test did the student do better? If we define 'better' as solely in terms of raw scores, then clearly the student did better on test A. However, test A might have been easier than test B, so that if the overall performances of all students on the tests are taken into account, the student's relative performance might be better on test B. Say:

$$\text{Test A: } \overline{X} = 65 \text{ and } s = 8$$
$$\text{Test B: } \overline{X} = 40 \text{ and } s = 8$$

Therefore, using the formula for calculating z scores, and looking up the corresponding areas in Appendix A (do this yourself) we obtain the results shown in Table 17.1. Thus, the student performed better on test B, by scoring higher than 93% of other students sitting the test.

This example illustrates that in some circumstances the meaning of specific scores has to be interpreted against 'standards'.

Another use of standard distributions is in interpreting the meaning of the results of investigations in the health sciences. Let us examine the following hypothetical example. An investigator measured levels of blood cholesterol in a sample of 300 adults who are meat eaters, and 100 adults who are vegetarians. The results of the investigation are summarized in Table 17.2.

Now, imagine that you are a clinician working with patients with cardiac disorders and you are interested in the following questions:

1. Approximately what percentage of vegetarians had blood cholesterol levels greater than the average meat eater?

2. Approximately what percentage of meat eaters had blood cholesterol levels lower than that of the average vegetarian?

The percentage of cases of vegetarians with blood cholesterol greater than 0.6 (the mean for the meat eaters) is represented by area A1 in Figure 17.6.

$$z = \frac{0.6 - 0.4}{0.1} = 2$$
$$\text{Area A1} = 0.0228$$

Therefore, approximately 2.3% of vegetarians had blood cholesterol levels higher than the average for meat eaters.

Figure 17.7 demonstrates the area (A2) corresponding to the percentage of meat eaters with lower blood cholesterol than the average vegetarian.

$$z = \frac{0.4 - 0.6}{0.15} = -1.33$$

$$\text{Area A2} = 0.0918$$

Therefore, approximately 9.2% of meat eaters had lower blood cholesterol levels than the average vegetarian.

Summary

We found that if the mean and standard deviation for a given distribution have been calculated, then we can transform any raw score into a standard (or z) score. The z score represents how many standard deviations a specific score is above or below the mean. The larger the value of the corresponding z score (whether it is positive or negative), the more deviant a given score is from the mean. A positive score means that it is above the mean and negative value means that is below the mean. We described how to calculate this transformed score for a population or a sample. Also, we outlined the essential characteristics of the normal and the standard normal curves.

If the original frequency distribution is approximately normal, then the table of standardized normal distributions (Appendix A) can be used to calculate percentile ranks of raw scores, or the percentage of scores falling between specified scores. Also, z scores are useful in comparing scores arising from two or more different normal distributions. The above information is applicable to clinical practice, for example in interpreting the significance of an individual's assessment in relation to known population norms.

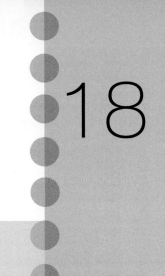

Correlation

CHAPTER CONTENTS

Introduction 139

Correlation 139

Correlation coefficients 141

   Selection of correlation coefficients 141

   Calculation of correlation coefficients . . . 141

Uses of correlations in the health sciences . . 143

   Estimating associations between variables 143

   Reliability and predictive validity
of assessment 144

   Estimating shared variance 145

Correlation and causation. 145

Summary. 146

Introduction

A fundamental aim of scientific and clinical research is to establish the nature of the relationships between two or more sets of observations or variables. Finding such relationships or associations can be an important step for identifying causal relationships and the prediction of clinical outcomes. The topic of correlation is concerned with expressing quantitatively the size and the direction of the relationship between variables. Correlations are essential statistics in the health sciences, used to quantitatively determine the validity and reliability of clinical measures (see Ch. 14) or expressing how health

problems are associated with crucial biological, behavioural or environmental factors (see Ch. 8). Having worked through this chapter you will be able to explain how correlation coefficients are used and interpreted in health sciences research and practice.

The specific aims of this chapter are to:

1. Define the terms correlation and correlation coefficient.
2. Explain the selection and calculation of correlation coefficients.
3. Outline some of the uses of correlation coefficients.
4. Define and calculate the coefficient of determination.
5. Discuss the relationship between correlation and causality.

Correlation

Consider the following two statements:

1. There is a positive relationship between cigarette smoking and lung damage.
2. There is a negative relationship between being overweight and life expectancy.

You probably have a fair idea what the above two statements mean. The first statement implies that there is evidence that if you score high on one variable (cigarette smoking) you are likely to score high on the other variable (lung damage). The second statement describes the finding that scoring high on the variable 'overweight' tends to be associated with lowered 'life expectancy'. The information

Table 18.1 Examination scores

| Student | Score (out of 10) | |
	Anatomy (X)	Physiology (Y)
1	3	2.5
2	4	3.5
3	1	0
4	8	6
5	2	1

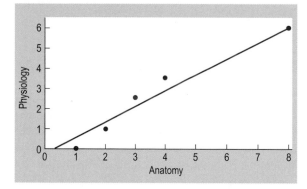

Figure 18.1 • Scattergram of students' scores in two examinations.

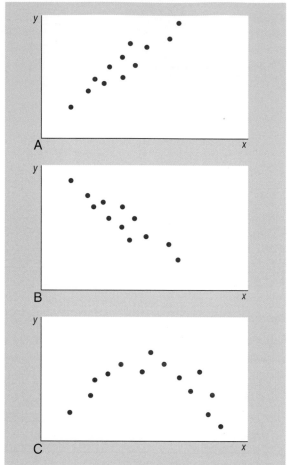

Figure 18.2 • Scattergrams showing relationships between two variables: (A) positive linear correlation; (B) negative linear correlation; (C) non-linear correlation.

missing from each of the statements is the numerical value for size of the association between the variables.

A *correlation coefficient* is a statistic which expresses numerically the magnitude and direction of the association between two variables.

In order to demonstrate that two variables are correlated, we must obtain measures of both variables for the same set of participants or events. Let us consider an example to illustrate this point.

Assume that we are interested to see whether student test scores for anatomy examinations are correlated with test scores for physiology. To keep the example simple, we will assume that there were only five ($n = 5$) students who sat for both examinations (see Table 18.1).

To provide a visual representation of the relationship between the two variables, we can plot the above data on a *scattergram* (also referred to as a *scatterplot*). A scattergram is a graph of the paired scores for each participant on the two variables. By convention, we call one of the variables x and the other one y. It is evident from Figure 18.1 that there is a positive relationship between the two variables. That is, students who have high scores for anatomy (variable X) tend to have high scores for physiology (variable Y). Also, for this set of data, we can fit a straight line in close approximation to the points on the scattergram. This line is referred to as a line of 'best fit'. This topic is discussed further in statistics under 'linear regression'. In general, a variety of relationships is possible between two variables; the scattergrams in Figure 18.2 illustrate some of these.

Figure 18.2A and B represent a linear correlation between the variables x and y. That is, a straight line is the most appropriate representation of the relationship between x and y. Figure 18.2C represents a non-linear correlation, where a curve best represents the relationship between x and y.

Figure 18.2A represents a *positive* correlation, indicating that high scores on x are related to high scores on y. For example, the relationship between cigarette smoking and lung damage is a positive correlation. Figure 18.2B represents a *negative* correlation, where high scores on x are associated with low scores on y. For example, the correlation between the variables 'being overweight' and 'life expectancy' is negative, meaning that the more you are overweight, the lower your life expectancy.

Correlation coefficients

When we need to know or express the numerical value of the correlation between x and y, we calculate a statistic called the correlation coefficient. The correlation coefficient expresses quantitatively the magnitude and direction of the correlation between the two variables.

Selection of correlation coefficients

There are several types of correlation coefficients used in statistical analysis. Table 18.2 shows some of these correlation coefficients, and the conditions under which they are used. As the table indicates, the scale of measurements used determines the selection of the appropriate correlation coefficient.

All of the correlation coefficients shown in Table 18.2 are appropriate for quantifying linear relationships between variables. There are other correlation coefficients, such as η (eta) which are used for quantifying non-linear relationships. However, the discussion of the use and calculation of all the correlation coefficients is beyond the scope of this text. Rather, we will examine only the commonly used Pearson's r, and Spearman's ρ (rho).

Regardless of which correlation coefficient we employ, these statistics share the following characteristics:

1. Correlation coefficients are calculated from pairs of measurements on variables x and y for the same group of individuals.
2. A positive correlation is denoted by $+$ and a negative correlation by $-$.
3. The values of the correlation coefficient range from $+1$ to -1, where $+1$ means a perfect positive correlation, 0 means no correlation, and -1 a perfect negative correlation.

Table 18.2 Correlation coefficient

Coefficient	Conditions where appropriate
φ (phi)	Both x and y measures on a nominal scale
ρ (rho)	Both x and y measures on, or transformed to, ordinal scales
r	Both x and y measures on an interval or ratio scale

4. The square of the correlation coefficient represents the coefficient of determination.

Calculation of correlation coefficients

Pearson's r

We have already stated that Pearson's r is the appropriate correlation coefficient when both variables x and y are measured on an interval or a ratio scale. Further assumptions in using r are that both variables x and y are normally distributed, and that we are describing a linear (rather than a curvilinear) relationship.

Pearson's r is a measure of the extent to which paired scores are correlated. To calculate r we need to represent the position of each paired score within its own distribution, so we convert each raw score to a z score. This transformation corrects for the two distributions x and y having different means and standard deviations. The formula for calculating Pearson's r is:

$$r = \frac{\Sigma z_x z_y}{n}$$

where z_x = standard score corresponding to any raw x score, z_y = standard score corresponding to any raw y score, Σ = sum of standard score products and n = number of paired measurements.

Table 18.3 gives the calculations for the correlation coefficient for the data given in the earlier examination scores example.

Therefore:

$$r = \frac{\Sigma z_x z_y}{n} = \frac{3.94}{5} = 0.79$$

(The z scores are calculated as discussed in Ch. 15.)

This is quite a high correlation, indicating that the paired z scores fall roughly on a straight line.

Table 18.3 Example calculations for correlation coefficient

Student	Raw scores		z scores		
	x	y	z_x	z_y	$z_x z_y$
1	3	2.5	−0.22	−0.04	+0.01
2	4	3.5	+0.15	+0.39	+0.06
3	1	0	−0.96	−1.12	+1.08
4	8	6	+1.63	+1.46	+2.38
5	2	1	−0.59	−0.69	+0.41
	$\overline{X} = 3.6$	$\overline{X} = 2.6$			$\Sigma z_x z_y = 3.94$
	$s_x = 2.7$	$s_y = 2.33$			

In general, the closer the relationship between the two variables approximates a straight line, the more r approaches 1.0. Note that in social and biological sciences, correlations this high do not usually occur. In general, we consider anything over 0.7 to be quite high, 0.3–0.7 to be moderate and less than 0.3 to be weak. The scattergrams in Figure 18.3 illustrate this point.

When n is large, the above equation is inconvenient to use to calculate r. Here we are not concerned with calculating r with a large n, although appropriate formulae or computer programs are available. For example, Coates & Steed (2003) described how to use the program 'SPSS' for calculating correlation coefficients. The printouts provide not only the value of the correlation coefficients but also the statistical significance of the associations.

Assumptions for using r

It was pointed out earlier that Pearson's r is used when the two variables are scaled on interval or ratio scales and when it is shown that they are linearly associated. In addition, the sets of scores on each variable should be approximately normally distributed.

If any of the above assumptions are violated, then the correlation coefficient might be spuriously low. Therefore, other correlation coefficients should be used to represent association between two variables. A further problem may arise from the truncation of the range of values in one or both of the variables. This occurs when the distributions greatly deviate from normal

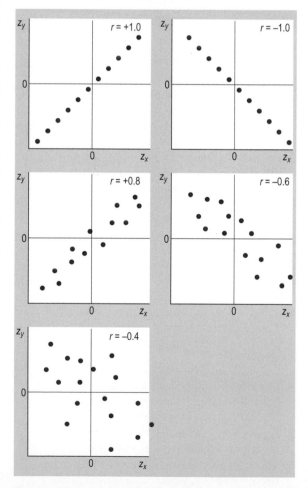

Figure 18.3 • Scattergrams and corresponding approximate r values.

Table 18.4 Rank-ordering of scores

Patient	Socioeconomic status (rank)	Severity of illness (rank)	d (difference between ranks)	d^2
1	6	5	1	1
2	7	8	−1	1
3	2	4	−2	4
4	3	3	0	0
5	5	7	−2	4
6	4	1	3	9
7	1	2	−1	1
8	8	6	2	4
				$\Sigma d^2 = 24$

shapes. The higher scale can be readily reduced to an ordinal scale.

If we measure the correlation between examination scores and intelligence quotients (IQs) of a group of health science students, we might find a low correlation because, by the time students present themselves to tertiary courses, most students with low IQs have been eliminated. In this way, the distribution of IQs would not be normal but rather negatively skewed. In effect, the question of appropriate sampling (see Ch. 5) is also relevant to selecting correlation coefficients.

Spearman's ρ

When the obtained data are such that at least one of the variables x or y was measured on an ordinal scale and the other on an ordinal scale or higher, we use ρ to calculate the correlation between the two variables. The higher scale can be readily reduced to an ordinal scale.

If one or both variables were measured on a nominal scale, ρ is no longer appropriate as a statistic.

$$\rho = 1 - \frac{6\,\Sigma\, d^2}{n^3 - n}$$

where d denotes the difference between paired ranks and n represents the number of pairs.

The derivation of this formula will not be discussed here. The 6 is placed in the formula as a scaling device; it ensures that the possible range of

ρ is from −1 to +1 and thus enables ρ and r to be compared. Let us consider an example to illustrate the use of ρ.

If an investigator is interested in the correlation between socio-economic status and severity of respiratory illness, and assuming that both variables were measured on, or transformed to, an ordinal scale, the investigator rank-orders the scores from highest to lowest on each variable (Table 18.4).

$$\text{Therefore: } \rho = 1 - \frac{6\,\Sigma\, d^2}{n^3 - n}$$

$$= 1 - \frac{6 \times 24}{8^3 - 8} = 0.71$$

Clearly, the association among the ranks for the paired scores on the two variables becomes closer the more ρ approaches +1. If the ranks tend to be inverse, then ρ approaches −1.

Uses of correlations in the health sciences

Estimating associations between variables

When the correlation coefficient has been calculated it may be used to estimate the value of one variable (y) given the value of the other variable (x). For instance, take a hypothetical example that the correlation between cigarette smoking and lung damage is $r = +1$. We can see from Figure 18.4

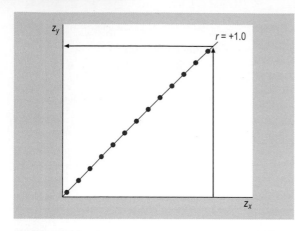

Figure 18.4 ● Hypothetical relationship between cigarette smoking and lung damage. $r = +1.0$.

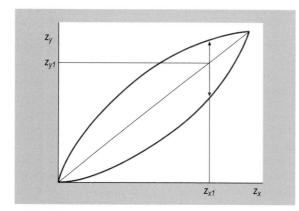

Figure 18.5 ● Hypothetical relationship between cigarette smoking and lung damage. $r = +0.7$. With a correlation of <1.0 the data points will cluster around rather than exactly on the line and may vary between the range of values shown for any given values of x or y and their corresponding z scores.

that, given any score on x, we can transform this into a z score (z_x) and then using the graph, we can read off the corresponding z score on y (z_y).

Of course, it is extremely rare that there should be a perfect ($r = +1$) correlation between two variables. In this case, the smaller the correlation coefficient, the greater the probability of making an error in estimation. For example, consider Figure 18.5, where the scattergram shown represents a hypothetical correlation of approximately $r = 0.7$. Here, for any transformed value on variable x (say z_{x1}) there is a range of values of z_y that correspond. Our best guess here is z_{y1}, the average

Table 18.5 Assessment of disability (%) by observers X and Y

Patient	Observer X	Observer Y	Rank X	Rank Y
1	85%	98%	1	1
2	75%	86%	2	2
3	74%	80%	3	3
4	72%	79%	4	4
5	69%	70%	5	5

value, but clearly a range of scores is possible, as shown in Figure 18.5. We will look at the issue of sampling error when we look at confidence intervals in Chapter 19. That is, as the correlation coefficient approaches 0, the range of error in prediction increases. A more appropriate and precise way of making estimations is in terms of regression analysis, but this topic is not covered in this introductory book.

Reliability and predictive validity of assessment

As you will recall, reliability refers to measurements using instruments or to subjective judgements remaining relatively the same on repeated administration (see Ch. 14). This is called test–retest reliability and its degree is measured by a correlation coefficient. The correlation coefficient can also be used to determine the degree of inter-observer reliability.

As an example, assume that we are interested in the inter-observer reliability (agreement) for two neurologists who are assessing patients for degrees of functional disability following spinal cord damage. Table 18.5 represents a set of hypothetical results of their independent assessment of the same set of five patients. There are many studies of inter-observer agreement in clinical judgements in the medical literature because such judgements are often very influential in decisions about treatment and diagnosis.

Observer Y clearly attributes greater degrees of disability to the patients than observer X. However, as stated earlier, this need not affect the correlation coefficient. If we treat the measurement as an ordinal scale, we can see from Table 18.5 that the ranks given to the patients by the two observers correspond, so that it can be shown that $\rho = +1$.

Clearly, the higher the correlation, the greater the reliability. If we had treated the measurements as representing interval or ratio data, we would have calculated Pearson's *r* to represent quantitatively the reliability of the measurement.

Predictive validity is also expressed as a correlation coefficient. For example, say that you devise an assessment procedure to predict how much people will benefit from a rehabilitation program. If the correlation between the assessment and a measure of the success of the rehabilitation program is high (say 0.7 or 0.8), the assessment procedure has high predictive validity. If, however, the correlation is low (say 0.3 or 0.4), the predictive validity of the assessment is low, and it would be unwise to use the assessment as a screening procedure for the entry of patients into the rehabilitation program.

Estimating shared variance

A useful statistic is the square of the correlation coefficient (r^2) which represents the proportion of variance in one variable accounted for by the other. This is called the *coefficient of determination*.

If, for example, the correlation between variable *x* (height) and variable *y* (weight) is $r = 0.7$, then the coefficient of determination is $r^2 = 0.49$ or 49%. This means that 49% of the variability of weight can be accounted for in terms of height. You might ask, what about the other 51% of the variability? This would be accounted for by other factors, say for instance, a tendency to eat fatty foods. The point here is that even a relatively high correlation coefficient ($r = 0.7$) accounts for less than 50% of the variability.

This is a difficult concept, so it might be worth remembering that 'variability' (see Ch. 16) refers to how scores are spread out about the mean. That is, as in the above example, some people will be heavy, some average and some light. So we can account for 49% of the total variability of weight (*x*) in terms of height (*y*) if $r = 0.7$. The other 51% can be explained in terms of other factors, such as somatotype. The greater the correlation coefficient, the greater the coefficient of determination, and the more the variability in *y* can be accounted for in terms of *x*.

Correlation and causation

In Chapter 7, we pointed out that there were at least three criteria for establishing a causal relationship. Correlation or co-variation is only one of these criteria. We have already discussed that even a high correlation between two variables does not necessarily imply a causal relationship. That is, there are a variety of plausible explanations for finding a correlation. As an example, let us take cigarette smoking (*x*) and lung damage (*y*). A high positive correlation could result from any of the following circumstances:

1. *x* causes *y*.
2. *y* causes *x*.
3. There is a third variable, which causes changes in both *x* and *y*.
4. The correlation represents a spurious or chance association.

For the example above, (1) would imply that cigarette smoking causes lung damage, (2) that lung damage causes cigarette smoking, and (3) that there was a variable (e.g. stress) which caused both increased smoking and lung damage. We need further information to identify which of the competing hypotheses is most plausible.

Some associations between variables are completely spurious (4). For example, there might be a correlation between the amount of margarine consumed and the number of cases of influenza over a period of time in a community, but each of the two events might have entirely different, unrelated causes. Also, some correlation coefficients do not reach statistical significance: that is, they may be due to chance (see Ch. 20).

Also, if we are using a sample to estimate the correlation in a population, we must be certain that the outcome is not due to biased sampling or sampling error. That is, the investigator needs to show that a correlation coefficient is statistically significant and not just due to random sampling error. We will look at the concept of statistical significance in the next chapter.

While demonstrating correlation does not establish causality, we can use correlations as a source for subsequent hypotheses. For instance, in this example, work on carcinogens in cigarette tars and the causes of emphysema has confirmed that it is probably true that smoking does, in fact, cause lung damage (*x* causes *y*). However, given that there is often multiple causation of health problems, option (3) cannot be ruled out.

Techniques are available which can, under favourable conditions, enable investigators to use correlations as a basis for distinguishing between competing plausible hypotheses. One such technique, called path analysis, involves postulating a probable temporal sequence of events and then establishing a correlation between them. This technique was borrowed from systems theory and has been applied in areas of clinical research, such as epidemiology.

Summary

In this chapter we outlined how the degree and direction between two variables can be quantified using statistics called correlation coefficients. Of the correlation coefficients, the use of two was outlined: Pearson's r and Spearman's ρ. Definitional formulae and simple calculations were presented, with the understanding that more complex calculations of correlation coefficients are done with computers.

Several uses for r and ρ were discussed: for prediction, for quantifying the reliability and validity of measurements, and by using r^2 in estimating the amount of shared variability. Finally, we discussed the caution necessary in causal interpretation of correlation coefficients. Showing a strong association between variables is an important step towards establishing causal links but further evidence is required to decide the direction of causality.

As with other descriptive statistics, caution is necessary when correlation coefficients are calculated for a sample and then generalized to a population. Generalization from a sample statistic to a population parameter must take into account the probability of sampling error, an issue which will be discussed in the following chapters.

Section 6

Data analysis and inference

19 Probability and confidence intervals. 149
20 Hypothesis testing: selection and use of statistical tests 159
21 Effect size and the interpretation of evidence 171
22 Qualitative data analysis 181

Statistical data analysis is an essential stage in conducting quantitative research (see Ch. 3). The principles of inferential statistics, as introduced in this section, are applied to decide if the obtained sample data show the differences and patterns we set out to demonstrate in the population. This is the case for all types of research where we are using sample data to make inferences concerning populations.

Quantitative research in the health sciences mostly involves working with samples drawn from populations. In order to generalize our findings, we must draw generalizations and inferences from sample statistics (e.g. $\overline{X}$, s) to the population parameters (e.g. μ, σ). Inferences are always probabilistic, because even with random samples there is always the chance of sampling error. The finite probability of sampling error implies that the differences or patterns identified in our sample data could represent random variations or chance patterns rather than 'real' ones which are true for the population as a whole.

As an illustration, imagine that we have collected data in a study aimed at identifying age-related differences in the use of sedatives and tranquillizers in a given population. Our participants ($n = 200$) kept diaries over a period of one year, recording each time they had taken a sedative or tranquillizer. The research question is: Is there a difference between sedative or tranquillizer use in older and younger people? Assume that the following hypothetical data were obtained:

Sedative and tranquillizer consumption			
Age group	n	$\overline{X}$	s
20–39	100	20	5
40–59	100	30	5

Three important and interrelated questions are examined in Section 6 concerning the evidence provided by sample data such as those shown in the above table.

1. Even if we used an adequate sampling procedure (see Ch. 5), how confident are we to infer that the true population parameters (μ) are the same as, or are at least close to, $\overline{X}$? For example, is it true that the mean tranquillizer intake for the 20–39 age group is $\mu = 20$?

2. It appears that there is a large difference between the two sample means; but is this difference also true for the populations? In other words, is this difference 'real' or significant, or is it simply due to sampling error?

3. What we are inferring is that μ(older) > μ(younger). In other words, are we justified in

concluding that the mean sedative/tranquillizer intake for the older age group is greater than for the younger group in the population?

The key issue here is that we are using sample data for decisions about populations. Sampling error refers to the difference between sample statistics and the actual state of the population. We cannot eliminate sampling error even with large and well-chosen samples. Rather, we can apply the principles of inferential statistics to calculate the probability of error. We then use this information to minimize the probability of making errors when we generalize from sample statistics to population parameters.

In Chapter 19, we examine how sampling distributions are derived and used for calculating the probability of obtaining a given sample statistic. This information can be applied to the calculation of confidence intervals, which represent a range of scores which contain the true population parameter at a given level or probability.

In Chapter 20, we outline the logic of hypothesis testing, using single sample z and t tests as exemplars. Hypothesis testing is a procedure used to decide if a difference or pattern identified in our sample data is statistically significant. If the outcome of our analysis is significant, then we are in a position to conclude that the patterns or differences found in our data may be generalized to the populations from which the samples were drawn.

There are numerous statistical tests available for analysing the significance of our data. In Chapter 20, we discuss criteria for selecting an appropriate statistical test, including (i) scale of measurement used to collect the data, (ii) the number of groups being compared and (iii) the dependence or independence of measurements. We will use the χ^2 (chi-square) test to demonstrate how statistical tests are selected and used to analyse the data.

Ultimately, statistical decision making is probabilistic, i.e. has some degree of chance and uncertainty, implying that the possibility of making decision errors cannot be eliminated. Statistical decisions may be correct, or involve what are called type I and type II errors. In Chapter 21, we examine how these errors may influence our interpretation of the results in relation to the aims or hypotheses guiding our research, and we will examine how to reduce the probability of making such errors.

The key concept discussed in Chapter 21 is effect size. Effect size determines the utility, i.e. the clinical significance, of the research findings. Also in this chapter we outline the relationship between effect size and the clinical or practical significance of research findings.

The aim of qualitative data analysis is to interpret the meaning of the experiences reported by the research participants. In Chapter 22, we will discuss the basic principles of qualitative data analysis including coding, content analysis and thematic analysis.

Probability and confidence intervals

19

CHAPTER CONTENTS

Introduction 149

Probability 149

Sampling distributions 151

Sampling distribution of the mean 152

Calculating confidence intervals 154

Confidence intervals using the *t* distribution. .155

Confidence intervals in health research 157

Summary. 157

Introduction

Sample statistics (such as $\overline{X}$, s) are estimates of the actual population parameters, in this case μ, σ. Even where adequate sampling procedures are adopted, there is no guarantee that the sample statistics are exactly the same as the true parameters of the population from which the samples were drawn. Therefore, inferences from sample statistics to population parameters necessarily involve the possibility of sampling error. As stated in Chapter 5, sampling errors represent the discrepancy between sample statistics (i.e. the results we obtain in a study sample) and true population parameters (i.e. what we would obtain if we accurately studied the whole population). Given that investigators usually have no knowledge of the true population parameters (because they are unable to study the entire population), inferential statistics are employed to estimate the probable sampling errors when using statistical data based on a study sample. While sampling error

cannot be completely eliminated, the probable size of sampling error can be calculated using *inferential statistics*. In this way investigators are in a position to calculate the probability of being accurate in their estimations of the actual population parameters.

The aims of this chapter are to examine how probability theory is applied to generating sampling distributions and how sampling distributions are used for estimating population parameters. Sampling distributions are used to estimate sampling error. This statistic is then used to calculate confidence intervals as well as testing hypotheses (see Ch. 20).

The specific aims of this chapter are to:

1. Define probability.
2. Demonstrate how sampling distributions are generated.
3. Show how sampling distributions of the mean are used to calculate the probability of a sample mean.
4. Explain how confidence intervals are calculated for continuous data.
5. Distinguish between *z* and *t* distributions.

Probability

The concept of probability is central to the understanding of inferential statistics. Probability is expressed as a proportion between 0 and 1, where 0 means an event is certain not to occur, and 1 means an event is certain to occur. Therefore if the probability (p) is 0.01 for an event then it is unlikely to occur (chance is 1 in 100). If $p = 0.99$

then the event is highly likely to occur (chance is 99 in 100). The probability of any event (say event A) occurring is given by the formula:

$$p(A) = \frac{\text{number of occurrences of A}}{\text{total number of possible occurrences}}$$

Sometimes the probability of an event can be calculated a priori (before the event) by reasoning alone. For example, we can predict that the probability of throwing a head (H) with a fair coin is:

$$p(H) = \frac{\text{number of occurrences of H}}{\text{total number of possible occurrences}}$$

$$= \frac{H}{H + T(\text{tails})} = \frac{1}{2} = 0.5$$

Or, if we buy a lottery ticket in a draw where there are 100 000 tickets, the probability of winning first prize is:

$$p(\text{1st prize}) = \frac{1}{100\ 000} = 0.00001$$

In some situations, there are no theoretical grounds for calculating the occurrence of an event (a priori). For instance, how can we calculate the probability of an individual dying of a specific condition? In such instances, we use previously obtained evidence to calculate probabilities a posteriori (after the event).

For example, if we have information for the mortality rates of a community (Table 19.1) we are in a position to calculate the probability of a selected individual over 65 years of age dying of any of the specified causes. For example, the probability of a given individual dying of coronary heart disease is:

$p(\text{dying of heart disease})$

$$= \frac{\text{\% of cases dying of heart disease}}{100\%}$$

$$= \frac{50\%}{100\%} = 0.5$$

Also, we can use the normal curve model, as outlined in Chapter 17, to determine the proportion or percentage of cases up to, or between, any specified scores. In this instance, probability is defined as the proportion of the total area cut off by the specified scores under the normal curve. As we discussed in Chapter 17, the greater the area under the curve, the higher the corresponding probability of selecting specified values.

Table 19.1 Causes of death for persons over 65

Cause of death	Percentage of deaths
Coronary heart disease	50
Cancer	25
Stroke	10
Accident	5
Infection	5
Other causes	5

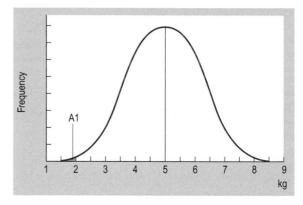

Figure 19.1 • Frequency distribution of neonate birth weights. Area A1 corresponds to $z < -2$.

For example, say that Figure 19.1 illustrates the birth weights of a large sample of neonates. Let us assume that the distribution is approximately normal, with the mean $(\overline{X})$ of 5.0 kg and a standard deviation (s) of 1.5. We can use the information to calculate the probability of any range of birth weights. Now, say that we are interested in the probability of a randomly selected neonate having a birth weight of 2.0 kg or under.

The area A1 under the curve in Figure 19.1 corresponds to the probability of obtaining a score of 2 or under. Using the principles outlined in Chapter 17 to calculate proportions or areas under the normal curve, we first translate the raw score of 2 into a z score:

$$z = \frac{x - \overline{X}}{s} = \frac{2 - 5}{1.5} = -2$$

Now we look up the area under the normal curve corresponding to $z = -2$ (Appendix A). Here we find that A1 is 0.0228. This area corresponds to a probability, and we can say that 'The probability of a neonate having a birth weight of 2 kg or less is 0.0228'. Another way of stating this outcome is that the chances are approximately 2 in 100, or 2%, for a child having such a birth weight.

We can also use the normal curve model to calculate the probability of selecting scores between any given values of a normally distributed continuous variable. For example, if we are interested in the probability of birth weights being between 6 and 8 kg, then this can be represented on the normal curve (area A2 on Fig. 19.2). To determine this area, we proceed as outlined in Chapter 15. Let $s = 1.5$.

$$z_1 = \frac{6-5}{1.5} = 0.67$$

$$z_2 = \frac{8-5}{1.5} = 2.0$$

Therefore the area between z_1 and $\overline{X}$ is 0.2486 (from Appendix A) and the area between z_2 and $\overline{X}$ is 0.4772 (from Appendix A). Therefore, the required area A2 is:

$$A2 = 0.4772 - 0.2486 = 0.2286$$

It can be concluded that the probability of a randomly selected child having a birth weight between 6 and 8 kg is $p = 0.2286$. Another way of saying this is that there is a 23 in 100, or a 23%, chance that the birth weight will be between 6 and 8 kg.

The above examples demonstrate that, when the mean and standard deviation are known for a normally distributed continuous variable, this information can be applied to calculating the probability of events related to this distribution. Of course, probabilities can be calculated for other than normal data but this requires integral calculus which is beyond the scope of this text. In general, regardless of the shape or scaling of a distribution, scores which are common or close to the average are more likely to be selected than those which are atypical located at the extreme ends of a distribution.

Sampling distributions

Probability theory can also be applied to calculate the likelihood of obtaining specific sample statistics from a specified population. These calculations are the basis for making probabilistic statistical inferences. Let us look at a hypothetical example of drawing samples for dichotomous outcomes.

Consider a container with a very large number of identically sized marbles. Imagine that there are two kinds of marbles present, black (B) and white (W), and that these colours are present in equal proportions, so that $p(B) = p(W) = 0.5$.

Given the above population, say that samples of marbles are drawn randomly and with replacement. (By 'replacement' we mean the samples are put back into the population, in order to maintain as a constant the proportion of B = W = 0.5.) If we draw samples of four (i.e. $n = 4$) then the possible proportions of black and white marbles in the samples can be deduced a priori as shown in Figure 19.3.

Ignoring the order in which marbles are chosen, Figure 19.3 demonstrates all the possible outcomes for samples of sample size $n = 4$. It is logically possible to draw any of the samples shown. However, only one of the samples (2B, 2W), is representative

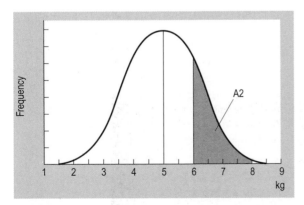

Figure 19.2 • Frequency distribution of neonate birth weights. Area A2 corresponds to probability of weight being 6–8 kg.

Possible outcomes	Number black	Number white	Proportions black
●●●●	4	0	1.00
●●●○	3	1	0.75
●●○○	2	2	0.50
●○○○	1	3	0.25
○○○○	0	4	0.00

Figure 19.3 • Characteristics of possible samples of $n = 4$, drawn from a population of black and white marbles.

of the true population parameter. The other samples would generate incorrect inferences concerning the state of the population. In general, if we know or assume (hypothesize) the true population parameters, we can generate distributions of the probability of obtaining samples of a given characteristic.

In this instance, when attempting to predict the probability of specific samples drawn from a population with two discrete elements, the binomial theorem can be applied. The expansion of the binomial expression $(P + Q)^n$ generates the probability of all the possible samples which can be drawn from a given population. The general equation for expanding the binomial expression is:

$$(P+Q)^n = P^n + \frac{n}{1}P^{n-1}Q + \frac{n(n-1)}{2}P^{n-2}Q^2 + \cdots Q^n$$

P is the probability of the first outcome, Q is the probability of the second outcome and n is the number of trials (or the sample size).

In this instance, P = proportion black (B) = 0.5, Q = proportion white (W) = 0.5, n = 4 (sample size). Therefore, substituting into the binomial expression:

$$(B+W)^4 = B^4 + 4B^3W + 6B^2W^2 + 4BW^3 + W^4$$

The following shows the composition of the samples which can be drawn from the specified population and the probability of obtaining a specific sample. For the present case:

Sample 1 $p(4B0W) = B^4$ $= (0.5)^4$ $= 0.0625$
Sample 2 $p(3B1W) = 4B^3W$ $= 4 \times (0.5)^3 (0.5) = 0.2500$
Sample 3 $p(2B2W) = 6B^2W^2$ $= 6 \times (0.5)^2(0.5)^2 = 0.3750$
Sample 4 $p(1B3W) = 4BW^3$ $= 4 \times (0.5)^3 (0.5) = 0.2500$
Sample 5 $p(0B4W) = W^4$ $= (0.5)^4$ $= 0.0625$

The calculated probabilities add up to 1, indicating that all the possible sample outcomes have been accounted for (because the probability of all possible events must equal 1.0). However, the important issue here is not so much the mathematical details but the general principle being illustrated by the example. For a given sample size (n) we can employ a mathematical formula to calculate the probability of obtaining all the possible samples from a population with known characteristics. The relationship between the possible samples and their probabilities can be graphed, as shown in Figure 19.4.

Taking the statistic 'number of black marbles in the sample', the graph in Figure 19.4 shows the

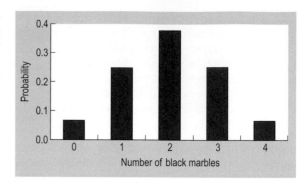

Figure 19.4 • Sampling distribution of black marbles, $n = 4$.

probability of obtaining any of the outcomes. The distribution shown is called a 'sampling distribution'. In general, a sampling distribution for a statistic indicates the probability of obtaining any of the possible values of a statistic.

Therefore, having obtained our sampling distribution we can see that some sample outcomes have low probability while others are more likely to occur. Although there is a finite chance of obtaining a sample such as 'all blacks', the probability of this happening is rather small ($p = 0.0625$). Conversely, a sample of 2B2W, which is equal to the true population proportions, is far more probable ($p = 0.375$).

The above example might be more meaningful in a health research context if we say that the black marbles represent unfavourable treatment outcomes and the white marbles successful treatment outcomes. What the example shows is that, even if there were no actual differences in the outcomes, in some extreme samples it might seem that all the patients benefited (5W) or that none had (5B). What was demonstrated is that the probability for such extreme outcomes was improbable ($p = 0.0625$). Generating sampling distributions for calculating the probability of given sample statistics is a basic practice in inferential statistics. The sampling distributions enable researchers to infer (with a determined level of confidence) the true population parameters from the sample statistics.

Sampling distribution of the mean

The binomial theorem is appropriate for generating sampling distributions for discontinuous nominal scale data. When measurements are continuous, the mean and standard deviations are appropriate as sample statistics are measured on interval or ratio scales. The sampling distribution of the mean represents the frequency distribution of sample means obtained from random samples drawn from the population. The sampling distribution of the mean enables the calculation of the probability of obtaining any given sample mean $(\overline{X})$. This is essential for testing hypotheses about sample means (see Ch. 20).

In order to generate the sampling distribution of the mean, we use a mathematical theorem called the central limit theorem. This theorem provides a set of rules which relate the parameters (μ, σ) of the population from which samples are drawn to the distribution of sample means $(\overline{X})$.

The central limit theorem states that, if random samples of a fixed n are drawn from any population, as n becomes large the distribution of sample means approaches a normal distribution, with the mean of the sample means $(\overline{X}_{\overline{x}}$ or $\mu_{\overline{x}})$ being equal to the population mean (μ) and the standard error of estimate $(s_{\overline{x}}$ or $\sigma_{\overline{x}})$ being equal to $\sigma/\sqrt{n}$. The standard error of the estimate is the standard deviation of the distribution of sample means.

Let us follow the above step by step.

1. Imagine we have a population of continuous scores or measurements with a mean of μ and a standard deviation of σ.
2. We select a very large number of random samples, each sample being of a size n.
3. Having obtained our samples, for each sample we calculate the sample mean $(\overline{X}_1, \overline{X}_2,...$ and so on).
4. Each sample mean, $\overline{X}$, is a number. The sampling distribution of the mean is a frequency distribution representing the large number of sample means.
5. The central limit theorem predicts theoretically the shape (normal for large n), mean $(\overline{X}_{\overline{x}}$ or $\mu_{\overline{x}})$ and standard deviation $(s_{\overline{x}}$ or $\sigma_{\overline{x}})$ of a large number of sample means.

It should be noted that:

1. The sampling distribution of the mean is a frequency distribution of a large number of sample means of size n drawn from a given population. When n increases, the sampling distributions approach normal.

2. The mean of the sample means $(\mu_{\overline{x}}$ or $\overline{X}_{\overline{x}})$ is the mean of the distribution of sample means. $\overline{X}_{\overline{x}}$ and $\mu_{\overline{x}}$ are equal to μ, the population mean.
3. The standard error of the mean $(s_{\overline{x}}$ or $\sigma_{\overline{x}})$ is the standard deviation of the frequency distribution of sample means drawn from a population. The magnitude of $s_{\overline{x}}$ or $\sigma_{\overline{x}}$ is equal to $\sigma/\sqrt{n}$, the population standard deviation divided by the square root of the sample size.
4. $\mu_{\overline{x}}$ and $\sigma_{\overline{x}}$ are used in reference to a sampling distribution based on all the possible samples drawn from a population (a population of samples, would you believe?), while $\overline{X}$ and $s_{\overline{x}}$ are used when the sampling distribution is based on a 'sample' of samples.

Let us have a look at an example. Assume for a hypothetical test of motor function that $\mu = 50$ and $\sigma = 10$. What is the probability of drawing a random sample from this population with $\overline{X} = 52$ or greater (i.e. $\overline{X} > 52$) given that $n = 100$? The central limit theorem predicts that, when we draw samples of $n = 100$ from the above population, the sampling distribution of the means will be as follows:

- The shape of the sampling distribution will be approximately normal.
- The mean of the sampling distribution will be equal to μ:

$$\mu_{\overline{x}} = \mu = 50$$

- The standard error of estimate $(\sigma_{\overline{x}})$ will be:

$$\sigma_{\overline{x}} = \frac{\sigma}{\sqrt{n}} = \frac{10}{\sqrt{100}} = 1$$

(We can show this as in Figure 19.5.)

Previously, we saw how we can use normal frequency distributions for estimating probabilities. Using the same principles as in Chapter 17, we can calculate the z score corresponding to $\overline{X} = 52$, and look up Appendix A to find out the area representing the probability in question:

$$z = \frac{\overline{X} - \mu_{\overline{x}}}{\sigma_{\overline{x}}} = \frac{52 - 50}{1} = 2$$

That is, $\overline{X} = 52$ is two standard error units above $\mu_{\overline{x}}$, the population mean for the sample means.

You may have noticed that the distribution of $\overline{X}$ is far less dispersed than X (i.e. the raw scores), as $\sigma_{\overline{x}} = 1$ and $\sigma = 10$.

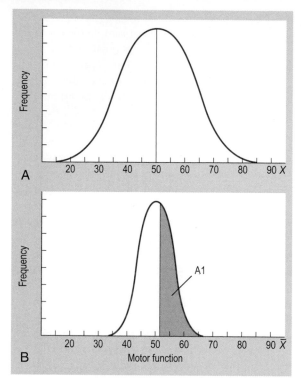

Figure 19.5 • Relationship between original population and sampling distribution of the mean, where μ = 50 and σ = 10: (A) original population; (B) sampling distribution of the mean.

Using Appendix A for establishing the probability, we find that the area representing $p(\overline{X} > 52)$, i.e. area A1 in Figure 19.5B, is:

$$p(\overline{X} > 52) = 0.5000 - 0.4772 = 0.0228$$

Therefore the probability of drawing a sample of $\overline{X} > 52$ is 0.0228. We will apply this notion to hypothesis testing in Chapter 20, but you might have noticed that it is a rather low probability. That is, it is unlikely ($p = 0.0228$) randomly to draw a sample with $\overline{X} > 52$ where $n = 100$ and $μ = 50$.

Calculating confidence intervals

Let us assume that you are asked to estimate the weight of a newborn baby. If you have experienced working with neonates, you should be able to make a reasonable guess. You might say 'The baby is 6 kg'. Someone might ask 'How certain are you that the baby is exactly 6 kg?' You might then say 'Well, the baby might not be exactly 6 kg, but I'm very confident that it weighs somewhere between 5.5 and 6.5 kg'. This statement expresses a confidence interval – a range of values that probably include the real value. Of course, the more certain or confident you want to be of including the true value, the bigger the range of values you might give: you are unlikely to be wrong if you guess that the baby weighs between 4 and 8 kg.

Confidence intervals can be calculated for a large range of statistics such as proportions, ratios or correlation coefficients. In this chapter we will look at confidence intervals for single samples as an illustration for using confidence intervals.

We have seen previously that if we know the population parameters we can estimate the probability of selecting from that population a sample mean of a given magnitude. Conversely, if we know the sample mean we can estimate the population parameters from which the sample might have come, at a given level of probability. Let us take an example to illustrate this point.

A researcher is interested in the systolic blood pressure (BP) levels of smokers of more than 10 cigarettes per day. She takes a random sample of 100 10+ smokers in her district and finds the mean BP = 148 mmHg for the sample, with a standard deviation of $s = 10$.

She wants to generalize to the population of smokers of more than 10 cigarettes per day in their district. The best estimate of μ (the population parameter) is 148, but it is possible that, because of sampling error, 148 is not the exact population parameter. However she can calculate a confidence interval (a range of blood pressures that will include the true population mean at a given level of probability). A confidence interval is a range of scores which includes the true population parameter at a specified level of probability. The precise probability is decided by the researcher and indicates how certain she can be that the population mean is actually within the calculated range. Common confidence intervals used in statistics are 95% confidence intervals, which offer a probability of $p = 0.95$ for including the true population mean, and 99% confidence intervals, which include the true population mean at a probability of $p = 0.99$.

Calculating the confidence interval requires the use of the following formula:

$$\overline{X} - zs_{\overline{x}} < \mu < \overline{X} + zs_{\overline{x}}$$

where $\overline{X}$ is the sample mean; z is the z score obtained from the normal curve table such that it cuts off the area of the normal curve corresponding to the required probability; $s_{\overline{x}}$ is the sample standard error, which is equal to the sample standard deviation divided by $\sqrt{n}$, i.e. $s_{\overline{x}} = s/\sqrt{n}$.

Let us turn to the previous example to illustrate the use of the above equation. Here $\overline{X} = 148$, and $s_{\overline{x}} = 10/\sqrt{100}$. Assume that we want to calculate a 95% confidence interval. We are looking for a pair of z scores which have 95% of the standard normal curve between them. In this case, 1.96 is the value for z which cuts off 95% of a normal distribution. That is, we looked up the value of z corresponding to an area (probability) of 0.4750, since the 0.05 has to be divided among the two tails of the distribution, giving 0.025 at either end. Substituting into the equation above we have:

$$148 - (1.96)\,(10/\sqrt{100}) \leq \mu \leq 148 + (1.96)$$
$$\times (10/\sqrt{100}) = 146.04 \leq \mu \leq 149.96$$

That is, the investigator is 95% confident that the true population mean, the true mean BP of smokers, lies between 146.04 (lower limit) and 149.96 (upper limit). There is only a 5% or 0.05 probability that it lies outside this range. If we chose a 99% confidence interval, then using the formula as above, we have:

$$148 - (2.58)\,(10/\sqrt{100}) \leq \mu \leq 148 + (2.58)$$
$$\times (10/\sqrt{100}) = 145.42 \leq \mu \leq 150.58$$

Here, 2.58 is the value of z which cuts off 99% of a normal distribution (Fig. 19.6). That is, the investigator is 99% confident that the true population mean lies somewhere between 145.42 and 150.58. Clearly, the 99% interval is wider than the 95% interval; after all, here the probability of including the true mean is greater than for the 95% interval. Conventionally, health sciences publications report 95% confidence intervals.

Confidence intervals using the *t* distribution

It was previously stated that 'as n becomes large, the distribution of sample means approaches a

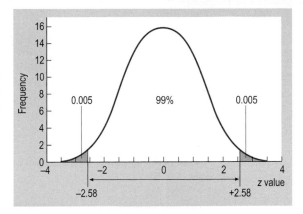

Figure 19.6 • *z* scores for 99% confidence interval.

normal distribution' (central limit theorem). The questions left to explain are:

- How large must the sample size, n, be before the sampling distribution of the mean can be considered a normal curve?
- What are the implications for the sampling distribution if n is small?

It has been shown by mathematicians that the sample size, n, for which the sampling distribution of the mean can be considered an approximation of a normal distribution is $n > 30$. That is, if n is 30 or more, we can use the standard normal curve to describe the sampling distribution of the mean. However, when $n < 30$, the sampling distribution of the mean is a rather rough approximation to the normal distribution. Instead of using the normal distribution, we use the *t distribution*, which takes into account the variability of the shape of the sampling distribution due to low n.

The *t* distribution (Fig. 19.7) is a family of curves representing the sampling distributions of means drawn from a population when sample size, n, is small ($n < 30$). A 'family of curves' means that the shape of the *t* distribution varies with sample size. It has been found that the distribution is determined by the *degrees of freedom* of the statistic.

The degrees of freedom (df) for a statistic represents the number of scores which are free to vary when calculating the statistic. Since the statistic we are calculating in this case is the mean, all but one of the scores could vary. That is, if you were inventing scores in a sample with a known mean, you would have a free hand until the very last score. There df is equal to $n - 1$ (the sample size

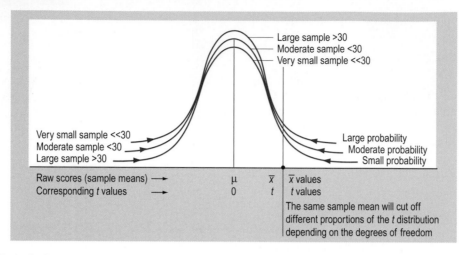

Figure 19.7 • *t* distributions.

minus one). Each row of figures shown in Appendix B represents the critical values of *t* for a given distribution.

1. The *t* distribution is symmetrical about the mean.

2. The values of *t* along the x-axis cut off specific areas under the curve, just as for *z*. These areas are given at the top of the page in Appendix B, under 'Directional' and 'Non-directional' probabilities.

3. The *t* distribution approaches a normal distribution as *n* becomes larger. As stated earlier, when *n* >30, for all practical purposes the *t* and *z* distributions coincide.

The *t* distribution, just as the *z* distribution, can be used to approximate the probability of drawing sample means of a given magnitude from a population; *t* can also be used for calculating confidence intervals. Let us re-examine the example relating to the blood pressure of smokers presented earlier. Let us assume that *n* = 25, with the other statistics remaining the same: $\overline{X} = 148$, *s* = 10. The general formula for calculating the confidence intervals for small samples is:

$$\overline{X} - ts_{\overline{x}} < \mu \; \overline{X} + ts_{\overline{x}}$$

You will note the similarity to the equation on p. 155; here *t* replaces *z*. If we want to show the 95% confidence interval, then we use the same logic as for *z* distributions (Fig. 19.8).

To look up the *t* values from the tables (Appendix B) consider (i) direction, (ii) probabilities and (iii) degrees of freedom (df).

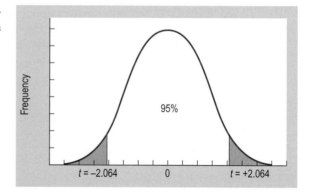

Figure 19.8 • The 95% confidence interval for sample size of 25.

We are looking at a 'non-directional' or 'two-tail' probability in the sense that the *t* values cut off 95% of the area of the *t* curve between them, leaving 5% distributed at the two tails of the *t* distribution: $p = 0.05$; df = 25 − 1 = 24. Therefore *t* = 2.064 (from Appendix B). Substituting into the equation for calculating confidence intervals:

$$148 - (2.1)\,(10/\sqrt{25}) \le \mu \le 148 + (2.1)\,(10/\sqrt{25})$$
$$148 - 4.2 \le \mu \le 148 + 4.2$$
$$143.8 \le \mu \le 152.2$$

Consider the width of the confidence interval defined as the distance between the upper and lower limits. Note that this is a wider interval than that which was obtained when *n* was 100. As

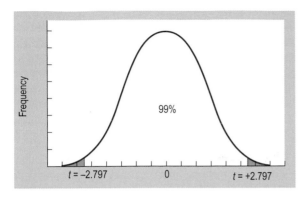

Figure 19.9 • The 99% confidence interval for sample size of 25.

sample size, n, becomes smaller, our confidence interval becomes wider, reflecting a greater probability of sampling error.

To calculate the 99% confidence interval (Fig. 19.9) we need to look up $p = 0.01$, non-directional, df = 24 in Appendix B to obtain the critical value of t, which is 2.797.

$$148 - (2.8)(10/\sqrt{25}) \leq \mu \leq 148 + (2.8)(10/\sqrt{25})$$
$$142.4 \leq \mu \leq 153.6$$

We can see that, when $n = 25$, the 99% confidence interval is wider than for $n = 100$. That is, the bigger our sample size, the narrower (more precise) our estimate of the range of values (which includes the true population parameter) becomes when our sample size is large.

Confidence intervals in health research

Confidence intervals can be calculated for all statistics obtained from sample data. For example, we can work out confidence intervals for proportions, percentages, odds ratios and other measures of effect size, as discussed in Chapter 15. In all these cases, the confidence interval represents an interval that includes at a given probability the true population value or parameter. To calculate the confidence interval we need to know the sampling distribution appropriate for the statistic and use this distribution to calculate the probable upper and lower values of the confidence interval. In general we use a 95% confidence interval which researchers abbreviate as 95% CI.

As an example, consider the study by Mostofsky et al (2010) which investigated the association between alcohol consumption and the relative risk of stroke. The authors found that the risk of stroke one hour after consuming alcohol was 2.3 (95% CI, 1.4 to 4.0; $p = 0.002$). These statistics indicate that:

1. The risk of stroke in those in the sample who consumed alcohol was 2.3 times the risk of stroke in those who did not have a drink.
2. We can be 95% confident that the population risk of consuming alcohol is between 1.4 and 4.0. In other words, the true value could be as little as 1.4 or as high as 4.0 times the risk for those who drink.
3. The value $p = 0.002$ represents the probability that the risk found in the sample is due to chance. In this case this probability is very small and the results are statistically significant, as we will discuss in Chapter 20.

Confidence intervals are of particular importance in evidence-based practice. The researcher or practitioner is able to see the range of values which contain the true value at a given level of probability, usually 95%. There are numerous websites available which you may want to consult for further information regarding the use and calculation of confidence intervals. This interval estimation is essential for determining the impact of a risk factor on health or the efficacy of a particular intervention. In general, a small sample size combined with highly variable results produces a wide confidence interval. Wide confidence intervals are undesirable in health research and practice because we are unable to be certain where the true population parameter lies. For example, if we say the percentage of patients improving following a treatment is 50% with a 95% CI of 25% to 75%, then we are very doubtful about the expected outcome. On the other hand, if we could say 50% with a 95% CI of 48% to 52% then we could be sure about the true benefit of the treatment. The narrower the 95% CI, the more accurate the inferences regarding actual population parameters.

Summary

It was argued in this chapter that, even with randomly selected samples, the possibility of sampling error must be taken into account when making inferences from sample statistics to population parameters. It was shown that probability theory can be applied to generating sampling distributions, which express the probability of obtaining a given sample from a population. With discontinuous, nominal data the binomial theorem provides a mathematical distribution for estimating the probability of obtaining possible samples. However, with continuous data, the central limit theorem is applied to generate the sampling distributions of the mean. The standard distribution of the mean enables the calculation of the probability-specified sample mean(s) by random selection. The sampling error of the mean ($s_{\bar{x}}$ or $\sigma_{\bar{x}}$), which expresses statistically the range of the sampling error, depends inversely on the sample size, such that the larger the n, the smaller the $s_{\bar{x}}$ or $\sigma_{\bar{x}}$.

One of the applications of sampling distributions is for calculating confidence intervals for continuous data. Confidence intervals represent a range of scores which specify, from sample data, the probability of capturing the true population parameters. Confidence intervals are essential statistics for the conduct of health research and evidence-based health care.

Health researchers usually report 95% confidence intervals. When sample sizes are small ($n < 30$), the t distribution is appropriate for calculating the sampling distribution of the mean. With large sample sizes, the two distributions merge together. As the next chapter will demonstrate, sampling distributions are essential for testing hypotheses, a procedure which uses inferential statistics to calculate the level of probability at which sample statistics support the predictions of hypotheses.

Hypothesis testing: selection and use of statistical tests

20

CHAPTER CONTENTS

Introduction 159
The logic of hypothesis testing 159
Steps in hypothesis testing 160
Illustrations of hypothesis testing 160
The relationship between descriptive and inferential statistics 162
Selection of the appropriate inferential test . . 163
The χ^2 test 164
χ^2 and contingency tables 165
Statistical packages 167
Summary 169

Introduction

Hypotheses are statements about the association between variables as pertaining to a specific person or population. For example, 'penicillin is an effective treatment for pneumonia' or 'obesity is a risk factor for heart disease'. Hypotheses addressing the state of populations are tested using sample data. Inferences are conclusions based on data using samples and are therefore always open to the possibility of error. In this chapter we will examine the use of inferential statistics for establishing the probable truth of hypotheses, as tested through sample data. Inferential statistics are based on applied probability theory and entail the use of statistical tests.

There are numerous statistical tests available that are used in a similar fashion to analyse clinical data. That is, all statistical tests involve setting up the relevant hypotheses, H_0 and H_A, and then, on the basis of the appropriate inferential statistics, computing the probability of the sample statistics obtained occurring by chance alone. We are not going to attempt to examine all statistical tests in this introductory book. These are described in various statistics textbooks or in data analysis manuals. Rather, in this chapter we will examine the criteria used for selecting tests appropriate for the analysis of the data obtained in specific investigations. To illustrate the use of statistical tests we will examine the use of the chi-square test (χ^2). This is a statistical test commonly employed to analyse categorical data. Finally, we will briefly examine the uses of the Statistical Package for Social Sciences™ (SPSS) for data analysis in general.

The aims of this chapter are to:

1. Discuss the criteria by which a statistical test is selected for analysing the data for a specific study.
2. Demonstrate the use of the χ^2 test for analysing nominal scale data.
3. Explain how statistical packages are used for quantitative data analysis.

The logic of hypothesis testing

Hypothesis testing is the process of deciding using statistics whether the findings of an investigation reflect chance or real effects at a given level of probability or certainty. If the results seem to not represent chance effects, then we say that the results are statistically significant. That is, when we say that our results are statistically significant we mean that the patterns or differences seen in the sample data are likely to be generalizable to the wider population from our study sample.

The mathematical procedures for hypothesis testing are based on the application of probability theory and sampling, as discussed previously. Because of the probabilistic nature of the process, decision errors in hypothesis testing cannot be entirely eliminated. However, the procedures outlined in this chapter enable us to specify the probability level at which we can claim that the data obtained in an investigation support experimental hypotheses. This procedure is fundamental for determining the statistical significance of the data as well as being relevant to the logic of clinical decision making.

Steps in hypothesis testing

The following steps are conventionally followed in hypothesis testing:

1. State the alternative hypothesis (H_A), which is the based on the research hypothesis. The H_A asserts that the results are 'real' or 'significant', i.e. that the independent variable influenced the dependent variable, or that there is a real difference among groups. The important point here is that H_A is a statement concerning the population. A real or significant effect means that the results in the sample data can be generalized to the population.

2. State the null hypothesis (H_0), which is the logical opposite of the H_A. The H_0 claims that any differences in the data were just due to chance: that the independent variable had no effect on the dependent variable, or that any difference among groups is due to random effects. In other words, if the H_0 is retained, differences or patterns seen in the sample data should not be generalized to the population.

3. Set the decision level, α (alpha). There are two mutually exclusive hypotheses (H_A and H_0) competing to explain the results of an investigation. Hypothesis testing, or statistical decision making, involves establishing the probability of H_0 being true. If this probability is very small, we are in a position to reject the H_0. You might

ask 'How small should the probability (α) be for rejecting H_0?' By convention, we use the probability of $\alpha = 0.05$. If the H_0 being true is less than 0.05, we can reject H_0. We can choose an α of 0.05, but not more, That is, by convention among researchers, results are not characterized as significant if $p > 0.05$.

4. Calculate the probability of H_0 being true. That is, we assume that H_0 is true and calculate the probability of the outcome of the investigation being due to chance alone, i.e. due to random effects. We must use an appropriate sampling distribution for this calculation.

5. Make a decision concerning H_0. The following decision rule is used. If the probability of H_0 being true is less than α, then we reject H_0 at the level of significance set by α. However, if the probability of H_0 is greater than α, then we must retain H_0. In other words, if:

   a. $p(H_0$ is true$) \leq \alpha$, reject H_0
   b. $p(H_0$ is true$) > \alpha$, retain H_0

   It follows that if we reject H_0 we are in a position to accept H_A, its logical alternative. If $p \leq 0.05$ then we reject H_0, and decide that H_A is probably true.

Illustrations of hypothesis testing

One of the simplest forms of gambling is betting on the fall of a coin. Let us play a little game. We, the authors, will toss a coin. If it comes out heads (H) you will give us £1; if it comes out tails (T) we will give you £1. To make things interesting, let us have 10 tosses. The results are:

Toss	1	2	3	4	5	6	7	8	9	10
Outcome	H	H	H	H	H	H	H	H	H	H

Oh dear, you seem to have lost. Never mind, we were just lucky, so send along your cheque for £10. Are you a little hesitant? Are you saying that we 'fixed' the game? There is a systematic procedure for demonstrating the probable truth of your allegations:

1. We can state two competing hypotheses concerning the outcome of the game:

   a. the authors fixed the game; that is, the outcome did not reflect the fair throwing of a coin. Let us call this statement the 'alternative hypothesis', H_A. In effect, the H_A claims that the sample of 10 heads came from a population other than P (probability of heads) = Q (probability of tails) = 0.5

b. the authors did not fix the game; that is, the outcome is due to the tossing of a fair coin. Let us call this statement the 'null hypothesis', or H_0. H_0 suggests that the sample of 10 heads was a random sample from a population where $P = Q = 0.5$.

2. It can be shown that the probability of tossing 10 consecutive heads with a fair coin is actually $p = 0.001$, as discussed previously (see Ch. 19). That is, the probability of obtaining such a sample from a population where $P = Q = 0.5$ is extremely low.

3. Now we can decide between H_0 and H_A. It was shown that the probability of H_0 being true was $p = 0.001$ (1 in a 1000). Therefore, in the balance of probabilities, we can reject it as being true and accept H_A, which is the logical alternative. In other words, it is likely that the game was fixed and no £10 cheque needed to be posted.

The probability of calculating the truth of H_0 depended on the number of tosses (n = the sample size). For instance, the probability of obtaining heads every times with five coin tosses is shown in Table 19.4. As the sample size (n) becomes larger, the probability for which it is possible to reject H_0 becomes smaller. With only a few tosses we really cannot be sure if the game is fixed or not: without sufficient information it becomes hard to reject H_0 at a reasonable level of probability.

A question emerges: 'What is a reasonable level of probability for rejecting H_0?' As we shall see, there are conventions for specifying these probabilities. One way to proceed, however, is to set the appropriate probability for rejecting H_0 on the basis of the implications of erroneous decisions.

Obviously, any decision made on a probabilistic basis might be in error. Two types of decision errors are identified in statistics as *type I* and *type II errors*. A type I error involves mistakenly rejecting H_0, while a type II error involves mistakenly retaining the H_0. Researchers can make mistakes about the truth or falsity of hypotheses using sample research data. Statistical method does not provide a guarantee against making a mistake, but it is the most rigorous way of making these decisions.

In the above example, a type I error would involve deciding that the outcome was not due to

chance when in fact it was. The practical outcome of this would be to falsely accuse the authors of fixing the game. A type II error would represent the decision that the outcome was due to chance, when in fact it was due to a 'fix'. The practical outcome of this would be to send your hard-earned £10 to a couple of crooks. Clearly, in a situation like this, a type II error would be more odious than a type I error, and you would set a fairly high probability for rejecting H_0. However, if you were gambling with a villain, who had a loaded revolver handy, you would tend to set a very low probability for rejecting H_0. We will examine these ideas more formally in subsequent parts of this chapter.

Let us look at another example. A rehabilitation therapist has devised an exercise program which is expected to reduce the time taken for people to leave hospital following orthopaedic surgery. Previous records show that the recovery time for patients had been $\mu = 30$ days, with $\sigma = 8$ days. A sample of 64 patients were treated with the exercise program, and their mean recovery time was found to be $\bar{X} = 24$ days. Do these results show that patients who had the treatment recovered significantly faster than previous patients? We can apply the steps for hypothesis testing to make our decision.

1. State H_A: 'The exercise program reduces the time taken for patients to recover from orthopaedic surgery'. That is, the researcher claims that the independent variable (the treatment) has a 'real' or 'generalizable' effect on the dependent variable (time to recover).

2. State H_0: 'The exercise program does not reduce the time taken for patients to recover from orthopaedic surgery'. That is, the statement claims that the independent variable has no effect on the dependent variable. The statement implies that the treated sample with $\bar{X} = 24$, and $n = 64$ is in fact a random sample from the population $\mu = 30$, $\sigma = 8$. Any difference between $\bar{X}$ and μ can be attributed to sampling error.

3. The decision level, α, is set before the results are analysed. The probability of α depends on how certain the investigator wants to be that the results show real differences. If he set $\alpha = 0.01$, then the probability of falsely rejecting a true H_0 is less than or equal to 0.01 (1/100). If he set $\alpha = 0.05$, then the probability of falsely rejecting a true H_0 is less than or equal to 0.05 or (1/20). That is, the smaller the α, the more confident the researcher is that the results support the alternative hypothesis. We also call α the level of significance. The smaller the α, the more significant the findings for a study, if we can reject H_0. In this case, say that the researcher sets α = 0.01. (Note: by convention, α should not be greater than 0.05.)

4. Calculate the probability of H_0 being true. As stated above, H_0 implies that the sample with $\bar{X} = 24$ is a random sample from the population with μ = 30, σ = 8. How probable is it that this statement is true? To calculate this probability, we must generate an appropriate sampling distribution. As we have seen in Chapter 17, the sampling distribution of the mean will enable us to calculate the probability of obtaining a sample mean of $\bar{X} = 24$ or more extreme from a population with known parameters. As shown in Figure 20.1, we can calculate the probability of drawing a sample mean of $\bar{X}$ = 24 or less. Using the table of normal curves (Appendix A), as outlined previously, we find that the probability of randomly selecting a sample mean of $\bar{X} = 24$ (or less) is extremely small. In terms of our table, which only shows the exact probability of up to z = 4.00, we can see that the present probability is less than 0.00003. Therefore, the probability that H_0 is true is less than 0.00003.

5. Make a decision. We have set α = 0.01. The calculated probability was less than 0.0001. Clearly, the calculated probability is far less than α, indicating that the difference is unlikely to be due to chance. Therefore, the investigator can reject the statement that H_0 is true and

accept H_A, that patients in general treated with the exercise program recover earlier than the population of untreated patients.

The relationship between descriptive and inferential statistics

As we have seen in the previous chapters, statistics may be classified as descriptive or inferential. Descriptive statistics describe the characteristics of data and are concerned with issues such as 'What is the average length of hospitalization of a group of patients?' Inferential statistics are used to address issues such as whether the differences in average lengths of hospitalization of patients in two groups are significantly different statistically. Thus, descriptive statistics describe aspects of the data such as the frequencies of scores, and the average or the range of values for samples, whereas inferential statistics enables researchers to decide (infer) whether differences between groups or relationships between variables represent persistent and reproducible trends in the populations.

In Section 5 we saw that the selection of appropriate descriptive statistics depends on the type of data being described. For example, in a variable such as incomes of patients, the best statistics to represent the typical income would be the mean and/or the median. If you had a millionaire in the group of patients, the mean statistic might give a distorted impression of the central tendency. In this situation the median statistic would be the most appropriate one to use. The mode is most commonly used when the data being described are categorical data. For example, if in a questionnaire respondents were asked to indicate their sex and 65% said they were male and 35% said they were female, then 'male' is the modal response. It is quite unusual to use the mode only with data that are not nominal. As a rule, the scale of measurement used to obtain the data and its distribution determine which descriptive statistics are selected.

In the same way, the appropriate inferential statistics are determined by the characteristics of the data being analysed. For example, where the mean is the appropriate descriptive statistic, the inferential statistics will determine if the differences between the means are statistically significant. In the case of ordinal data, the appropriate inferential

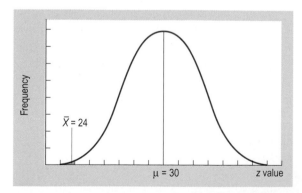

Figure 20.1 • Sampling distribution of means. Sample size = 64, population mean = 30, standard deviation = 8.

statistics will make it possible to decide if either the medians or the rank orders are significantly different. With nominal data, the appropriate inferential statistic will decide if proportions of cases falling into specific categories are significantly different.

Thus, when the data have been adequately described, the appropriate inferential statistic will follow logically. However, when selecting an appropriate statistical test, the design of the investigation must also be taken into account.

Selection of the appropriate inferential test

Before addressing the issue of the selection of the appropriate inferential statistical test, it is useful to reiterate the reason why a statistical test should be employed in research.

In some studies, inferential statistical tests are not required. For example, if a health care needs-assessment survey is conducted in a particular community, using a full population, the investigator might not be overly concerned with generalizing the results to other communities, or demonstrating that certain relationships between variables are reliable. It may be enough to be able to say, for example, that '35% of the respondents indicated that they were dissatisfied with the existing level of medical services'. In this instance, descriptive statistics are all that the investigator requires to do the job since the complete population was studied. If, however, the investigator wishes to argue that certain differences between groups or certain correlations between variables for a sample are generalizable to the population, then inferential statistical tests are necessary.

The inferential statistic provides the investigator with a means of determining how reproducible the obtained results are, by enabling access to a probability. The probability associated with the value of an inferential statistic informs the investigator of the likelihood that the results obtained were due to chance factors, or if they are significant at a given level of probability.

As noted earlier, we are not going to examine all of the numerous statistical tests available for decision making. Rather, the aim of this chapter is to examine the criteria used for selecting tests appropriate for the analysis of data obtained in investigations. To illustrate the use of statistical tests we will look at the χ^2 test, commonly employed for analysing nominal data. We examine the interpretation of findings that do not reach statistical significance and the relationship between statistical and clinical significance. In Chapter 21 we will consider some of the determinants of making decisions concerning the actual adoption and use of treatments and diagnostic tests in clinical settings.

There are a variety of statistical tests, some of which are named in Table 20.1. The selection of the appropriate statistical test is determined by the following considerations:

1. The scale of measurement used to obtain the data (nominal, ordinal, interval, or ratio).
2. The number of groups used in an investigation (one or more).
3. Whether the measurements were obtained from independent participants or from related samples, such as those involving repeated measurements of the same participants.
4. The assumptions involved in using a statistical test, such as the distribution of the scores or the minimum required sample size.

Table 20.1 shows a number of statistical tests in order to illustrate how statistical tests are selected for analysing data. Several points are worth noting.

Table 20.1 Selection of tests of significance

Scale	Two groups		Three or more groups	
	Independent	Dependent	Independent	Dependent
Nominal	χ^2 test	McNemar's test	χ^2 test	Cochran's Q test
Ordinal	Mann–Whitney U test	Sign test	Kruskal–Wallis H test	Friedman two-way analysis of variance
Interval or ratio	t test (independent groups)	t test (dependent groups)	ANOVA (F) (independent groups)	ANOVA (F) (dependent groups)

1. It can be seen that appropriate tests are selected on the basis of the four criteria outlined above. When we have determined these four criteria for a given investigation, the 'cell' containing the appropriate test can be readily selected. Although not shown in Table 20.1, there are instances when there are a number of statistical tests available in a particular cell. Here we need additional criteria for deciding between two tests within a cell. For instance, we saw in the previous section that, if $n < 30$, we use the t test rather than the z test.

2. The tests appropriate for analysing ordinal and nominal data are non-parametric, or distribution-free. The tests for analysing interval or ratio data are called parametric tests. The parametric tests (e.g. z, t or F) require that certain assumptions (such as normality and equal variance) be valid for the populations from which the samples were drawn. The non-parametric tests (e.g. χ^2, Mann–Whitney U) require few, if any, assumptions about the underlying population distributions.

3. Even before the data are collected, an investigator should have a good idea of which statistical test is appropriate for analysing the data. Sometimes, however, the distribution of the data is such that the test that was initially selected is found to be inappropriate.

Let us look at some examples to illustrate how statistical tests are selected.

An investigator wishes to evaluate the effectiveness of a new treatment in contrast to a conventionally used treatment. Assume that the outcome (dependent variable) is measured on a five-point ordinal scale. Each participant is assigned to one of the two treatment groups. Which test would the investigator use to analyse the significance of sample data when:

1. The measurement was ordinal?
2. There were two groups (new treatment, conventional treatment)?
3. Participants were independently assigned to a specific group?

By inspection of Table 20.1 the investigator would select the Mann–Whitney U test to analyse the significance of the data.

If we change the above example by stating that the dependent variable was measured on an interval scale, the appropriate test would now be a t test (for independent groups). Let us say that three groups were used (by the inclusion of a placebo group) by the investigator. Now, if the outcome measurement remained ordinal, the appropriate test for analysing the data is the Kruskal–Wallis H test. If, however, the outcome measures were interval, it follows from Table 20.1 that the appropriate test for analysing the results would be the ANOVA (analysis of variance).

Finally, say that in the original example each of the participants was treated with both the new and old treatments. Now, the data would have been obtained from the repeated measurement of the same participants, and the appropriate statistical test would be the Sign test (ordinal, two groups, dependent).

Table 20.1 does not include all the available statistical tests and their uses. In fact, mathematical statisticians can generate inferential tests appropriate for a whole variety of designs. The basic idea is to use probability theory to generate appropriate sampling distributions in terms of whether the probability of H_0 being true can be calculated, and the statistical significance of the findings evaluated (Schwartz & Polgar 2003).

Rather than examining all the tests and their underlying assumptions, we will look at the use of the χ^2 test in some detail. As well as being a very useful test for analysing nominal data, it (along with the z and t) illustrates how statistical tests are carried out to test hypotheses.

The χ^2 test

As shown in Table 20.1, χ^2 (chi-square) is appropriate for statistical analysis when:

- Variables are measured on a nominal scale.
- Measurements are of independent participants.

The χ^2 test is appropriate for deciding if proportions of cases falling into categories are different at a given level of significance.

The statistic, χ^2, is given by the formula:

$$\chi^2 = \sum \frac{(f_o - f_e)^2}{f_e}$$

where f_o = observed frequency for a given category and f_e = expected frequency for a given category, assuming H_0 was true.

The sampling distribution for χ^2 is a family of curves, which, like t, vary with degrees of freedom. The use of this inferential statistic is best illustrated by an example.

Suppose that an investigator is interested in finding out whether there is a difference in the

Table 20.2 Treatments offered

Psychotherapy	Drugs	Electroconvulsive therapy
$n = 45$	$n = 40$	$n = 65$

Table 20.3 Treatments (f_e is shown in parentheses)

Psychotherapy	Drugs	Electroconvulsive therapy
45	40	65
(50)	(50)	(50)

relative frequency of different kinds of treatments currently offered to extremely depressed patients. A random sample of 150 patients is selected from a population of patients in Australia, and the type of treatment offered to them is determined from their medical records, as shown in Table 20.2.

The entries in each cell represent the frequency with which patients were given the various treatments. Thus, 45 patients were offered psychotherapy, 40 patients offered drugs and 65 patients offered electroconvulsive therapy. The χ^2 is the appropriate test for analysing these data. Let us follow the steps involved in hypothesis testing, as outlined previously.

1. H_A: there is a difference in the population proportions for the three treatments. H_A is nondirectional when we use χ^2.

2. H_0: there is no difference in the population proportions of the three treatments. The frequencies shown in each cell in the table occurred through random sampling from a population where there is an equal frequency of the three treatments.

3. Decision level, α: say the investigator sets a significance level of 0.05 for rejecting H_A ($\alpha = 0.05$).

4. Calculation of the statistic: χ^2_{obt} is the value of χ^2 calculated from the data obtained. To calculate χ^2_{obt}, we must determine f_e for each cell (f_o is, of course, determined by the data). If the null hypothesis (H_0) is true, then our expectation is that the frequencies in each cell should be the same. In this case, $n = 150$, so that f_e should be $150/3 = 50$, given that there are three cells. Let us show this in tabular form (Table 20.3). We can now calculate χ^2_{obt}, by calculating $(f_o - f_e)^2/f_e$ for each cell, and then summing the values.

$$\chi^2_{obt} = \sum \frac{(f_o - f_e)^2}{f_e}$$
$$= \frac{(45 - 50)^2}{50} + \frac{(40 - 50)^2}{50} + \frac{(65 - 50)^2}{50}$$
$$= 0.5 + 2.0 + 4.5$$
$$= 7.0$$

The greater the discrepancy between f_e and f_o, the greater the calculated value of the chi-square statistic (χ^2_{obt}). The direction of the difference is of no significance as the difference between f_e and f_o is squared.

5. Making decisions concerning H_0: the decision rule for χ^2 is similar to that of the z and t tests, as shown in the previous chapter:

$$\chi^2_{obt} \geq \chi^2_{crit}, \text{ reject } H_0$$
$$\chi^2_{obt} < \chi^2_{crit}, \text{ retain } H_0$$

Here, χ^2_{crit} is the critical value of the statistic χ^2, which cuts off a proportion of the sampling distribution equal to α. The value of χ^2_{crit} is obtained from the tables in Appendix C. To look up this statistic, we need to know:

  a. α, which was set at 0.05 for this example
  b. the degrees of freedom, df.

Note that with χ^2 the degrees of freedom with one variable is $k - 1$, where k stands for the number of categories or groups. In this instance, we have $k = 3$ (three treatments) so that df $= 3 - 1 = 2$. Now we can look up the tables in Appendix C. In this case, $\alpha = 0.05$ and df $= 2$, therefore $\chi^2_{crit} = 5.99$.

Here, since $\chi^2_{obt} > \chi^2_{crit}$ we can reject H_0 at a 0.05 level of significance. The investigator is in a position to accept H_A (that the three treatments are offered at different frequencies to depressed patients). Clearly, electroconvulsive therapy is given most frequently for the condition (in this hypothetical example).

χ^2 and contingency tables

In the previous example of χ^2 we had clear expectations of the expected frequencies (f_e) and were dealing with only one variable. The χ^2 test is also relevant for analysing nominal data where f_e is not known, and where we are interested in the effects of more than one variable. Thus, χ^2 is a statistical test appropriate for deciding whether two variables are significantly related.

For example, an investigator compares the effectiveness of drug therapy with coronary artery surgery in males 55–60 years old, suffering from coronary heart disease. A sample of 40 patients consenting to the investigation is selected from this population, and randomly divided into the two treatment groups (drugs only or coronary artery surgery). The treatment outcome is measured in terms of survival over 5 years. The outcome of this hypothetical study is shown in Table 20.4.

Table 20.4 is called a contingency table. A contingency table is a two-way table showing the relationship between two or more variables. Note that the levels of the variables have been classified into mutually exclusive categories ('drugs or surgery' for the independent variable, and 'dead or alive' for the dependent variable, in this instance). The cells in the contingency table show the frequency of cases falling into each joint category (for example, 11 people in the 'drugs only' category had died during the 5 years). The row and column marginal scores are the sums of the frequencies. The row and column marginals necessarily add up to n, the sample size ($n = 40$ for this example).

Table 20.4 is called a two-by-two (2×2) contingency table. Depending on the number of categories (or levels) in each of the two variables, we might have 3×2 tables, 3×3 tables, etc. Let us now turn to analysing the data.

1. H_A: there is a difference in the proportion of patients surviving for 5 years following the two types of treatment.
2. H_0: there is no difference in the frequency of survival rates; any difference between observed and expected frequencies in the sample is due to chance.
3. Decision level: $\alpha = 0.05$.
4. Calculation of the statistic χ^2_{obt}

$$\chi^2_{obt} = \sum \frac{(f_o - f_e)^2}{f_e}$$

To make our explanation of the calculation easier, let us label the cells and the marginal values, as shown in Table 20.5. We calculate χ^2_{obt} by calculating f_e for each of the cells and then substituting this value into the equation for χ^2_{obt}. In order to calculate the expected frequencies, f_e, for each of the cells, we use the formula:

$$\frac{\text{Row total} \times \text{column total}}{n}$$

Substituting into the above formula for each of the cells:

$$A: f_e = \frac{j \times l}{n} \qquad B: f_e = \frac{j \times m}{n}$$

$$C: f_e = \frac{k \times l}{n} \qquad D: f_e = \frac{k \times m}{n}$$

Now f_o are the observed frequencies as in the data, summarized in contingency Table 20.5. Substituting the values for f_e and f_o for each cell is shown in Table 20.6.

5. Making decisions concerning H_0: the degrees of freedom for a contingency table are calculated by the following formula:

$$df = (r-1)(c-1)$$

where r = the number of rows and c = the number of columns. In this instance, given a 2×2 contingency table:

$$df = (2-1)(2-1) = 1$$

Now we can look up χ^2_{crit} for $\alpha = 0.05$ and $df = 1$. From Appendix C, $\chi^2_{crit} = 3.84$.

Table 20.5 General format for 2 × 2 contingency table

A	B	j
C	D	k
l	m	n

Table 20.4 Contingency table showing obtained frequencies for a hypothetical study comparing survival after treatments

	Drugs	Surgery	*Row marginal*
Dead	11	8	*19*
Alive	9	12	*21*
Column marginal	*20*	*20*	*n = 40*

Table 20.6 Sample calculation of chi-square (χ^2)

	f_o	f_e	$(f_o - f_e)^2$	$(f_o - f_e)^2/f_e$
A	11	9.5	2.25	0.236
B	8	9.5	2.25	0.236
C	9	10.5	2.25	0.214
D	12	10.5	2.25	0.214
n	40			$\chi^2 = 0.90$

Therefore, since $\chi^2_{obt} < \chi^2_{crit}$ we must retain H_0: there is no statistically significant difference in the frequencies of survival over 5 years following the two kinds of treatments. Our data show that either there is no difference in the outcomes of the two treatments or we made a type II error.

The χ^2 test can be used to analyse the statistical significance of nominal data arising from experimental or non-experimental investigations. This non-parametric test can be used provided that two simple assumptions are met:

1. Each participant has provided only one entry into the χ^2 table; that is, each of the entries is independent.
2. The expected frequency (f_e) in each cell is at least 5. Therefore, if the sample size is too small, χ^2 may not be used.

If either of these assumptions is violated, the use of χ^2 is inappropriate for statistical decision making. Assumption 2 is particularly important when the degrees of freedom is 1 (df = 1) for a contingency table.

Statistical packages

We have considered several examples of establishing the statistical significance of the results. These calculations were presented only for teaching purposes. Some older applied statistics textbooks are crammed with complicated formulae for calculating dozens of different inferential statistics. Researchers now use statistical packages which have made statistical analysis simpler and more accessible to all researchers. The following steps are followed when using statistical packages:

1. *Select a statistical package*. There are many packages on the market, including Statistical Package for Social Sciences ('SPSS™'), 'STATISTICA™', 'Statsview™' or various spreadsheets with useful statistical functions. Each program has its strengths and weaknesses and some researchers have formed strong attachment to specific programs. If you are a beginner, you should be guided by your thesis supervisor or your workplace mentor about the availability of packages.
2. *Training*. It is useful to learn how to use a package before you begin data analysis. Depending on your aptitude and experience, training sessions take one or two days. With more complex

scientific packages such as 'STATISTICA' it might require long-term usage before one feels like an expert user.

3. *Encode the raw data*. We begin by encoding the data. You have to be clear about issues such as which are the independent or dependent variables, or the scaling of the data (continuous/discontinuous). That is, designs and measurement procedures used in your research project influence the encoding process.
4. *Identifying the statistical analysis required*. Some degree of statistical knowledge is required beyond that covered in this book to enable you to confidently select and interpret the appropriate statistical analyses. Keep in mind that our book is introductory; it is expected that you will complete a more advanced statistics subject. For more complex analyses it might be useful to seek expert help.
5. *Printout*. You will select the appropriate statistical analysis from the 'menu' and print out the results of the analysis.
6. *Interpretation*. Finally you will need to interpret the 'printout' in relation to your research questions and/or hypotheses.

Let us look at a simple example. Say we are interested in the benefits of exercise for improving mobility in nursing home residents. A sample of 24 ($n = 24$) residents with reduced mobility are selected and have given informed consent to participate. The participants are randomly assigned to either of two groups: 'E', which involves them undertaking an exercise program suitable for improving mobility in elderly patients, and 'C', which involves undertaking alternative activities of equal duration. The outcome or dependent variable is measured as the distance in metres safely walked by the residents unassisted at the completion of the exercise and control programs. The research hypothesis here is: exercise improves mobility in nursing home residents. We will look at a set of created data to illustrate hypothesis testing using a statistical package (SPSS).

Let us follow the steps for analysing the data:

1. Assume that the SPSS package is readily available in your workplace and you are informed by your computing expert or supervisor.
2. You have had some training. Even if no formal training is available, self-help books such as

SPSS: analysis without anguish. Version 11.0 for Windows (Coates & Steed 2003) are very useful.

3. After accessing the spreadsheet for the program, we encode the data in the two columns representing 'E' and 'C'. We inform the program that the data are 'continuous' (ratio-scale data).

4. We refer to Table 20.1 to identify the required statistical analysis. Here we have:

   a. two groups

   b. independent groups

   c. ratio-scale data.

   Therefore, we select the independent t test for analysing the data from the 'menu' of inferential tests available.

5. Printouts: Tables 20.7 and 20.8 for SPSS are based on printouts presented in Coates & Steed (2003, p 73). We changed the original example which contains additional information: the interested reader might wish to examine it further in Coates & Steed (2003).

Table 20.7 shows key descriptive statistics:

- n refers to the sample size for each group
- mean ($\bar{X}$) for each group
- standard deviation (s) for each group
- standard error mean ($s_{\bar{x}}$) for each group. You will recall from Chapter 19 that $s_x = s/\sqrt{n}$. Here, for the control group, 'C' is the standard error of the mean and is equal to $2.864/\sqrt{11} = 0.863$, as shown in Table 20.7.

The group mean for the exercise group does in fact indicate a better overall performance. However, we are justified in concluding that exercise in general produces improved mobility in nursing home residents. To answer this question we must look at the results of the t test, as shown in Table 20.8.

The following information was presented:

- The t obtained was -0.695, the minus sign simply reflecting that the mean for the exercise group was less than the mean for the control group. A t value of 0.695 is quite 'small' in relation to the critical values for t shown in Appendix B.
- 'df' refers to degrees of freedom. For the control group's t test, df = $n_1 + n_2 - 2$. Here, df = $11 + 11 - 2 = 20$, as shown in Table 20.8.
- 'Sig. (2-tailed)' refers to the probability of a difference between the means being obtained by chance, i.e. $p(H_0$ is true). The decision rule is that we reject H_0 if $p<0.05$. Here the calculated probability is 0.495 and therefore we retain H_0. We conclude that the results were not statistically significant.
- The 'mean difference' refers to the difference between the two sample means; i.e. $8 - 9 = -1$, as shown in Table 20.8.
- 'Standard error difference' refers to the standard error of the distribution of sample means. We will not discuss this statistic in detail. However, as shown in Chapter 17, the standard error enables us to calculate a 95% confidence interval; in this case for $\bar{X}_C - \bar{X}_E$.
- The lower and upper limits show that the true (i.e. population) difference ($\mu_C - \mu_E$) probably ($p = 0.95$) falls between -4.003 and 2.003. This is a wide range for a confidence interval and therefore indicates that residents who exercise might be able to walk either four extra metres or two metres less than those who don't exercise. Of course, any other difference between the two limits is possible. Clearly, such

Table 20.7 Printout for descriptive statistics

Treatment	n	Mean	Standard deviation	Standard error mean
Control (C)	11	8.00	2.864	0.863
Exercise (E)	11	9.00	3.821	1.152

Table 20.8 t test for equality of means

Treatment	t	df	Sig. (2-tailed)	Mean difference	Standard error difference	95% confidence interval Lower	Upper
Control (C)	−0.695	20	0.495	−1.00	1.440	−4.003	2.003
Exercise (E)	−0.695	18.539	0.496	−1.00	1.440	−4.018	2.013

results are far too variable to attribute any clinical benefits to the exercise program.

Summary

In this chapter we examined the use of statistical tests for analysing and interpreting the results of quantitative research. There are a variety of statistical tests available for analysing the significance of the obtained data. The statistical test appropriate for analysing a given set of data is selected on the basis of:

1. The scaling of the data.
2. The dependence/independence of the measurements.
3. The number of groups being studied.
4. Specific requirements for using a statistical test.

Generally, parametric and non-parametric statistical tests were distinguished on the grounds of the scaling of the data and the assumptions underlying the sampling distributions.

None of the individual statistical tests was discussed in detail, except the χ^2 test, which was presented as an example. The χ^2 test illustrates the principle that theoretical sampling distributions can be generated, and the probability of obtaining specific outcomes can be calculated. If the obtained value of the inferential statistic is greater than or equal to the critical value, the null hypothesis can be rejected at the level of significance specified by the type I error rate (α). This is the case regardless of which particular statistical test is being used. The retention of H_0 might reflect a correct decision, or a type II error. Effect size and sample size are the key factors that determine type II error rate, as will be discussed in Chapter 21.

Effect size and the interpretation of evidence

21

CHAPTER CONTENTS

Introduction 171

Effect size 171

   Effect size with continuous data 172

   Effect size with discontinuous data 173

Confidence intervals and effect size 173

   Calculating confidence intervals 174

   Confidence intervals and statistical
significance 174

How to optimize statistical inferences 175

How to interpret null
(non-significant) results 175

Statistical power analysis 176

Clinical decision-making 177

Overview of conducting data analysis 178

   Descriptive statistics 178

   Inferential statistics 178

Summary 178

Introduction

When researchers have demonstrated statistical significance within the results of a study, what have they actually done? Statistical significance indicates that the results obtained in the study are probably not just due to chance but represent support for the study research hypothesis. However, it is not correct to assume that having established statistical significance means that the results are clinically important or useful for guiding our practices. We

must also establish the *clinical* or *practical significance* of our results following the step of demonstrating statistical significance.

So how do we do that? The practical significance of the results depends on a statistic referred to as the 'effect size'; the larger the 'effect size', the more likely it is that the results will be clinically useful. As we will see in this chapter, effect size is the most relevant statistic for establishing the efficacy of an intervention.

The aims of this chapter are to discuss the following:

1. Effect size, that is how large the relationships or differences observed in the data are.
2. The relationship between effect size and statistical and clinical significance.
3. The determinants of statistical power.
4. Basic principles of clinical decision making.

Effect size

Effect size expresses the size of the change or degree of association that can be attributed to a health intervention. The term *effect size* is also used more broadly in statistics to refer to the size of the phenomenon under study. For example, if we were studying gender effects on how long people live, a measure of effect size could be the difference in life expectancy between males and females. On average, this difference is actually around 5 years, which has real implications! In a correlational study, the effect size is the size of the correlation between the selected variables under study (e.g. r^2 as discussed in Chapter 18). There are many measures or indicators of effect size; the one which is relevant to analysing the results of a study is selected on the basis of the scaling of the outcome or dependent variable (Sackett et al 2000).

Effect size with continuous data

The concept of effect size for continuous data (i.e. an interval or ratio measurement scale) can be illustrated by results from two student research projects supervised by one the authors.

Study 1: Test–retest reliability of a force measurement machine

In this first study, the student was concerned with demonstrating the test–retest reliability of a device designed to measure maximum forces being produced by patients' leg muscles under two conditions (flexion and extension). Twenty-one patients took part in the study and the reliability of the measurement process was tested by taking two readings for the same patients an hour apart and then calculating the Pearson correlation between the readings obtained from the machine in question during two trials separated by an hour for each patient. The results are shown in Table 21.1. Both results reached the $p = 0.01$ level of significance.

The student was ecstatic when the computer data analysis program informed that the correlations were statistically significant at the 0.01 level (indicating that there was less than a 1 in 100 chance that the correlations were illusory or actually zero). We were somewhat less ecstatic because, in fact, the results indicated that approximately 69% (1 – 0.56^2) and 71% (1 – 0.54^2) of the variation was not shared between the measurements of the first and second trial. In other words, the measures were 'all over the place', despite statistical significance being reached. Thus, far from being an endorsement of the measurement process, these results were somewhat of a condemnation. This is a classic example of the need for careful interpretation of effect size in conjunction with statistical significance.

Study 2: A comparative study of improvement in two treatment groups

The second project was a comparative study of two groups: one group suffering from suspected repetition strain injuries (RSI) induced by frequent computer data entry and a group of 'normals'. An activities of daily living (ADL) assessment scale was used and yielded a 'disability' index of between 0 and 50. There were 60 people in each group. The results are shown in Table 21.2.

The appropriate statistic for analysing these data happens to be the independent groups t test, although this is not important for understanding this example. The t value for these data was significant at the 0.05 level. Does this finding indicate that the difference is clinically meaningful or significant? There are two steps in interpreting the clinical significance of the results.

First, we calculate the effect size. For interval or ratio-scaled data the effect size 'd' is defined as:

$$d = \frac{\mu_1 - \mu_2}{\sigma}$$

where $\mu_1 - \mu_2$ refers to the difference between the population means and σ refers to the population standard deviation.

Since we rarely have access to population data we use sample statistics for estimating population differences. The formula becomes:

$$d = \frac{\overline{X}_1 - \overline{X}_2}{s_1}$$

where $\overline{X}_1 - \overline{X}_2$ indicates the difference between the sample means and s_1 refers to the standard deviation of the 'normal' or 'control' group. Therefore, for the above example, substituting into the equation yields:

$$d = \frac{30.4 - 33.2}{1.2} = -2.33$$

In other words, the average ADL score of the people with suspected RSI was 2.33 standard deviations under the mean of the distribution of

Table 21.1 Pearson correlations between trials 1 and 2

Flexion	Extension
0.56	0.54

Table 21.2 Mean ADL disability scores

	RSI group	Normals
Mean	33.2	30.4
Standard deviation	1.6	1.2

'normal' scores. The meaning of d can be interpreted by using standardized scores. The greater the value of d, the greater the standardized difference between the means and therefore the larger the effect size.

Second, we need to consider the clinical implications of the evidence. It might be that the difference of 2.8 units in the ADL scores is important and clinically meaningful. However, if one inspects the means, the differences are slight, notwithstanding the statistical significance of the results. This example further illustrates the problems of interpretation that may arise from focusing on the level of statistical significance and not on the effect sizes shown by the data.

When we say that the findings are clinically or practically significant we mean that the effect is sufficiently large to influence clinical practices. It is the health workers rather than statisticians who need to set the standards for each health and illness determinant or treatment outcome. After all, even relatively small changes can be of enormous value in the prevention and treatment of illnesses. There are many statistics currently in use for determining effect size. The selection, calculation and interpretation of various measures of effect are beyond our introductory book, but interested readers can refer to Sackett et al (2000).

Effect size with discontinuous data

For a randomized controlled trial (RCT), cohort or case-control study with two groups, effect sizes correspond to the size of the difference between the two groups. For dichotomous data, measures of effect size include the odds ratio, the absolute risk reduction and the relative risk reduction.

As we discussed in Chapter 15, odds ratio (OR) compares the odds of the occurrence of an event for one group with the odds of the event for another group. For an RCT, the odds ratio compares the odds of an event for the intervention group with the odds for the control group. For example, the odds for each group, of having type 2 diabetes, in the hypothetical RCT of an exercise program for obese men, are given in Chapter 15. So, using these numbers, the odds ratio is:

$$OR = \frac{0.25}{0.67} = 0.37$$

So, this means that the odds of developing type 2 diabetes in the intervention group are about a third of those for the control group. An OR of this size could well be interpreted as evidence for the efficacy of the exercise program.

Absolute risk reduction (ARR) is a simple and useful measure of effect size. It is calculated by subtracting the percentage of people in the control group who experience the event, from the percentage of people in the intervention group who experience the event. The percentage values for each group for the hypothetical RCT of the exercise program for obese men are given above. Using these numbers, the absolute risk reduction is:

$$ARR = 20\% - 40\% = -20\%$$

This means that the risk of type 2 diabetes was reduced by 20% in the intervention (exercise) group.

Relative risk reduction (RRR) is calculated by dividing the absolute risk reduction by the value corresponding to the percentage of people in the control group who experience the event. For the hypothetical RCT of the exercise program for obese men, the ARR and the percentage of the control group who experience the event (develop type 2 diabetes) are given above. Using these numbers the relative risk reduction is:

$$RRR = \frac{20\% - 40\%}{40\%} = -0.5 \text{ or } 50\%$$

In other words, the risk of developing type 2 diabetes is reduced by half (by 50%) in the intervention (exercise) group, relative to the control group. This finding also indicates that the hypothetical treatment was effective; however, we will need to demonstrate the statistical significance of the results.

Confidence intervals and effect size

The calculation of confidence intervals is an essential step in analysing and reporting effect sizes. Effect sizes and associated confidence intervals constitute the most important research findings for conducting evidence-based practice (Sackett et al 2000; 'CONSORT').

Calculating confidence intervals

Calculated from the sample data, the confidence interval (CI) is represented by a range of values which contain, at a given level of probability, the true population parameter (see Ch. 19). For example, the 95% CI for an OR will include, at a probability of $p = 0.95$, the actual OR for the population. There is only a small probability ($p \leq 0.05$) that the population OR will fall outside the lower or upper limits of the 95% CI.

For example, consider the hypothetical RCT discussed earlier in the chapter. The OR for the sample was found to be 0.37. Can we infer in general that the exercise program reduces the odds of type 2 diabetes by *exactly* this number? Of course not; rather the researcher will need to calculate and report the 95% CI. Say that the researchers calculated and reported the following results:

$$OR = 0.37 \ (0.32; \ 0.42)$$

The above results would indicate that the odds of type 2 diabetes in the population could be reduced to 0.32 (lower limit) or 0.42 (upper limit) by the exercise program. That is, we are not absolutely confident in the actual population effect size (OR), but we can be 95% confident that it is between 0.32 and 0.42. Similarly, confidence intervals (usually but not always 95% CI) are reported for other measures of effect size including relative risk ratios, Cohen's d, or r^2.

The calculation of confidence intervals for effect sizes is beyond the scope of this introductory text. However, interested readers may consult Hicks (2009) for details of conducting these calculations. In general, the calculated width of a confidence interval depends on the degree of variability of the data and the sample size. The larger the sample size, the narrower the confidence interval. Large sample sizes enable us to collect more information than small samples and then enable us to make precise estimates of the true effect size for the population.

Confidence intervals and statistical significance

As for other statistics (see Ch. 20), we can calculate the probability of an effect size being just due to chance or an actual effect. An effect size, such

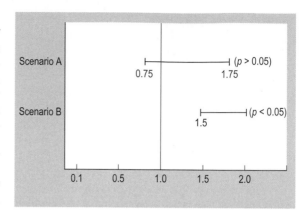

Figure 21.1 • Decision criterion: risk of type II error (miss).

as 'OR' or 'd' is reported as statistically significant if the probability of it occurring by chance is less than 0.05 ($p \leq 0.05$). There is a close relationship between the confidence interval for an effect size and statistical significance as illustrated by the results of a hypothetical RCT (Figure 21.1).

Figure 21.1 illustrates the results of a study where the outcome measure was on a nominal scale and the results were analysed using OR as the measure of effect size. For 'Scenario A', OR is equal to 1.25 with a lower limit of 0.75 and upper limit of 1.75. This range includes OR = 1.0, indicating that the true population value of no effect is included in the range of the confidence interval. These findings indicate that we would retain H_0: OR = 1.0 at a 0.05 level of significance.

For 'Scenario B', the results were OR = 2.0 with a lower limit equal to 1.5 and an upper limit equal to 2.5. Here the OR = 1.0 indicating no *effect* is not included in the 95% CI. Therefore, we can reject the null hypothesis and accept the alternative H_A:

$$OR \neq 1.0 \ (p < 0.05)$$

These examples apply to other measures of effect size linking 95% CI and statistical significance. If the confidence interval does not include the null value then the results are deemed to be statistically significant. As discussed further in Chapter 24, effect sizes with 95% CI are the key statistics for determining the efficacy of interventions in the context of conducting evidence-based health care.

How to optimize statistical inferences

It should be evident from the previous discussion that statistical decision making can result in incorrect decisions. There are two main types of inferential error: type I and type II.

A type I error occurs when we mistakenly reject H_0; that is, when we claim that our experimental hypothesis was supported when it is, in fact, false. The probability of a type I error occurring is less than or equal to α. For instance, if we set $\alpha = 0.01$, then the probability of making a type I error is less than or equal to 0.01; the chances are equal to or less than $1/100$ that our decision in rejecting H_0 was mistaken. The smaller the α, the less the chance of making a type I error. We can set α as low as possible, but by convention it must be less than or equal to 0.05.

A type II error occurs when we mistakenly retain H_0; the probability of a type II error is denoted by β (beta). If n is large we are more likely to reject H_0 and conclude that the results are statistically significant.

Type I errors represent a 'false alarm' and type II errors represent a 'miss'. Figure 21.2 illustrates that, if we reject H_0, we are making either a correct decision or a type I error. If we retain H_0, we are making either a correct decision or a type II error. While we cannot, in principle, eliminate type I and type II errors from scientific decision making, we can take steps to minimize their occurrence.

We minimize the occurrence of type I error by setting an acceptable level for α. In scientific research, editors of most scientific journals require that α should be set at 0.05 or less. This convention helps to reduce false alarms to a rate of less than $1/20$. Replication of the findings by other independent investigators provides important evidence that the original decision to reject H_0 was correct.

How do we minimize the probability of type II error?

1. Increase the sample size, n.
2. Reduce the variability of measurements ($s_{\bar{x}}$, either by increasing accuracy or by using samples that are not highly variable for the measurement producing the data).
3. Use a directional H_A, on the basis of previous evidence about the nature of the effect.

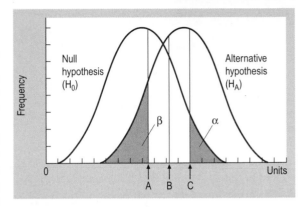

Figure 21.2 • Decision criterion: risk of type I error (false alarm).

4. Set a less demanding α, type I error rate. There is a relationship between α and β, such that the smaller α, the greater β. This relationship is illustrated in Figure 21.2. Figure 21.2 shows that, as α decreases, β increases. Inevitably, as we decrease the type I error rate, we increase the probability of type II error. This is the reason why we do not normally set α lower than $p = 0.01$. Although a significance level such as $\alpha = 0.001$ would reduce 'false alarms' it would also increase the probability of a 'miss'.
5. Finally, a large effect size reduces the probability of making a type II error

How to interpret null (non-significant) results

As we discussed in previous chapters, the researcher will sometimes analyse data using a statistical method and the results show no statistically significant relationships or differences. In other words, the researcher cannot reject the null hypothesis. There are several reasons why the researcher may obtain a null result.

1. The trend or difference that the researcher originally hypothesized is incorrect (i.e. there is no effect).
2. The sample included in the analysis is unrepresentative, so the effect does not show up, although it exists in the wider population (i.e. the data collected are flawed).
3. There are insufficient cases in the sample to detect the trend; this is especially a problem

Table 21.3 Statistical decision outcomes

Reality	Decision: effect	Decision: no effect
Effect	Correct	Type II error (miss)
No effect	Type I error (false alarm)	Correct

if the trends are subtle (i.e. the effect size is small; the study sample is not big enough).

4. The measurements chosen have very high or inherent random variability (i.e. the measurement tools used are not good enough).

Therefore, if the researcher obtains a null result, one or more of the above explanations may apply. There are, however, actions that can be taken to minimize the chance of missing real effects. In order to understand these actions, it is necessary again to examine the table illustrating the possible outcomes of a statistical decision (as shown in Table 21.3).

Table 21.3 shows the four possible decision outcomes described above. On the basis of the statistical evidence you may:

1. Correctly conclude there is an effect when there really is an effect.
2. Decide that there is an effect when there really is not (this is a 'false alarm' or type I error).
3. Decide that there is not an effect when there really is (this is a 'miss' or type II error).
4. Correctly decide there is not an effect when indeed there is not.

Statistical power analysis

The statistical power of a statistical analysis is defined as 1 – probability of a miss (type II error or β).

$$\text{Power} = 1 - \beta$$

That is, the lower the probability of making a type II error, the more likely that we are to make a correct decision. For example, if the power of a particular analysis is 0.95, for a given effect size we will correctly detect the existence of the effect 95 times out of 100. Power is an important concept in the interpretation of null results. For example, if a researcher compared the improvements of two groups of only five patients under different treatment circumstances, the power of the analysis would almost certainly be low, say 0.1. Thus 9 times out of 10, even with an effect really present, the researcher would be unable to detect it. Contemporary health research requires that the power for a study should be at least 0.8. What this means is that we should be 80% certain that we will identify an effect if it is actually true for the population.

It is essential to be careful in the interpretation of null results where they are used to demonstrate a lack of superiority of one treatment method over another, especially when there is a low number of cases. This may be purely a function of low statistical power rather than the equivalence of the two treatments. Unfortunately the calculation of statistical power is complicated and beyond the scope of this text. However, there are technical texts, such as Cohen (1988) and Ellis (2010), that are available to look up the power of various analyses. There are also statistical programs that perform the same function. The best defence against low statistical power is a good-sized sample. Before quantitative research projects are approved by funding bodies or ethics committees, there is the requirement that sufficient data will be collected to identify real effects.

Effect size is also an important consideration for identifying both statistical and clinical significance. We are more likely to detect a significant pattern or trend in our sample data when a factor has a strong influence on health or illness outcomes. A very powerful treatment such as the use of antibiotics for bacterial infections could be demonstrated even in a small sample. Table 21.4 shows the association between effect size and sample size for determining statistical and clinical significance for the results of research and evaluation projects. The most useful results for clear decision making occur when both effect size and sample size are large. Where the effect size is large but the results are not statistically significant, it might be useful to replicate the study with a larger sample size. Unfortunately, in real research it might be difficult to obtain a large sample and the effect size, we discover, might be disappointingly small. It is for this reason that researchers make the best use of previous research and, if possible, complete pilot studies. The evidence from previous research and the results of pilot studies enable us to conduct power analyses for estimating the minimum sample size for detecting an effect if it is really there.

Table 21.5 shows how evidence for statistical and clinical significance can be combined to interpret the findings of a study. A clear positive outcome is when there is strong evidence for both

Table 21.4 The relationship between effect size, sample size and decision making

Effect size	Sample size	
	Large	*Small*
High	Both statistical and clinical significance are likely to be demonstrated	Statistical significance might not be demonstrated, but clinical significance would be indicated
Low	Statistical significance would be likely, but the results might not indicate clinically applicable outcomes	Neither statistical nor clinical significance is likely. Statistically significant results might result in a type I error

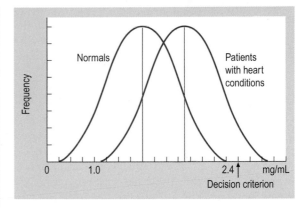

Figure 21.3 • Decision criterion: risk of type II error (miss)

Table 21.5 How to interpret findings

Clinical significance	Statistical significance	
	Yes	No
Yes	Clear: strong evidence for treatment effect	Inconclusive: need for further research (e.g. with larger samples)
No	Inconclusive: suggests findings might not be meaningful – need further research	Clear: strong evidence for lack of a treatment effect

Acknowledgement: We are grateful to Dr. Paul O'Halloran (La Trobe University) for this table.

Table 21.6 Clinical decision outcomes

Reality	Decision: pathology	Decision: no pathology
No pathology	Type I error (false alarm)	Correct decision
Pathology	Correct decision	Type II error (miss)

clinical and statistical significance. In this case we are confident that the information obtained is clinically useful and generalizable to the population. Another clear finding, provided that the sample size was adequate, is the lack of clear treatment effect. Such negative findings can be very useful in eliminating false hypotheses or ineffectual treatments.

Clinical decision-making

The decisions confronting a clinician making a diagnosis on the basis of uncertain information are similar to the scientist's hypothesis-testing procedure. As a hypothetical example, assume that a clinician wishes to decide whether a patient has heart disease on the basis of the cholesterol concentration in a sample of the patient's blood. Previous research of patients with heart disease and 'normals' has shown that, indeed, heart patients tend to have a higher level of cholesterol than 'normals'.

When the frequency distributions of cholesterol concentrations of a large group of heart patients and a group of 'normals' are graphed, they appear as shown in Figure 21.3. You will note that, if patients present with a cholesterol concentration between 1.0 and 2.4 mg/mL, it is not possible to determine with complete certainty whether they are normal or have heart disease, due to the overlap of the normal and heart disease groups in the cholesterol distribution.

Therefore, the clinician, like the scientist, has to make a decision under uncertainty: to diagnose pathology (i.e. reject the null hypothesis) or normality (i.e. retain the null hypothesis). The clinician risks the same errors as the scientist, as shown in Table 21.6.

The relative frequency of the type of errors made by the clinician can be altered by moving the point above which the clinician will decide that pathology is indicated (i.e. the decision criterion). For example, if clinicians did not bother their colleagues or patients with false alarms (type I errors), they might shift the decision criterion to 2.5 mg/mL (Fig. 21.1). Any patient presenting with a cholesterol level below 2.5 mg/mL would be considered normal. In this particular case, with a decision point of 2.5 mg/mL, no 'false alarms' would occur. However, a huge number of people with real pathology would be missed (type II errors).

If clinicians value the sanctity of human life (and their bank balance after a successful malpractice suit) they will probably adjust the decision criterion to the point shown in Figure 21.2. In this case, there would be no misses but lots of false alarms.

Thus, most clinicians are rewarded for adopting a conservative decision rule, where misses are minimized, by receiving lots of false alarms. Unfortunately, this generates a lot of useless, expensive and sometimes even dangerous clinical interventions.

Overview of conducting data analysis

Let us have a look at a hypothetical example for illustrating how the use of descriptive and inferential statistics is applied when analysing quantitative data. There is evidence that exposure to heavy metals, such as lead, may result in changes in the cognitive abilities of young adults. A researcher selects the design referred to as a *cohort* study (see Ch. 8), for guiding data collection to answer the research question 'How does significant exposure to lead influence the IQ in young people between 18 and 20 years of age?' Assume that a sample of 100 volunteers between 18 and 20 years are identified as having high serum lead levels. This group is tested and compared on IQ with a control group matched on age, gender and socio-economic background.

The research hypothesis is therefore:

> The group of 16–19-year-olds exposed to lead will have lower IQs on the Wechsler Adult Intelligence scale than a matched group with no exposure to lead.

Say that the statistical package SPSS is used to analyse the data (see Ch. 20).

Descriptive statistics

Having entered the data, the first step is to calculate the relevant descriptive statistics. Given that the variable, IQ, is an interval scale (see Ch. 14), the appropriate statistics for representing the results are the mean and the standard deviation. *Graphing* the frequency distribution would help to visualize the difference between the IQs of the exposed group and the non-exposed (control) group. Say that the following results are calculated:

Exposed group: $\overline{X}_e = 90$, $S_e = 15$, $n_e = 100$

Non-exposed comparison group:
$$\overline{X}_c = 105, S_e = 15, n_c = 100$$

where $\overline{X}$ is the mean, S the standard deviation and n the sample size for each of the exposed and non-exposed groups. Clearly, there is a 15-point difference between the two groups. This would be a large difference; however, we need to establish if it was due to random error/chance (see Ch. 20).

Inferential statistics

To establish the probability of the null hypothesis H_0, $\mu_e = \mu_c$, we would select the independent groups t test (see Ch. 20). The hypothetical results would be $t = 7.1$, df $= 198$, $p < 0.001$. Therefore, we reject the null hypothesis and say that our results are statistically significant at the 0.001 level. In other words, the findings can be generalized to the population; that is, we infer that young people exposed to lead have lower IQs than those who are not exposed.

The effect size enables us to estimate the size of the effect. In this case, there was a large 15-point difference in the IQs. Using Cohen's d to calculate the standardized effect size results in $d = 1.0$ (0.8; 1.2); 0.8 and 1.2 are the approximate lower and upper limits for the 95% CI. This is a large effect size indicating that the exposure to lead is having serious impact on the cognitive development of young people. Of course, this is just a hypothetical example, but such a large effect size in real life would be a cause for concern that is of practical significance.

Summary

In the interpretation of a statistical test, the researcher calculates the statistical value and then compares this value against the appropriate table to obtain the probability level. If the probability is below a certain value (0.05 is a commonly chosen value), the researcher has established the statistical significance of the analysis in question. The researcher must then interpret the implications of the results by determining the actual size of the effects observed. If these are small, the results may be statistically significant but clinically unimportant. Statistical significance does not imply clinical importance.

A null result (indicating no effects) must be carefully interpreted. It is possible that the researcher has missed an effect because of its small size and/or insufficient cases in the analysis. The statistical analysis measures the chance of correctly detecting a real effect of a given size. Thus, a null result may be a function of low statistical power, rather than there being no real effect. It is necessary to carry out a statistical power analysis *before* undertaking a research project.

There are several criteria, beyond statistical significance, which need to be considered before making decisions concerning the clinical relevance of investigations. The most important criterion is a large and consistent effect size. In addition to effect size, the determination of clinical or practical significance is influenced by negative side-effects of treatments and economic limitations concerning the administration of health care in a given community.

Qualitative data analysis

22

CHAPTER CONTENTS

Introduction 181

Understanding meaning in everyday life 181

Coding qualitative data 182

   Predetermined coding 182

   Coding and thematic analysis 182

Content analysis. 183

Thematic analysis, 'verstehen' and grounded theory 184

Interpretation and social context 185

The accuracy of qualitative data analysis . . .187

Summary. .188

Introduction

As we discussed in Chapters 2, 3 and 10, the aim of qualitative research is to provide evidence for understanding experiences of health and illness from the perspective of the participants. Qualitative data are collected through techniques such as in-depth interviews, focus groups and participant observation (Chs 11–13). Qualitative data analysis refers to the processes by which researchers organize the information collected and analyse the meanings of what was said and done by the participants. When conducting qualitative data analysis we bring our values, experiences and theories when analysing and constructing the meaning of what our respondents are telling us about their lives.

The specific aims of this chapter are to:

1. Describe the process of interpreting qualitative research data.
2. Describe the basic procedures involved in conducting content analysis, thematic analysis and semiotic analysis.
3. Discuss the comparative advantages and disadvantages of using different types of qualitative analyses.
4. Explain basic strategies for ensuring the accuracy of interpretations.

Understanding meaning in everyday life

Understanding people involves discovering their beliefs, desires, intentions. We do this by listening to them and observing what they say and do, taking into account the social settings in which these actions occur.

For instance, one person says to another: 'Would you like to come in for a coffee?' What are the intentions of the speaker? Does he or she simply want to prepare the coffee and consume it in silence? Or should we look for 'hidden' or 'latent' meanings in order to understand the speaker's true intentions? Consider these two everyday scenarios:

1. You have been given a lift by a workmate who had to go out of his way to drive you home. Although you are tired, it seems the right thing to offer the driver refreshments. However, your intention is to be polite and acknowledge the colleague's effort; in fact you are hoping

that the invitation will be refused. The 'hidden message' here is 'Thank you and goodbye!' The worst-case outcome is that the colleague is too insensitive to read your intentions and stays around gossiping until midnight. Bad luck!

2. The British film 'Brassed Off' (1996) has a scene where a young woman is escorted home after a date by a young man. A dialogue was (approximately) as follows:

She: Come up for a cup of coffee.

He: I don't drink coffee.

She: That's alright; I don't have any.

The above dialogue shows the nuances in the everyday use of language. Just as we sometimes misunderstand meanings and intentions in everyday life, we can also misinterpret the data produced by qualitative data collection. To avoid error we need to cross-check the accuracy of our interpretation.

Coding qualitative data

At the conclusion of the data collection process, qualitative researchers are confronted by transcripts which record the narratives expressed by the participants. The first step of analysis is to thoroughly read the transcripts, that is to 'immerse' oneself in the text. Once we have acquired an overall understanding of the narratives the next step is to code the text. To do this the researchers develops a coding system which is used to organize the data (what was said) into categories based on similarities of words, concepts and themes. There are two main approaches to coding: predetermined and emerging with thematic analysis.

Predetermined coding

Predetermined coding uses predetermined categories to organize and analyse the transcripts.

For example, you might do a survey to study clients' experiences of a rehabilitation program at your workplace. Say that you conducted 20 in-depth interviews and produced a 100-page transcript representing what people said in these interviews. Considering your research aims, you might code the statements into three categories:

1. Satisfaction with the rehabilitation program.
2. Dissatisfaction with the rehabilitation program.
3. Neutral statements.

At the simplest level, analysing the first two categories would enable us to understand the reasons why the clients found the rehabilitation programs to be satisfactory or unsatisfactory. This information could be useful for improving the program. In most studies the coding system would be more elaborate.

Coding and thematic analysis

An alternative approach to using predetermined codes is to develop a coding system that identifies common themes as they emerge from the text. Different qualitative researchers advocate different approaches to coding but it typically involves the following steps. The researchers first study their transcripts, and develop a close familiarity with them. During this process, all the concepts, themes and ideas are noted to form major categories. Often, the researcher will then attach a label and/or number to each category and record their positions in the transcript. Coding is an iterative process (we retrace our steps), with the researcher coding and re-coding as the interpretation progresses. The researchers, having developed the codes and coded the transcripts, then attempt to interpret their meanings in the social context of the participants (see Ch. 10).

Coding is rather like cutting and pasting together similar things; it is an essential process for identifying segments of a text which convey similar meanings. There are a number of units of analysis that can be used to examine meanings in the text. These units reflect the way language is structured and used for communication and can be the bases for coding.

Words: can be identified in the way they have been used, whether descriptively or as expletives.

Concepts: these are words or phrases that convey complex ideas or meanings such as 'disability' or 'stigma'.

Sentences: are grammatically correct sequences of words which convey meaning in a language. Sentences conveying similar meanings can be coded and grouped together.

Themes: are ideas that are represented in a pattern or with a certain degree of frequency within a text. They are made up of a number of concepts which represent experiences and meanings the individuals attach to them. For example, references to hostile intentions in other people that often emerge in the discourses of people having being diagnosed with paranoid schizophrenia.

Consider the following (Polgar & Swerissen 2000):

Difficulties with moving, walking and shifting weight can be part of the everyday experience. The inability to move when others are moving, to join in group activities that involve some mobility, and the inability to participate in sport are characteristic of the problems faced by individuals with disabilities. When identity can be gained from joining in physical group activities, people with disabilities can face disadvantage. If it is participation or just companionship that is desired, physical activities do not provide opportunities for some of those with disabilities and can lead to a sense of separation.

We can identify in the above text, words, phrases and sentences that contain synonyms (words that mean the same thing). These terms can be coded together and are therefore grouped. *Moving, walking, shifting weight*: these are aspects of the same concept, as representing aspects of physical activity not achievable by those who are severely disabled. In this text, these terms have been used several times. *Move when others are moving; join in group activities that involve some mobility; participate in sport*: these are phrases conveying synonyms of physical disadvantage that can reduce the ability of some people with severe disabilities to participate. Also, there are sentences about physical activities with others. *When identity can be gained from joining in physical group activities, people with disabilities can face disadvantage. If it is participation or just companionship that is desired, physical activities do not provide opportunities for some of those with disabilities and can lead to a sense of separation.* These sentences convey similar themes about the disadvantage faced by some people with disabilities through their inability to participate in physical activity. *Disadvantage* and *separation* are two emotive terms signifying problems faced by some people with disabilities. These terms can be coded together, demonstrating the way concepts can be used to code qualitative data.

Content analysis

Content analysis enables the identification of units of meaning occurring in a text. Content analysis is a technique which can be seen as a blending of quantitative and qualitative methods. The recognition and coding of meaning are qualitative, while the counting of the meaningful 'chunks' is quantitative. The 'meaningful chunks' can be words, sentences or paragraphs: that is, the units of language that were coded by the researchers from the narratives and dialogues.

To illustrate content analysis, consider the following unpublished study. One of the authors was interested in how leading newspapers were representing the use of stem cells in medical research. The following research questions were asked:

1. How extensive was the newspaper coverage of the medical use of stem cells?
2. What was the attitude of the newspapers (positive, negative or neutral) to the use of stem cells?

In relation to question 1, the data were collected by identifying relevant newspaper articles published on the topic and measuring the length of the columns. They were quantified by counting the number of articles published per month across the selected time interval. The data relevant to question 2 were obtained by identifying statements supportive or critical of using stem cells or simply 'neutral' descriptions of the nature and possible uses of stem cells. The column lengths for each of the three categories were measured and the percentages devoted to each were graphed across the months. Therefore, the content analysis provided evidence for the level of interest and changing attitudes of the media towards the use of stem cells. This evidence was relevant to understanding the cultural context in which government policy for using stem cells was being formulated.

The discussion of content analysis provides a good opportunity for raising the issue of computer-assisted data analysis. As the texts are often transcribed using PCs, the text is available in electronic form. This means that the text can be fed into a software package, such as NVivo to assist with its analysis. For example, say that the data representing the contents of a hundred newspaper articles were transcribed into a software package. We could now introduce our codes and identify the segments of the whole text which use the relevant words/phrases/sentences. The segments can then be retrieved, examined or modified (cut and paste) on screen. Also, various frequency counts can be readily performed using software tools.

A detailed discussion for selecting and using computer packages is beyond the scope of the present book. Interested readers might find Rice (2009) a useful introduction to selecting and using currently available software packages for expediting and improving qualitative data analysis in general (not only for content analysis). There is an ambivalent attitude among qualitative researchers to computer-assisted data analysis. A key objection has been the distancing of the researcher from the creativity and surprising insights afforded by the more hands-on approaches. Another objection is that meanings of words and sentences sometimes do not follow dictionary definitions but rather have to be understood in the general context. The true meaning of certain subtle and ambiguous communications can be missed in crude and electronically conducted data analyses.

Content analysis is a technique that combines elements of both qualitative and quantitative approaches. We interpret the meaning of the text for developing our coding strategy for organizing or 'chunking' the text and then we use statistics to describe the quantities of text devoted to a specific point of view. Content analysis can be used to test hypotheses, for example hypotheses addressing the positive and negative media perspectives at a given point in time on embryonic stem cell research.

Thematic analysis, 'verstehen' and grounded theory

Counting and hypothesis testing is not the essence of the qualitative approach. What we are trying to do is to see things from the perspectives of our informants and to explain their actions from their points of view. The German word *verstehen* is often used in phenomenological research to express the notion of 'putting ourselves in someone else's shoes' or attaining a strong empathy with their situation. Empathy with other people might seem quite simple, just something we do as human beings. It is worthwhile remembering, however, that sometimes we misunderstand how people feel or think, even when they are our close friends or family. In the same way, we might misunderstand the points of view of persons who are very different to us in age, gender, education, language and culture. Yet, it is essential to understand the points of view of the people to whom we offer health services. So how does 'verstehen' arise through qualitative health research?

First, as we described earlier, our data collection must use a technique (in-depth interviews, written materials, focus groups, etc.) that enables our

respondents to express their point of view. Second, we can adopt a theoretical framework for explaining our understanding of the respondents' experiences. The key point, in the context of *grounded theory*, is that our explanations or theories must emerge inductively from the information provided by our informants. The theory is constructed gradually as more evidence is provided by additional informants. Third, the data are often analysed by coding and thematic analysis as we outlined earlier in this chapter.

A theme is a grouping of ideas or meanings which emerge consistently in the text. The themes emerging from the data illuminate the experiences of the informants and enable us to understand their points of view ('verstehen'). Let us consider an example of thematic analysis.

In a study titled 'The plight of rural parents caring for adult children with HIV', McGinn (1996) studied the experiences of parents caring for their adult children with acquired immunodeficiency syndrome/human immunodeficiency virus (AIDS/HIV). In-depth interviews were conducted with eight mothers and two fathers from rural families involved in this task. The interview transcripts were analysed using a thematic analysis/grounded theory approach (Miles & Huberman 1984).

McGinn extracted three major themes:

1. *Physical and mental problems related to HIV/AIDS.* Here the parents discussed their experiences of their children's problems and the emotional consequences of physical decline and death. For example:

He would fall over, so I would sit him in the wheelchair. And then from within a week in November he went from not being able to sit in the wheelchair to not getting out of bed. And he went from eating little bits of food along with taking a liquid nutrition to just liquid nutrition… and then he got to where he wouldn't swallow the liquid nutrition and he subsisted on just water and juices and Pepsi… and then in the end he even refused them: he wouldn't take anything… He just wasted away.

2. *Stigma associated with having AIDS.* Because of the mode of transmission of AIDS and superstitious fears of contracting the condition, many of the parents found themselves socially isolated at such a very difficult time of their lives. For example:

That Sunday, I never will forget. I asked him, 'Do you want anybody to know?' And I don't remember if he said no, but his head... he almost shook it off. No way did he want anybody to know what the real problem was. But I want you to know that that was a terrible, stressful time. People who came, who normally would be support for me... weren't. It was a real traumatic experience.

3. *Health care.* This theme summarizes the difficulties of accessing necessary health services in rural settings. Even though there were serious deficiencies in health services, one mother reported:

> As for the hospital, I couldn't have asked for a better hospital. There may have been nurses who refused to work with him, I don't know, but the nurses that did come in were great... They even hugged and kissed him goodbye whenever he got well and left. They didn't act like they didn't want to be around him and I appreciated that. I think that's important.

These three themes enable us to understand and empathize with the parents of these very sick young people. Also, they were the bases for recommending improvements in rural health care which directly address the needs of AIDS sufferers and their families in non-metropolitan environments.

Also, we must note that McGinn's paper reported the experiences of people in the mid-1990s, living in rural Canada. With improvements in the treatment and prevention of AIDS and a decrease in the stigma attached to the condition, the experiences of families caring for sufferers have improved. Because of differences and changes in practices and the cultural context, it is always important to note the time and place at which interpretive research was carried out.

Interpretation and social context

As we have seen, qualitative data analysis is a systematic way of interpreting texts. There are many areas of study (e.g. history, politics, theology) where the interpretation of texts is an essential part of the research process. What these diverse disciplines have in common with qualitative health research is the recognition that the meaning of language and texts must be interpreted in a cultural context.

An example is *hermeneutics*, which is a method that was originally used to analyse the meaning of religious texts. Consider the meaning of the term 'god'. When the Romans spoke of Augustus Caesar as a 'god', they were referring to him as a hero who was immortal in the history of Rome. The use of the term 'god' by a polytheistic is quite different to meanings in the context of contemporary Judaeo-Christian or Muslim traditions. The meaning of the term must be interpreted in the context of the religious tradition (polytheistic, monotheistic) and the position of the speaker (believer, non-believer).

An important issue in reading texts is that they might have implicit (in addition to explicit) meanings. *Semiotics* is a method of textual interpretation which seeks to uncover the hidden, omitted meanings implicit in a text. In order to do this, we must adopt a theoretical framework in terms of which we can 'deconstruct' a text. The theoretical framework reflects our understanding of the culture within which the text was produced. You have probably read the book *Animal Farm* by George Orwell. There are several levels at which one can read this story; for example:

- A fairy tale about the imaginary lives of farm animals where animals have human traits and concerns.
- A morality tale in Aesop's style about how power corrupts and leads to betrayal.
- A critique of Stalinism and a re-telling of the bloody history of the Bolshevik revolution and its social consequences in the Soviet Union.

In order to identify Orwell's book as a political critique, one needs to understand the historical/cultural context in which the author worked and lived.

To illustrate these points, we will examine a letter to the editor in a Melbourne newspaper by a woman writer who was apparently concerned about the physical and mental health of young men:

> They're just asking for it.
>
> Since the weather improved, it seems that young men all over the place are discarding their shirts and going about half-naked. I worry for them. Do they have any idea of what a provocative and inviting image they put across?
>
> To my mind, they would be doing themselves a far greater service if they would just compromise a little and get dressed properly. It might not seem fair, and it might be less comfortable, but at least then there wouldn't any longer be the danger of urge-driven women raping young men because of the confusing visual signals they so often put across.

Let us analyse the text consistent with a procedure outlined in Daly et al (1997). First, let us analyse the explicit content of the letter.

1. *Tone.* Serious and condescending as that used by authority figures such as teachers and magistrates; '...now, see here young man, this is for your own benefit...' type of communication.

2. *Language.* Moralistic (e.g. 'dressed properly', 'going about half-naked') and calling for responsibility ('compromising a little'). Also the language is alarmist, predicting that men non-compliant to a dress code will be assaulted.

3. *The aim.* The explicit aim of the letter is to warn young men of the dire consequences of dressing immodestly and thereby inviting attention by 'urge-driven women'.

4. *Repetition of ideas.* The main idea seems to be that a scantily dressed man is sexually provocative to women. Another notion is that women are struggling to control powerful sexual urges. It is implied that men should accept responsibility for suppressing these urges in women. If men dress immodestly then they have to accept the consequences.

5. *Themes.* The first basic explicit theme is the importance of men taking responsibility in projecting a safe, chaste image. The second is the power and danger of women's sexual urges which can explode into assault when provoked by scantily dressed males. An underlying theme which you might have detected is one of 'blaming the victim'; if men are assaulted it is their fault, they should have been more careful.

6. *Oppositional elements.* If men ignore the letter writer's message and move towards the choice of scanty dress, then they are putting themselves at risk. That is, modest dress means safety while immodest dress means assault. Another dichotomy is gender: women are sexually powerful and dangerous; men are presented as naive victims lacking any defined sexuality. In different ways the overt themes emerging from the text are demeaning of both males and females.

You may have different views about how best to interpret the text. As Daly and colleagues (1997, p 183) noted: 'Let us now make some basic semiotic moves across the data'. Let us interrogate the 'data' further using the six points suggested by Daly et al (1997).

- Is the content of the letter preposterous? Are there scantily dressed male construction workers being dragged into alleys by out-of-control schoolgirls? Are there gangs of libidinous females cruising our streets with evil purposes on their minds? Preposterous! The incidence of assault by women is, to all intents and purposes, very low, regardless of how men choose to dress. Therefore, the letter is unsound or it may be a parody.

- In order to understand the meaning of the letter, we play a language game as follows: read 'male' for 'female' in the text. The story now reads quite differently; in fact it resembles a more usual story told to women concerning their responsibility for ensuring that men don't assault them.

- One might propose that the latent agenda for the letter was to ridicule the notion that victims are in some way responsible for the violence of the perpetrator.

- The apparent hero of the explicit story was the author, the caring woman dispensing advice to young men to keep themselves safe by dressing in a chaste fashion. In the implicit story the villains are people who blame women for contributing to violence simply by the clothes they wear.

- What is missing from the original story? Or what was introduced? The writer introduced the notion of female sexuality as an urge that could transform at the slightest provocation into violence. If this notion is ludicrous for females, the question is, how can it be tenable for males? You might ask that if the true intention of the author was to denounce myths of male sexuality then why didn't she say so directly? This is like asking why George Orwell wrote a fairy tale with talking farm animals rather than a direct denouncement of totalitarianism and Stalinist terror. It is a question of how we use language; we use metaphors, parables, hyperboles and so on for expressing ourselves in an interesting, colourful fashion. Semiotics is one of the ways for interpreting the meanings that might be hidden or camouflaged in the original narrative.

- A basic principle for semiotic analysis is selecting a theoretical framework in terms of which we can deconstruct the original narrative and identify its hidden, repressed or mystifying elements. The key to the previous analysis was that the basic idea underpinning the argument (that immodestly dressed males are in danger of being assaulted by out-of-control women) was false and absurd. Our interpretation of the meaning is that the text is a parody of the victim-blaming discourses in patriarchal societies. By adopting a feminist theoretical framework we are in a position to identify the hidden meaning of the text and infer the intentions of the author.

- There is always the possibility that we have misinterpreted the text and misrepresented the intentions of the author. What if she was genuinely concerned about the welfare of young men? The fact of the matter is that there are no absolute guarantees. It might be that, regardless of his well-known interest in political affairs, George Orwell was simply intending to create a children's story when he wrote *Animal Farm*.

In the next part of this chapter we will outline some strategies for ensuring validity and reliability for qualitative research.

The accuracy of qualitative data analysis

How can we be sure that the themes we identified in a text accurately reflect the actual views of the participants? Also, how do we know that similar themes would emerge from the reports of other people who had similar experiences to our sample?

There are a number of qualitative researchers who ensure that the collection and interpretation of their evidence are carried out in a rigorous fashion. The following represent some of the key methodological criteria for conducting qualitative research (Lincoln & Guba 1985):

1. *Data saturation*. This refers to ensuring that we have collected sufficient data from our respondents. Saturation occurs when the themes and ideas emerging from the text become repetitive and we are confident that the inclusion of new participants or further engagement with current participants will not lead to novel themes or interpretations.
2. *Credibility*. Checking if the interpretation of the evidence is judged as accurate by both the research participants and also independent clinicians or scholars. In other words, does your interpretation make sense and if not, why not?

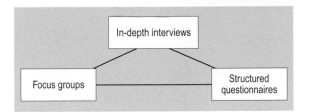

Figure 22.1 • Triangulation using different approaches to data collection.

3. *Auditability*. This refers to each of the steps of the research process being clearly described, so that an independent scholar can critique the research process from its beginning to the analysis and interpretation of the data. The auditor confirms or rejects the researcher's methodology.
4. *Triangulation*. This strategy involves the use of multiple independent methods for collecting data and checking if the themes and interpretations emerging from these different methods are consistent and matching. For example, in order to evaluate client satisfaction with a health service you might use three different data collection strategies (Fig. 22.1). It is useful (but not essential) to use three different data collection methods. The researcher might, if appropriate, use both qualitative (e.g. in-depth interviews) and quantitative (e.g. structured questionnaires) methods for data collection. These are called 'mixed' designs (see also Chs 1 & 9).

As you can see, the methodological concerns in qualitative research are parallel to those of quantitative research (i.e. reliability and validity). However, because of the differences in the way the two types of research are conducted, the terminology for describing the methodological principles is somewhat different. There is another difference to keep in mind; some of the facts about the world discovered by physical, biological and behavioural scientists are held as universal truths, even if the laws and theories integrating these facts are open to revision (see Ch. 1). For example, the structure of human DNA as discovered over the last 50 years is assumed to be true for all humans. In contrast, qualitative evidence depends on time, place and socio-economic circumstances. For instance, the experiences of rural parents caring for adult children with HIV/AIDS is specific to the mid-1990s when the data were collected by McGinn (1996). Things have changed; the treatment of people with

HIV/AIDS is far more effective and the stigma associated with this illness has become less prejudicial, at least in some communities. Therefore, the experiences of people caring for those with HIV/AIDS 20 years after this research are likely to be different.

Summary

There are different approaches to analysing qualitative data depending on the theoretical framework and data collection strategies adopted by the researchers. However, as we saw in this chapter, there are several common aspects to qualitative data analysis:

- 'Immersion' in the data: reading and re-reading the texts to develop a sense of what it is that respondents are trying to say.
- Developing a coding system and identifying the themes emerging from the text.
- Using these themes as a basis for insight, empathy (verstehen) with the experiences, emotions and thinking of the respondents.
- Interpreting and theorizing the respondents' experiences in the context of cultural or historical settings.
- Ensuring the accuracy of the interpretations by cross-checking themes and explanations with other sources of data, other researchers' interpretations of the data, and the respondents.

Section 7

Evaluation and dissemination of research results

23 Critical evaluation of published research 191

24 Synthesis: systematic reviews and meta-analyses 199

As discussed in Chapter 3, having completed our project, we need to communicate our research results to the community of health scientists and health professionals. The most acceptable way of communicating research findings by established researchers is first to report the results at a professional conference and then to write a more formal publication in a peer reviewed journal. Each journal has its particular set of rules and requirements for how research projects should be written up for publication. In general, at least for quantitative research, the format for presenting our research follows the sequential stages of the research process outlined in the present book. This general format is outlined in Chapter 3, which includes a detailed discussion of the specific sections of a research paper and outlines some 'stylistic' considerations required by journal editors.

In Chapter 23, we outline how we evaluate the quality of a research paper and its results. We also discuss what happens if we find serious problems with the design, data collection and analysis and interpretations of a research project.

We discussed in Chapter 1 how, as clinicians using evidence-based health care, we need to be able to critically evaluate research publications.

For clinical researchers it is an ethical requirement that we report our results in an accurate and honest fashion. Before a paper is published in a reputable journal, it is critically evaluated by experts in the area (called referees or peer reviewers) for errors or problems. However, even though reviewers do their best, sometimes serious problems can remain unidentified. Ultimately, it is our task as health professionals to read important publications critically. We owe it to our patients and clients to be cautious and critical concerning the research we use to back up our clinical practice. However, being critical does not mean we must be cynical or derogatory towards the work of health researchers. It is difficult to do good quality research.

In reality, a single research project is rarely sufficient either to verify or falsify a theory, or to convincingly demonstrate the effectiveness of a treatment. Rather, we need to evaluate and summarize the literature as a whole: that is, conduct a literature review. Conflicting findings or gaps in the knowledge for a given area of health care identified in our literature review encourage further research. In Chapter 24, we discuss how systematic reviews and meta-analyses are conducted in health sciences. Well-conducted systematic reviews provide the foundations for evidence-based health care.

Critical evaluation of published research

23

CHAPTER CONTENTS

Introduction 191

Guidelines for critical appraisal of research
publications 192

Critical evaluation of the introduction
in a research paper 192

   Adequacy of the literature review 192

   Clearly defined aims or hypotheses 192

   Selection of an appropriate research
   strategy 194

   Selection of appropriate
   variables/information to be collected . . . 194

Critical evaluation of the methods section
in a research paper 194

   Research participants 194

   Instruments/apparatus/tools. 194

   Procedure 195

Critical evaluation of the results section in a
research paper 196

Critical evaluation of the discussion
section in a research paper. 196

Summary. .197

Introduction

By the time a research report is published in a peer-reviewed journal, it has been critically reviewed by experts. Usually, changes have been made to the initial draft by the author(s) responding to the reviewers' comments. Nevertheless, even a thorough evaluation procedure doesn't guarantee the validity of the design or the conclusions presented in a published paper. Ultimately, you as a health professional must be responsible for judging the validity and relevance of published material for your own clinical activities (which is why you are studying health sciences). Evidence-based practice focuses on the ways in which practitioners can improve their clinical practice by using research evidence. The systematic review processes employed by bodies such as the Cochrane Collaboration are intended to assist clinicians in the selection of interventions that are well proven and safe (see Ch. 24).

The proper attitude to take with published material, including systematic reviews, is one of hard-nosed scepticism, whatever the status of the publication. This attitude is based on our understanding of the uncertain and provisional nature of scientific and professional knowledge, as outlined in Chapter 1. In addition, health researchers deal with the investigation of complex phenomena, where it is often impossible for ethical reasons to exercise the desired levels of control or to collect crucial information required to arrive at definitive conclusions. The conduct of a valid critique requires that we compare the methods used by the researchers with the rules of evidence in the context of a research project. Critical evaluation identifies the strengths and weaknesses of a research publication, to ensure that patients receive assessment and treatment based on the best available evidence.

The aim of this chapter is to discuss the evaluation of published research. The chapter is organized around the evaluation of the specific sections of research publications.

The specific aims of this chapter are to:

1. Examine the criteria used for the critical evaluation of a research paper.
2. Discuss the implications of identifying problems in design and analysis in a given publication.
3. Outline briefly strategies for summarizing and analysing evidence from a set of papers.
4. Discuss the implications of critical evaluation of research for health care practices.

Guidelines for critical appraisal of research publications

Many textbooks on health research methodology or evidence-based health care provide guidelines for the critical appraisal of published research. For example, Hicks (2009) suggested a list of questions relevant for conducting rigorous appraisals and provided a detailed sample critique of a health research publication. Critical appraisal is an essential step in conducting evidence-based health care (see Ch. 24). Consequently, textbooks in this area devote chapters to explaining critical evaluations. For example, Dawes et al (2005) provide detailed guidelines for critiquing publications based on different types of designs, including randomized controlled trials (RCTs), case-control and cohort studies and systematic reviews.

There are also numerous websites hosted by reputable organizations for facilitating the appraisal of published evidence. A useful online example is the University of South Australia Division of Health Sciences International Centre for Allied Health (http://www.unisa.edu.au/cahe/resources/cat/defa ult.asp) which is dedicated to the critical evaluation of published research.

Some groups created critical appraisal schemes which attempt to produce numerical scores to represent methodological quality. For example, the Downs and Black quality index generates an overall score out of 21 to represent the quality of a publication. Publications with low scores may be excluded from systematic reviews or attributed with poor credibility. While such quantitative approaches are followed by some reviewers to identify risk of bias (e.g. Soares-Weiser et al 2010; see Ch. 4) it is worth noting that the critical appraisal of published research is not easily qualified. Rather, health researchers or practitioners need to make critical judgements based on their personal knowledge, experience and work contexts.

Table 23.1 summarizes some of the potential problems, and their implications, which might emerge in the context-critical evaluation of an investigation. A point which must be kept in mind is that, even where an investigation is flawed, useful knowledge might be drawn from it. The aim of critical analysis is not to discredit or tear down published work, but to ensure that the reader understands its implications and limitations with respect to theory and practice. In this chapter we will focus on the constructive, critical evaluation of each stage of the research process as identified in Chapter 3.

Critical evaluation of the introduction in a research paper

The introduction of a paper essentially reflects the planning of the research. Inadequacies in this section might signal that the research project was erroneously conceived or poorly planned. The following issues are essential for evaluating this section.

Adequacy of the literature review

The literature review must be sufficiently complete, including all relevant publications, so that it accurately presents the current state of knowledge in the area. Key papers should not be omitted, particularly when their results could have direct relevance to the research hypotheses or aims. Researchers must be unbiased in presenting evidence that is unfavourable to their personal points of view. This is why we now have systematic review procedures, such as those utilized by the Cochrane Collaboration, so as to avoid inappropriate and biased exclusion or inclusion of work that supports or challenges a point of view favoured by the researcher or other researchers who hold contrary opinions. Poor review of the literature could lead to needlessly repeating research or making mistakes that could have been avoided if the previous works' findings had been incorporated into formulation of the research design.

Clearly defined aims or hypotheses

As stated in Chapter 4, the aims or hypotheses of the research should be clearly stated. If this clarity

Table 23.1 Checklist for evaluating published research

Problems which might be identified	Possible implications in a research article
1. Inadequate literature review	Misrepresentation of the conceptual basis for the research
2. Vague aims or hypotheses	Research might lack direction; interpretation of evidence might be ambiguous
3. Inappropriate research strategy	Findings might not be relevant to the problem being investigated
4. Inappropriate variables selected	Measurements might not be related to concepts being investigated
5. Inadequate sampling method	Sample might be biased; investigation could lack external validity
6. Inadequate sample size	Sample might be biased; statistical analysis might lack power
7. Inadequate description of sample	Application of findings to specific groups or individuals might be difficult
8. Instruments lack validity or reliability	Findings might represent measurement errors
9. Inadequate design	Investigation might lack internal validity; i.e. outcomes might be due to uncontrolled extraneous variables
10. Lack of adequate control groups	Investigation might lack internal validity; size of the effect difficult to estimate
11. Biased participant assignment	Investigation might lack internal validity
12. Variations or lack of control of treatment parameters	Investigation might lack internal validity
13. Observer bias not controlled (Rosenthal effects)	Investigation might lack internal and external validity
14. Participant expectations not controlled (Hawthorne effects)	Investigation might lack internal and external validity
15. Research carried out in inappropriate setting	Investigation might lack ecological validity
16. Confounding of times at which observations and treatments are carried out	Possible series effects; investigation might lack internal validity
17. Inadequate presentation of descriptive statistics	The nature of the empirical findings might not be comprehensible
18. Inappropriate statistics used to describe and/or analyse data	Distortion of the decision process; false inferences might be drawn
19. Erroneous calculation of statistics	False inferences might be drawn
20. Drawing incorrect inferences from the data analysis (e.g. type II error)	False conclusions might be made concerning the outcome of an investigation
21. Protocol deviations	Investigation might lack external or internal validity
22. Over-generalization of findings	External validity might be threatened
23. Confusing statistical and clinical significance	Treatments lacking clinical usefulness might be encouraged
24. Findings not logically related to previous research findings	Theoretical significance of the investigation remains doubtful

in expression of the aims is lacking, then the rest of the paper will be compromised. In a quantitative research project, it is usual to see a clear statement of the hypotheses as well as the research aims. All research, whether qualitative or quantitative, should have a clear and recognizable statement of aim(s).

Selection of an appropriate research strategy

In formulating the aims of the investigation, the researcher must consider the best research strategy. For instance, if the demonstration of causal effects is required (e.g. the treatment caused the improvement), a survey method may be inadequate for the aims of the research. If the purpose of the study is to explore the personal interpretations and meanings of participants then a qualitative strategy will be best. Some researchers now advocate mixed designs where multiple studies using different methods are performed to examine different perspectives of the same issues. Essentially, the critical appraisal of research is an examination of the extent to which researchers have selected the appropriate research method.

Selection of appropriate variables/information to be collected

In a quantitative study, if the selection of the variables is inappropriate to the aims or questions being investigated, then the investigation will not produce useful results. Similarly, in a qualitative study, the information to be collected must be appropriate to the research aims and questions.

Critical evaluation of the methods section in a research paper

A well-documented methods section is a necessary condition for understanding, evaluating and perhaps replicating a research project. In general, the critical evaluation of this section will allow a judgement of the validity of the investigation to be made.

Research participants

This section shows if the study participants were representative of the intended target group or population and the adequacy of the sampling model used.

Sampling model used

In Chapter 5, we outlined a number of sampling models that can be employed to optimize the representativeness of a study sample. If the sampling model is inappropriate, then the sample might be unrepresentative, raising questions concerning the external validity of the research findings. In qualitative research, although the participant sampling method may be less formal than in a quantitative study, the issue of representativeness is still pertinent in terms of being able to apply the results.

Sample size/number of participants

Use of a small sample is not necessarily a serious problem, provided the sample is representative. However, given a highly diverse population, a small sample may not be adequate to ensure representativeness of the study sample when compared to the population (see Ch. 5). A small sample size decreases the power of the statistical analysis in a quantitative study (see Ch. 21). As discussed in Chapter 5, unlike in quantitative sampling procedures, sometimes there is disagreement among qualitative researchers as to the issue of how many participants are needed.

Description of the study participants

A clear description of key participant characteristics (e.g. age, sex, type and severity of their condition) should be provided. When necessary and possible, demographic information concerning the population from which the participants have been drawn should be provided. If not, the reader cannot adequately judge the representativeness of the sample.

Instruments/apparatus/tools

The validity and reliability of observations and/or measurements are important for good research. In this section, the investigator must demonstrate the adequacy of the tools used for the data collection.

Validity and reliability

A quantitative investigator should use standardized tools, or establish the validity and reliability of new tools used. A lack of proven validity and reliability will raise questions about the adequacy of the research findings (see Ch. 14). A full description of the structure and use of novel tools should be presented so that they can be replicated.

Procedure

A full description of how the investigation was carried out is required for both replication and for the evaluation of its internal and external validity. The requirement of providing a clear and explicit rationale for the research applies to both qualitative and quantitative studies.

Adequacy of the research design

It was stated previously that a good design should minimize alternative conflicting interpretations of the data collected. For quantitative research aimed at studying causal relationships, poor design will result in uncontrolled influences by extraneous variables, muddying the identification of causal effects. In Section 3, we looked at a variety of threats to internal validity which must be considered when critically evaluating an investigation. In a qualitative study the theoretical approach taken in the study design or approach should be clearly stated (see Chs 4 & 10).

Control groups in causal research

When the aim is to identify causal factors in quantitative research, a common way of controlling for bias and confounding effects is the use of control groups (e.g. placebo, no treatment, conventional treatment). If control groups are not employed, then the internal validity of the investigation might be questioned. Also, if placebo or untreated groups are not present, the size of the effect due to the treatments might be difficult to estimate (see Ch. 7).

Participant assignment

When using experimental designs such as RCTs, care must be taken in the assignment of participants so as to avoid significant initial differences between treatment groups. Even when quasi-experimental or natural comparison strategies are used, care must be taken to establish the equivalence of the groups. Whenever possible, intervention studies should use double- or single-blind procedures. If the participants, researchers or observers are aware of the aims and predicted outcomes of the investigation, then the validity of the investigation will be threatened through bias and expectancy effects. In qualitative research, it is very important that the research findings are not unduly influenced by the personal positions of the researchers in a way that obscures the meanings and interpretations of the research participants. Of course, the position of the researcher in any study, whether qualitative or quantitative, will to some extent influence the findings but this needs to be kept to a minimum.

Treatment parameters

It is important to describe all the treatments or interventions given to the different groups. If the treatments differ in intensity, or the administering personnel take different approaches, the internal validity of the project is threatened. The adherence of the study in the delivery of the intervention to the intended intervention is sometimes called *treatment fidelity*. In studies aiming to demonstrate the efficacy, the sequence of any treatments and observations must be clearly indicated, so that issues such as confounding variables and bias can be detected (see Ch. 7). Identification of variability in treatment and observation times can influence the internal validity of experimental, quasi-experimental or $n = 1$ designs, resulting in inaccurate decisions (see Chs 7–9).

Settings

The setting in which a study is carried out has implications for external (ecological) validity. An adequate description of the setting is necessary for evaluating the generalizability of the findings. The context of the investigation may have important effects on the study outcomes. Research conducted in the investigator's lab or office may yield different results to the same work conducted in the field (see Ch. 5). The accurate description of settings is a particularly important consideration when appraising qualitative research. The meaning of personal experiences is very much dependent on time, place and culture (see Chs 2, 10 & 22).

Critical evaluation of the results section in a research paper

The results of quantitative studies are analysed using descriptive and inferential statistics (see Chs 15–21). Inadequacies in statistical analysis result in misinterpretation of the research findings.

Tables and graphs

Data should be correctly tabulated or drawn and adequately labelled for interpretation. Complete summaries of all the relevant findings should be presented.

Selection of statistics

Where appropriate both descriptive and inferential statistics must be selected according to specific rules. The selection of inappropriate statistics could distort the findings and lead to inappropriate inferences.

Calculation of statistics

Clearly, both descriptive and inferential statistics must be correctly calculated. The use of computers generally ensures this, although some attention must be paid to gross errors when evaluating the data presented. Effect sizes and confidence intervals are essential statistics for evaluating the clinical significance of the results. If these statistics are not provided the reader may be unable to apply the results to a practical setting (see Ch. 21).

Methods of qualitative analysis

The methods chosen must complement the theoretical approach taken in the study and be performed according to the specified protocols (see Ch. 22).

Critical evaluation of the discussion section in a research paper

In the discussion section the investigators interpret the evidence with reference to the initial aims, research question and hypotheses of the investigation. Incorrect interpretation of the evidence may lead to distortions of knowledge and ineffective practices being offered to clients.

Drawing correct inferences from the collected information/data

The inferences from the collected information or data must take into account the limitations of the study and the analytical methods used to analyse them. In the quantitative domain we have seen, for instance in Chapter 18, that correlations do not necessarily imply causation, or that a lack of significance in the statistical analysis could imply a type II error or incorrect missing of a real trend or finding (see Ch. 21). In the qualitative domain, the findings must follow reasonably from the information collected in the investigation according to the paradigm used (see Ch. 22).

Logically correct interpretations of the research findings

Interpretations of the findings must follow from the information collected, without extraneous evidence being introduced. For instance, if the investigation used a single-participant design, the conclusions should not claim that a procedure is generally useful for the entire population.

Research protocol deviations

In interpreting the data or information collected in a study, the investigator must indicate, and take into account, unexpected deviations from the intended research protocols. For instance, in a quantitative study a placebo/active treatment code might be broken, or 'contamination' between control and experimental groups might be discovered. In a qualitative study, it could be that participants have conversed with each other about the research prior to one of the participants completing participation. If such deviations are discovered by investigators, they are obliged to report these, so that the implications for the results might be taken into account.

Generalization from the findings to the population

Strictly speaking, the data obtained from a given sample are generalizable only to the population from which the participants were drawn. This point is sometimes ignored by investigators and the findings are generalized to participants or situations which were not considered in the original sampling plan. Qualitative researchers may vary in their willingness to claim generalizability of their findings outside the actual research participants, but this must also be systematically considered.

Statistical and clinical significance of the results

As explained in Chapter 21, in quantitative studies, obtaining statistical significance does not necessarily imply that the results of an investigation are clinically applicable or useful. In deciding on clinical significance, factors such as the size of the effect, side effects and cost-effectiveness, as well as value judgements of patients concerning outcome, must be considered.

Theoretical significance of the evidence

It is necessary to relate the results of an investigation to previous relevant findings that have been identified in the literature review. Unless the results are logically related to the literature, the theoretical significance of the investigation remains unclear. The processes involved in comparing the findings of a set of related papers are introduced in Chapter 24.

Summary

A critical approach to appraisal refers to making *judgements* concerning the validity of research projects and evaluating their contribution to knowledge and practice. Our judgements are based on the application of the principles of research to analysing a specific research paper or as a set of related research papers. This is obviously the reason why you need to understand the basic principles before you can conduct a valid critique. The critical approach is not at all negative or destructive but is an essential component of constructing knowledge based on the best available evidence. Being capable of conducting a methodological critique is an essential skill for practitioners committed to evidence-based health care.

Even when some problems are identified with a given research report, it is nevertheless likely that the report will provide some useful additional knowledge. Given the problems of generalization, an individual research project is usually insufficient for firmly deciding upon the truth of an hypothesis or the usefulness of a clinical intervention. Rather, as we will see in Chapter 24, the reader needs to scrutinize the range of relevant research and summarize the evidence using qualitative and quantitative review methods. In this way, individual research results can be evaluated in the context of the research area. Disagreements or controversies are ultimately useful for generating hypotheses for guiding new research and for advancing theory and practice.

Synthesis: systematic reviews and meta-analyses

24

CHAPTER CONTENTS

Introduction 199

Basic principles 200

Narrative reviews of research evidence 200

Systematic reviews 201

   Research questions 201

   Theoretical framework
for systematic reviews 201

   Search strategy for systematic reviews . . 201

   Appraisal and selection
of key papers for the review 202

   Coding the included research studies . . . 202

   Interpretation of the research evidence . . 203

Meta-analysis 203

   Extracting data from individual studies . . 204

   Combining data from diverse studies . . . 204

   Interpreting the results of a meta-analysis. 204

Validity of systematic reviews. 206

   Sampling. 206

   Extracting the data. 207

   The state of the research program. 207

The Cochrane Collaboration 207

   Evidence-based practice 207

Summary. 208

Introduction

The research papers published in scientific and professional peer-reviewed journals are the most important source of research for driving evidence-based health care. Each research publication contributes to the overall knowledge base for describing, understanding and solving health problems. However, an individual research project is usually insufficient for firmly deciding the truth of a research hypothesis or determining the efficacy of a clinical intervention. In order to have more soundly based evidence we need to compare, contrast and synthesize the results of research papers dealing with the same topic. Consistent results across diverse research studies provide a sounder basis for justifying the evidence-based delivery of health services.

The term 'research literature' refers to the set of publications containing the network of theories, hypotheses, practices and evidence representing the current state of knowledge in a specific area of the health sciences. A literature review contains both the critical evaluation of the individual publications and the identification of emergent trends and patterns of evidence based upon these studies. The literature review is a synthesis of the available knowledge in an area and therefore constitutes the strongest foundation for initiating further advances in theory and practice.

The overall aim of this chapter is to outline the basic strategies used for synthesizing evidence and producing a literature review.

The specific aims of the chapter are to:

1. Identify the basic methodological principles relevant to writing a health sciences review.
2. Describe the process for conducting a narrative review.

3. Describe the process for conducting a systematic review.
4. Explain how to interpret the findings of a published meta-analysis.
5. Explain the uses and limitations of systematic reviews and meta-analyses.

Basic principles

The first thing to consider is that writing a literature review is a demanding intellectual challenge. The facts do not 'speak' for themselves. Rather, the evidence has to be extracted, critically evaluated, organized and synthesized into a logical, coherent representation of the current state of knowledge. For example, consider the review by Olanow (2004) titled 'The scientific basis for the current treatment of Parkinson's disease'. This relatively brief 15-page review is based on only 75 references, although there are thousands of research papers, articles and reports available on the anatomy, physiology and treatment of Parkinson's disease. In writing the review, the author had to make a series of expert judgements regarding which were the nine key papers, containing the most salient, up-to-date information for understanding the medical treatment of Parkinson's disease. Many papers were rejected.

Second, the outcome of the review process is influenced by the theoretical orientation and professional background of the reviewer. Olanow, a leading neurologist, provided an authoritative review written from a biomedical perspective. In contrast, a physiotherapist working in neurological rehabilitation might take a different conceptual approach to the causes and treatment of Parkinson's disease. He or she might place more emphasis on psychological and social factors as integral components of the aetiology and treatment of Parkinson's disease.

Third, the selection, analysis, critique and synthesis of the materials is an active, interpretive process drawing on the personal experiences, interests and values of the reviewer. Even if their professional backgrounds are identical, there are no guarantees that two reviewers interpreting the evidence from the same set of publications will arrive at exactly the same conclusions. Depending on how these reviewers approached the subject matter, they might emphasize different aspects of the evidence or select different patterns in the data as being important, resulting in different syntheses. In Chapter 1, we discussed the post-positivist position that theories

and preconceptions can influence our perceptions of what is happening in the world, and therefore shape the way in which we construct knowledge.

Last, the notion that we all have our experiences, opinions and prejudices does not imply that 'anything goes' when writing health sciences reviews. On the contrary, we need to apply the principles of scientific methodology to ensure that we provide an accurate overview of the literature. In other words, there are principles that we must follow in preparing a literature review.

As stated before, in preparing literature reviews and evaluating research findings, a multiplicity of papers must be considered, at least according to the following general steps:

1. Identify relevant literature; select key papers.
2. Critically evaluate key papers, as discussed in this section. You might decide to discard some papers if irreparable problems are discovered.
3. Identify general patterns of findings in the literature. Tabulate findings, where appropriate.
4. Identify crucial disagreements and controversies.
5. Propose valid explanations for the disagreements. Such explanations provide a theoretical framework for resolving controversies and proposing future research.
6. Provide a clear summary concerning the state of the literature, identifying progress, obstacles and further research.

Narrative reviews of research evidence

There are several approaches to conducting health sciences reviews. For example, the previously mentioned review by Olanow (2004) can be classified as a 'narrative' review. This approach entails producing a 'story-like' overview of the state of current evidence and theories. A narrative approach to reviewing literature means that the review is conducted in a story-telling fashion. Narrative reviews are basically of two kinds: those where the review constitutes the entirety of the paper, and those which are only part of the paper, and are integrated into the introductory section of a paper that reports a research study. Narrative reviews have an important place in the evidence base for health practice. For instance:

- A narrative review is an essential part of the 'Introduction' section of all reports of research studies. The review outlines the current state of knowledge, identifies gaps in that knowledge, justifies the research in terms of its capacity to advance knowledge and practice, and provides that background and the rationale for the research questions.

- A narrative review is also an essential first step for constructing models and theories. The review is used to identify and synthesize available evidence and then to demonstrate the 'fit' between the proposed conceptual framework (theory) and the facts.
- A narrative review can also be of use for the purpose of identifying current best practice in preventing and treating a particular health problem.

The quality of narrative reviews varies, given that the analysis, critique and synthesis of the material is an active process, which draws on the creativity and intellectual style of the reviewer. There is no guarantee that two people interpreting the evidence from the same set of papers will produce identical syntheses. Depending on how individuals approach the subject matter of a field, they may emphasize different aspects of the evidence or select different patterns in the data, resulting in a potentially different overall conclusion. In the extreme, some health workers hold biased theoretical and ideological positions to such an extent that the meaning of the evidence could be completely distorted (e.g. a medical scientist employed by a tobacco company, who reviews literature relating to the health risks). There are various sources explaining how to conduct reviews (see, for example, http://www.prisma-statement.org/).

Systematic reviews

Although reviewers generally adhere to the principles of science and logic in conducting a narrative review, there have been concerns about bias in the selection of evidence to be included and lack of clarity. More recently, systematic reviews and meta-analyses have been introduced to enhance the rigour for combining and interpreting the state of the literature. Systematic reviews rely on the explicit use of the methodological principles discussed in previous chapters. In effect, systematic reviews follow the problem-solving approach as used for conducting empirical research as outlined

in Chapter 3. Let us examine a published example (Polgar et al 2003) to illustrate the logic and principles underlying the conduct of systematic reviews.

Research questions

When conducting a systematic review, we are expected to formulate a clear review research question that will be answered by the outcomes of the review. You might have read about the research using embryonic or stem cells for reconstructing the brains of people suffering from neurological conditions such as stroke and Parkinson's disease. We were interested in reviewing the evidence for answering the research question 'How effective is reconstructive neurosurgery (i.e. the grafting of immature cells) for improving the signs and symptoms of Parkinson's disease?' (Polgar et al 2003).

Theoretical framework for systematic reviews

Although this principle is not adhered to by all reviewers, it is very useful to specify the theoretical framework(s) which guides a specific review. The theoretical framework used for conducting the review was identified as the 'Repair Model'. This is a purely biomedical, quantitative view of neural reconstruction based on the notion that recovery is due to the replacement of dopaminergic cells damaged in Parkinson's disease. An explicit theoretical framework is essential for understanding a given area of health as a coherent research program (see Ch. 1).

Search strategy for systematic reviews

The next step is to identify the relevant publications. Several issues are relevant to devising a search strategy. First, a number of different sets of key terms are used to conduct the electronic search in order to 'match' these terms with those in the papers in the different online databases (e.g. Medline, Embase, CINAHL, etc.). A 'hand search' of current conference proceedings is conducted as a double check for key authors. In general the reviewer should have available at least two to three key papers that can be included in the review. For example, in Polgar et al (2003) we conducted the following search:

> A search of Medline (1994–2000 and 2000/01–2000/10) using the exploded terms 'fetal tissue transplantation', 'Parkinson's disease, human or fetal tissue transplants', 'Parkinson's disease, human', also using the author 'Kopyov' was conducted. In conjunction with this search, abstracts from the American Society for Neural Transplantation and Repair conferences (1999, 2000) were hand searched for authors that may have been overlooked. The reference lists of key papers were searched to identify papers that might not have been identified through on-line search mechanisms. An additional electronic search was conducted using the following databases: Medline (1966–March Week 2, 2001), Embase (1994–April Week 1, 2001), CINAHL (1982–March Week 2, 2001).

The general point here is that reviewers must be diligent in identifying all the publications which constitute the literature in the area targeted for review. The search should include both 'electronic, on-line searches' and 'hand' searches of key journals for cross-checking if the relevant papers were identified by the search engines. It is essential to have a working knowledge of who the key researchers are in a particular field and what critical issues exist in a research program before we can undertake a formal published review.

Appraisal and selection of key papers for the review

Critical appraisal refers to applying the principles of design, sampling, measurement and analysis to make judgements about the quality of research evidence (see Ch. 23). Depending on the area of health sciences being reviewed, literature searches might yield any number of publications, from one or two to many hundreds. Relying on the outcome of the search, the reviewers might re-state the research questions and redefine the scope of the proposed systematic review. This will expand or restrict the number of studies for further searchers. In addition, explicit inclusion/exclusion criteria are used to identify the most relevant sources. For example, Polgar et al (2003) used the following criteria for including a study in a review. In order to be included in the review, a study had to:

- be published in a peer-reviewed journal
- have transplantation surgery performed after 1993, following consensus for optimal donor characteristics

- have grafted human or embryonic cells
- have followed 'best practice' stereotactic surgery procedures
- have followed standard post-surgical assessment protocols.

It would be tedious in the present context to explain the specific reasons for each of the above selection criteria; interested readers will find that they were justified in the original review. The point is that we must have explicit, objective criteria for including or excluding studies.

The key papers function as a sample of the best available information accessible in the literature. Parallel to empirical research, we use the evidence from key papers to draw inferences about the state of knowledge in the area under review. The use of diagnostic searches and explicit inclusion/exclusion criteria ensure that the 'sample' of papers produces a representative, rather than a biased, sample of the overall knowledge.

Coding the included research studies

When the process of selecting and collecting the publications is complete, we have the available evidence relevant to answering our research question. The information that we seek is embedded in the text of research publications. We need to extract the key information from the text of each of the papers selected for the review. We can approach the analysis of the meaning of this information in a way that is similar to qualitative data analysis (see Ch. 22). Similarly to the predetermined codes used in content analysis, reviewers use the constant features of quantitative research for identifying the categories appropriate for analysing the key papers. These features include:

1. The design of the studies.
2. The sampling strategies used and the sample characteristics.
3. The ways in which the treatment or intervention was administered.
4. The data collection strategy used (i.e. the measurement strategy).
5. The statistical and clinical significance of the results.

Other dimensions or features might also be coded or the above features can be modified according

Table 24.1 Compliance with insulin use by diabetics (hypothetical example)

Publication	Sample size	Average age of patients (years)	Method of measuring compliance	Percentage of patients compliant
Smith (2000)	50	55	Self-report	85
Jones (2001)	60	58	Self-report	82
Brown (2001)	50	59	Blood sugar level	40
Miller (2002)	55	56	Blood sugar level	35

to the judgements of the authors. These aspects of the research process are often presented in a table form, as shown in Table 24.1. We used a hypothetical example rather than the previous published review.

To illustrate coding, consider a set of four hypothetical studies reporting on levels of diabetic patients' compliance to self-injection of insulin. The results and key features of the hypothetical studies are tabulated in Table 24.1.

Table 24.1 represents how findings from several publications might be tabulated. Key information about each study, as well as the outcomes, is presented in the table, enabling the emergence and demonstration of an overall pattern to be seen.

Interpretation of the research evidence

The coding of the hypothetical studies enables the reviewer to answer the research question: 'How compliant are patients with diabetes with using insulin?' The hypothetical summarized evidence illustrates that sometimes no clear overall trends emerge from the tabulated findings.

In the simple hypothetical example shown in Table 24.1, the percentage of compliance reported by Smith (2000) and Jones (2001) is over twice that reported by Brown (2001) and Miller (2002). Clearly, there is an inconsistency in the literature. A possible explanation for this discrepancy might emerge by inspection of Table 24.1. Neither differences in sample size nor the average ages of the patients provide an explanation for the difference. However, the method by which compliance was measured emerges as a plausible explanation. The investigators Smith and Jones relied on the patients' self-reports and might have overestimated compliance levels, in contrast to Brown and Miller,

who used a more objective method and found poor levels of compliance. Of course, this explanation is not necessarily true, but is simply an hypothesis to guide future investigations of the problem. There are other possibilities which might account for the pattern of findings. It appears that more research is needed.

Meta-analysis

Dooley (2001) discussed the availability of different strategies for summarizing research findings from multiple studies:

1. *Qualitative*. A qualitative review involves the selection of key features of related publications such as designs, participant characteristics or measures used in the studies. These features are presented in a table form, such that differences in the features of the research can be related to outcomes. The qualitative reviews identified by Dooley (2001) are related to the systematic reviews, as we discussed above.

2. *Quantitative*. A quantitative review calls for the condensation of the results from several papers into a single statistic. This statistic represents an overall or pooled effect size. These procedures are meta-analyses which are systematic procedures for summarizing the results published in a set of research papers.

Although many statistical procedures can be used for synthesizing data, meta-analysis also refers to an active area of statistics examining strategies most suitable for synthesizing published evidence. Statisticians have developed software packages such as 'Comprehensive Meta-Analysis' which expedite the computational difficulties entailed in synthesizing evidence from diverse studies (http://www.metaanalysis.com).

Extracting data from individual studies

The basic requirement for a meta-analysis is extraction of equivalent results from the individual studies. If the studies have different outcome measures, then the meta-analysis is difficult (although not necessarily impossible) to perform. The clearest approach is to extract data which is measured in exactly the same way, across these studies. For example, pain can be assessed in a number of different ways. These include: in terms of a dichotomy (e.g. whether the person is experiencing pain or is pain free); by rating the self-perceived intensity of the pain on a scale of 1–10; by rating the intensity on a visual analogue scale from zero to 100; by measuring the amount of analgesia required to remain pain free. The optimal situation for synthesizing results across two or more related studies on pain is one where the pain outcomes were measured in the same way in each of the studies.

The size of the effect of the intervention (or the effect size) is of primary interest when synthesizing the results of randomized controlled trials (RCTs) using a meta-analysis. There are a number of measures of effect size for both dichotomous outcomes (e.g. experiencing pain, pain free) and continuous outcome measures (e.g. ratings of pain on a scale of 1–10). Some of these measures of effect size are discussed below. When synthesizing the results of several RCTs, the same effect size measures are preferable.

Combining data from diverse studies

How are results synthesized? Let us look at a simple example for combining data. Say that you are interested in the average age of the participants in three related studies: A, B and C (Table 24.2).

Say we wish to calculate the average age for all the 230 participants in the three studies. Could we calculate the overall mean, $\overline{X}$, simply by adding up the three means and dividing by three? The answer is no, because there are different numbers of participants across the groups. We must give a weight to each of the statistics depending on 'n', the sample size for each study. The equation which we use is:

$$\overline{X} = \frac{(\overline{X}_A \times n_A) + (\overline{X}_B \times n_B) + (\overline{X}_C \times n_C)}{n_A + n_B + n_C}$$

$$= \frac{(40 \times 80) + (45 \times 50) + (60 \times 100)}{80 + 50 + 100}$$

$$= 49.8$$

The point here is that, in order to calculate the correct overall statistics, we must give a weight to each study. In general, the weight assigned to a study represents the proportion of information the study contributes to the overall analysis. For the above calculation, weight was determined by the sample size used in each study. In general the weight assigned to a study represents the proportion of the information contributing to the calculation of the overall statistic.

Even the calculation of a simple statistic like 'average overall age' can be useful for understanding the state of a research program. For instance, in Polgar et al (2003) we found that the mean age of Parkinson's disease sufferers was 56 years, with the mean overall duration of the illness being 13 years. These results indicated that the average age of onset of the disease was only about 43 years, indicating that experimental reconstructive neurosurgery has been offered to an unrepresentative sample of Parkinson's disease sufferers. Typically people with Parkinson's disease are in their late sixties or early seventies.

Of course we need to synthesize other clinically and theoretically relevant statistics appearing across the papers constituting a research program, including the overall pooled standard deviation, the overall statistical significance, the overall effect size and the confidence intervals for the overall effect sizes. These analyses are best carried out using statistical software packages. You can check the Internet for further information regarding the logic of meta-analysis and currently available software packages.

Interpreting the results of a meta-analysis

There are different ways for conducting and reporting the results of meta-analyses which have become quite frequent in the health sciences literature. A

Table 24.2 Participants' ages in three hypothetical studies

Study	Number of participants (n)	Average age ($\overline{X}$)
A	80	40
B	50	45
C	100	60

typical way of presenting the results is shown in Figures 24.1 and 24.2, which show the hypothetical outcome of a computer-assisted meta-analysis (modified from www.metaanalysis.com). The graphics shown in these figures are referred to as 'forest plots'. A forest plot is a visual representation of the results of a meta-analysis.

Say that the printout showed the results of five randomized double-blind trials (see Ch. 5) aiming to demonstrate the effectiveness of a vaccine for influenza. In each of the studies volunteers were given either the vaccine (treated) or a placebo (control) injection. The following features of Figures 24.1 and 24.2 are important for interpreting the outcomes of a meta-analysis.

Studies

Following searching and critical analysis of the relevant literature, as discussed previously, the reviewer selected the five papers shown. If you look carefully at the sample sizes in each of the groups under treated (odds) and control (odds), you will find that the sample sizes are not equal. If they represent randomized trials, you might ask why the groups were unequal in the studies. Sometimes unequal groups represent people dropping out because of harmful side effects to the treatment.

Effect

The effect size was represented as an odds ratio (OR), which is a commonly used statistic for outcomes measured on a nominal scale. For this measure the outcome is diagnosed with influenza following vaccination or placebo over, say, 6 months: 'yes' or 'no'. Looking at the first (English) study, the odds of 'yes' to 'no' are 30/530 for the treated group and 40/540 in the control group. The statistical software package computed an OR of 0.750, indicating a slight reduction in the odds of contracting influenza. Note that an OR = 1 means equal odds or no difference at all, while decreasing OR under 1.0 favours treatment. For example, an OR of 0.5 would indicate that the vaccination halved the odds for contracting influenza in the sample.

Confidence intervals

As we discussed in Chapter 17, a 95% confidence interval contains the true population parameter at $p = 0.95$. The lines produced from the 'squares' containing the sample OR represent the 95% confidence intervals. You can see in Figure 24.1 that all the confidence intervals for the five studies overlap with 1.0, indicating that we cannot infer that the studies favour the treatment.

Weights and totals

When you look at the 'odds' columns in Figures 24.1 and 24.2, you can see that there is a variation in the sample sizes used in the hypothetical studies. For example, the 'Scottish' study included 12 200 participants, while the 'US' study included only 300 participants. These differences

Study	Year	Effect size	Treated (odds)	Control (odds)	0.1	0.2	0.5	1.0	2	5	10
English study	2000	0.750	30 / 530	40 / 540							
Canadian study	2001	1.406	45 / 445	40 / 540							
Scottish study	2002	0.833	500 / 5500	600 / 5600							
Australian study	2002	0.875	210 / 2210	240 / 2240							
US study	2000	0.667	20 / 120	30 / 130							
Total		0.857	805 / 8805	950 / 9050			Favours treatment		Favours placebo		

Figure 24.1 • Results of a hypothetical meta-analysis: negative findings.

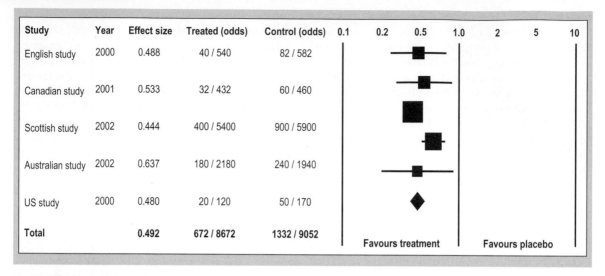

Study	Year	Effect size	Treated (odds)	Control (odds)
English study	2000	0.488	40 / 540	82 / 582
Canadian study	2001	0.533	32 / 432	60 / 460
Scottish study	2002	0.444	400 / 5400	900 / 5900
Australian study	2002	0.637	180 / 2180	240 / 1940
US study	2000	0.480	20 / 120	50 / 170
Total		0.492	672 / 8672	1332 / 9052

Figure 24.2 • Results of a hypothetical meta-analysis: positive findings.

contribute to the relative 'weight' of the study represented graphically by the area of the 'squares' in the forest plots. Clearly, the larger the square, the greater the sample size. You will also note that the confidence intervals are wider with the smaller squares in comparison to the larger squares. As discussed in Chapter 20, the larger the sample size, the more 'power' we have for making accurate inferences.

The 'Totals' in Figures 24.1 and 24.2 refer to the overall statistics synthesized from the results of the five hypothetical studies. These statistics are represented by the diamond shapes on the forest plots. In Figure 24.1 the total OR was 0.857, indicating a very weak effect for the vaccination. The OR is close to 1 or equal 'odds' for having influenza. For the results shown in Figure 24.2, the total OR was 0.492. This represents a strong effect, indicating that the odds for contracting influenza would have been more than halved by the vaccination. Such results are suggestive of the clinical or practical significance of introducing the treatment.

Validity of systematic reviews

The interpretation of the results of published meta-analyses is far more difficult than indicated in the above example. Let us look at some of the sources of difficulties.

Sampling

The results reported in the papers selected for review generally represent a sample of the total information published in a field. This leads us to the first problem: studies that do not report statistically significant findings are often not submitted or accepted for publication. By not having access to these 'negative' findings, the selection of papers becomes biased towards those with reported 'positive' outcomes. Also, in published research papers where outcomes for multiple dependent variables are reported, only the statistically significant outcomes are reported, undermining attempts to synthesize the evidence accurately (Polgar et al 2003).

In addition, the exclusion/inclusion criteria used for selecting the studies can result in a sampling bias. Some practitioners of evidence-based medicine (e.g. Sackett et al 2000) are reluctant to include studies which have not adopted a randomized experimental design. While this approach has strong methodological justifications, valuable information can be lost by using highly selective inclusion criteria. Of course, the more information that is lost, the weaker the external validity of the review or meta-analysis in relation to the 'population' of research results constituting a research program. The reduced external validity is a trade-off for including only methodologically stronger studies in the review.

Extracting the data

Another source of error arises when extracting the data from an individual meta-analysis. Some authors report very clear, descriptive statistics but others report their results in an obscure, uninterpretable fashion. Also, some journals and authors only discuss the statistical significance of the results. Obscure and incomplete reporting of the evidence leads to errors in synthesizing overall statistics.

The state of the research program

The validity of a systematic review or meta-analysis is limited by the methodological rigour and statistical accuracy of the studies selected for review. To put it bluntly, many health-related problems cannot be resolved and questions cannot be answered on the basis of the currently available evidence. An inconclusive systematic review or meta-analysis is not necessarily a waste of time. Although inconclusive attempts to synthesize data cannot be used to make valid clinical decisions, they provide strong evidence for gaps in knowledge and provide objective grounds for identifying further research required to advance the research program (e.g. Polgar et al 2003). Until better evidence becomes available we simply provide the best practices suggested by tradition and experience.

The Cochrane Collaboration

Cochrane (1972), a Scottish medical practitioner, was one of the first influential practitioners in the modern era to advocate the systematic use of evidence to inform clinical practice.

In recognition of Cochrane's pioneering work, the Cochrane Collaboration, the Cochrane Library and the Cochrane Database of Systematic Reviews were established. The Cochrane Collaboration is now a large international venture with a series of special-interest groups commissioning and maintaining reviews on a wide range of topics. There are also detailed protocols that have been established for the conduct and presentation of Cochrane systematic reviews. Although the scope of the Cochrane Database is very broad, much of it is quite focused on intervention research; that is,

what intervention approaches work best for specific health problems and populations. The database is now expanding into other areas but there is a strong intervention focus.

The Cochrane approach adheres to a hierarchy of evidence. There are five levels of evidence, with systematic reviews of multiple randomized controlled trials at the top, followed by single randomized controlled trials, evidence from trials without randomization but with pre-post, cohort or time-series measurement, evidence from non-experimental studies and, at the bottom level, opinions of respected authorities. Many reviews, however, only focus on the top two levels of the evidence categories. Obviously, because of the intervention-oriented nature of many Cochrane reviews, qualitative research, case study and policy research do not yet figure prominently in this system.

The Cochrane Database of Systematic Reviews is available on a wide range of websites in different countries. Access arrangements for the reviews vary widely from country to country. In some countries some fees are payable, but in others, such as Australia, the government has taken out a national subscription so that access may be freely available. In order to access the database, we suggest that you use a search engine to search for 'Cochrane Collaboration' and follow the links or consult your librarian.

Evidence-based practice

Although the name of evidence-based medicine or evidence-based practice is relatively new, the idea of using research evidence to inform the design of clinical interventions is very old. Muir Gray (2009) provides a very good review of this approach. Evidence-based health care has been influential in promoting the need for the systematic use of evidence to promote the delivery of high-quality health care (Sackett et al 2000).

As Muir Gray (2009) noted, evidence-based practice has at its centre three linked ideas. These are how to find and appraise evidence, how to develop the capacity for evidence-based decision-making and how to get research evidence implemented in practice. The finding and appraising of evidence draw heavily upon systems such as the Cochrane Collaboration approach where evidence is systematically collected and appraised according to pre-defined principles and protocols. However, the facilitation and implementation elements of evidence-based practice are important additions to the basic establishment of research evidence to support particular approaches in the provision of health services. The evidence-based practice movement is based upon the recognition that the mere existence of evidence for the effectiveness of particular interventions does not mean that it will necessarily be effectively implemented. This is the new element of evidence-based practice: the systematic implementation of programs based upon sound research evidence.

Summary

We have seen in this chapter that the advancement of knowledge and practice depends not only on the results of individual research projects but also on the information provided by the synthesis of the results across the literature. Where the projects share the same clinical aims and theoretical frameworks, they are said to constitute a research program. In this chapter we outlined the process of identifying and selecting publications which contain theoretically or practically relevant research findings. We argued that reviewing a research program is an active, creative process which is influenced by our expectations and attitudes. While absolute objectivity is not a realistic requirement of a reviewer, there are basic rules to ensure that the review of the evidence is carried out with a minimal degree of bias.

A systematic review of the literature proceeds by identifying the basic components of research papers for organizing the evidence. We use these dimensions to identify patterns or trends which enable us to synthesize the information and answer the research questions. When studies are sufficiently similar, their results can be condensed into single statistics such as overall effect size. In this chapter, we examined how the results of meta-analyses are interpreted.

The relationships between the state of a research program and practice are very complex. We examined hypothetical situations where there was a strong consistency in the research findings and clear trends emerging in the literature could be identified. In these cases, applying the results is relatively straightforward in that we can either adopt or reject the use of a treatment on the basis of the evidence. Systematic reviews and meta-analyses are essential means for identifying best practices available for our patients. However, even well-conceived reviews and meta-analyses can fail to identify clear trends or clinically meaningful effect sizes. When the evidence is inconclusive, we simply continue with traditional practices and identify further research required for resolving unanswered questions concerning improved efficacy. In this way research in the health sciences is a continuous process, producing better information for advancing theory and practice, as we discussed in Chapter 1 of this book.

Glossary of research terms

AB design A type of experimental design in which the participant is monitored during a baseline phase followed by an intervention phase.

ABAB design A type of experimental design in which the participant is monitored during a baseline phase followed by an intervention phase which, in turn, is followed by further baseline and intervention phases.

Abstract An abbreviated summary of a research report, generally found at the beginning of the report.

Acquiescent response mode A style of answering questions which results in the respondent choosing the middle category in a response scale.

Alternative hypothesis Sometimes also known as the experimental hypothesis. This is the hypothesis for which the researcher is trying to gain support in a statistical analysis, by rejecting the null hypothesis. The alternative hypothesis is represented by the symbol H_A or H_1.

Apparatus Any equipment or special facilities used in a research project.

Area sample A type of sampling procedure in which the units of the sample are where people live or work, rather than who they are. The researcher divides the target area into sections and then samples the sections.

Assignment The process in an experiment where the researcher allocates subjects to the various groups. Matching and random assignment are the two most common methods. The goal of assignment is to achieve identical groups.

Assignment errors A situation that arises in an experiment where the assignment or allocation of people to groups results in groups with different characteristics.

Authority An appeal to authority argument is based on the proposition that someone of high status knows best, not whether the argument is soundly based.

Bar graph A method of displaying data where the frequency of a particular category is reflected in the height of the bar in the graph.

Baseline A phase in an intervention study where the participant is receiving no intervention.

Bell-shaped curve This is the characteristic shape of the normal distribution.

Bias As all humans, health and medical researchers have hopes and expectations regarding the outcomes of a research project. We have an emotional investment in whether the data support our hypotheses or demonstrate that our interventions are effective for our patient. Bias represents the conscious or unconscious ways in which researchers influence participations and the research process resulting in the distortions of the results and drawing erroneous conclusions about the implications of the research project.

Biased sample A biased sample is one that is not representative. It does not reflect the composition of the population to which the researcher is attempting to generalize.

Case-control designs These designs involve identifying people with a targeted disease or condition (cases) and comparing them to people who do not have the disease or condition (controls). The aim is to identify relevant health-related differences between the groups.

Causal explanation An attempt to explain the occurrence of a particular phenomenon or event by identifying the cause(s).

Causality An event or factor (A) is generally argued to have caused another one (B) if the following conditions are met: (i) if (A) occurs then (B) occurs; (ii) if (A) does not occur then (B) does not occur; (iii) if (A) precedes (B) in time.

Central tendency The central tendency of a frequency distribution is the average, middle or most common score. Measures of central tendency include the mean, the median and the mode.

Chi-square (χ^2) A statistical test often used with categorical data. It is based on a comparison of the frequencies observed and the frequencies expected in the various categories.

Clinical significance Refers to the practical or applied relevance of the results. Whether or not an outcome is clinically significant is judged by health practitioners, but statistically it is expressed by the effect size. The greater the effect size, the more likely it is that a health-related factor has an impact on clinical decision making such as the selection of an intervention.

Closed-response format A method of eliciting answers from people in a questionnaire in which the researcher provides fixed response categories, e.g. yes or no.

Coding A qualitative method of analysis of materials such as interviews where categories are formed and their interrelationships examined.

Cohort studies Two or more groups (cohorts) of participants are compared over a period of time on a number of health-related outcomes. The aim of these studies is to identify factors (exposure) which are different across the groups and may be causally associated with the differences in health outcome. For example, two cohorts may differ on diet cholesterol intake (exposure) resulting in differences in the prevalence of heart disease (outcome). The internal validity of cohort studies is often problematic, as factors other than the identified exposure may be the causes of the outcome.

Complete observer A type of research strategy in which the researcher observes social interactions with no direct personal input; for example, observation via a one-way mirror or through the analysis of a video tape.

Complete participant A research strategy in which the researcher completely participates in the research setting in order to experience its characteristics.

Confidence interval The confidence interval of a sample statistic is the expected range in which the actual population value will be found, at a given level of confidence or probability.

Content validity The extent to which a test or assessment matches the real requirements of the situation' for example, a living skills assessment would have high content validity if it measured cooking, self-care, etc.

Contingency table A method of presenting the relationship between two categorical variables in the form of a table.

Continuous data Data with values that do not fall into discrete categories, e.g. measures of temperature and mass.

Control In an experiment, the researcher attempts to control or eliminate the influence of extraneous variables so that any changes or differences may be attributed solely to the intervention.

Control group In an experiment, a control group is generally a non-treatment group which is compared with the experimental group to study the effects of the intervention.

Correlation coefficient A statistic designed to measure the size and direction of the association between two variables. The values vary between 0.0 and +1.0 or −1.0.

Correlational studies Studies that are concerned with investigating the associations between variables.

Critical theory In qualitative research, critical theory explains how personal meanings and actions are influenced by the person's social environment.

Critical value of a statistic The value of the statistic (obtained from appropriate tables) that the calculated value for a given result must exceed in order to attain statistical significance.

Curvilinear correlation coefficient A measure of association between variables designed to investigate curved rather than straight-line relationships.

Data The information collected by a researcher.

Deduction A process where a general principle is applied to a particular case to explain it. For example, all humans die; this is a human, therefore he/she will die.

Deontological ethics A system of ethics which holds that some actions are, in principle, right, while others are wrong. According to this view, we must do the right thing, even when the consequences of our actions are not the best possible outcomes. For example, as health professionals we must do our best to save the life of an evil person even when we are certain that he will continue to do bad things.

Descriptive statistics Statistics designed to describe characteristics of a sample. For example, the most common or typical value or the extent of variation among such values.

Determinism The view that all events are caused by other events.

Directional hypothesis A directional hypothesis is one that asserts that differences between groups in the data will occur in a particular direction. For example, the hypothesis 'smokers die younger than non-smokers' is a directional hypothesis.

Discontinuous data Sometimes termed discrete data; variables that have discrete categories, e.g. male versus female.

Discussion A section of a research report in which the research findings are discussed.

Dispersion Sometimes known as variability: the extent to which scores in a group of scores vary. This may be measured by statistics such as the standard deviation, variance, range and semi-interquartile range.

Ecological validity The extent to which the results of a study may be generalized to the real world.

Effect size The amount of change created by an intervention, especially in an experimental study.

Empathy In qualitative research, the ability to understand the perspectives of others.

Epidemiology The study of the distribution and determinants of disease within a community.

Ethics A project is ethical to the extent that its design and execution conform to a set of standards or conventions guiding research.

Ethics committees These are groups appointed by institutions, such as a university or a hospital, consisting of professional members such as researchers, ethicists and statisticians as well as people from the community. The role of the committee is to scrutinize the ethical and methodological standards of all research proposals which involve the institution. No research can be initiated until the committee decides to approve the project. It is essential that an explicit research protocol is presented to the committee, and that researchers scrupulously implement the protocol.

Ethnography A descriptive qualitative study, often of an individual or situation, usually written from the perspective of the participant(s) in the first person.

Ethnomethodology A qualitative approach to research which involves the study of social processes associated with the ways in which people perceive, describe and explain the world.

Evidence-based health care Defined as identifying and applying currently available and methodologically valid research evidence for selecting the best available practice for assessing or treating patients.

Expected frequency In the analysis of categorical data, the expected frequency is the one that would be expected in a particular category, under certain theoretical conditions. The expected frequency of women in a sample of 100 people would be 50, if equal proportions of sexes were assumed.

Experiment A research design involving the random allocation of subjects to groups and the application of different interventions to these groups. A non-intervention control group is often employed in an experimental design. The aim of an experiment is to be able to conclude validly that differences in outcomes for the groups were caused by the different interventions.

External validity The extent to which the results of the study may be generalized to the population.

Extreme response mode A method of responding to questions in which the respondent chooses the most extreme available response categories.

Factorial design A type of research design in which combinations of several independent variables are manipulated concurrently. A 2×2 factorial design involves the manipulation of two independent variables, each with two levels.

False negative The situation that occurs when a diagnostic test indicates that the person being assessed does not have a disease when he/she actually does.

False positive The situation that occurs when a diagnostic test indicates that the person being assessed has a disease when he/she does not.

Forced-response format A method of eliciting responses to a questionnaire in which there is no middle response category. This is sometimes done to avoid acquiescent response mode.

Forest plot A graph representing the outcomes of a meta-analysis. Typically, a forest plot shows the effect size and 95% confidence intervals for the individual trials and the overall or 'pooled' effect size.

Frequency distribution The way in which scores within a given sample or population are distributed.

Frequency polygon A method of graphing frequency distributions.

Grounded theory A qualitative research approach that advocates the development of theories to explain social phenomena grounded in data, following a process of induction, deduction and verification.

Hawthorne effect An effect which results in the improvement of subjects' performances through being observed and/or social contact. An example of a placebo effect.

Hermeneutics An approach to analysing the meaning of texts in the cultural contexts in which they were originally produced.

Histogram A method of graphing frequency distributions.

History A threat to the validity of studies in which unforeseen and uncontrolled events occur to the participants during the study that are outside the control of the researcher and which may be responsible for changes in the participants.

Hypothesis A proposition advanced by the researcher which is evaluated using the data collected.

Incidence rate The occurrence of new cases of a disease or condition within a specified time frame. See also *Prevalence*.

Incidental sample A method of sampling in which the researcher takes the most conveniently available cases.

Independent variable In an experiment an independent variable is the variable or condition manipulated by the researcher.

Induction The process in which a set of observations is made and a general principle formed to explain them. For example, 'Every human I have read about eventually dies; this is a human, therefore I expect him/her to die'.

Informed consent The situation where a competent person, in possession of all the relevant facts, has agreed to participate in a research study.

Instrumentation In a study, instrumentation may be a threat to internal validity. It refers to the situation when the instrumentation changes over the period of the study, thus invalidating comparison of measured results.

Internal validity In a study, internal validity refers to the ability of the researcher to attribute differences in the groups or participants to the independent variable.

Inter-observer reliability The extent to which observers rating a particular phenomenon agree with each other.

Interrupted time series A type of research design in which a case is repeatedly measured over time to produce a series of measurements. The series is interrupted by an intervention or event, the effects of which may then be monitored by continuing the measurement series.

Interval scale A type of measurement scale with the following properties: (i) the values are distinguishable; (ii) they are ordered; (iii) the intervals between the points on the scale are equal; (iv) the zero point is not absolute, i.e. does not represent the absence of the quantity.

Interview A conversation between one or more interviewers and interviewees with the purpose of eliciting certain information.

Intra-observer reliability The extent to which an observer rating a particular phenomenon agrees with his/her own rating when presented with the same task on two different occasions.

Likert scales Likert scales are used in 'closed response' format questionnaires to quantify subjective beliefs and attitudes. Likert-like formats include a statement, e.g. 'I love statistics', followed by a five-or seven-point scale, with a neutral, middle choice; e.g. (1) strongly agree, (2) agree, (3) undecided, (4) disagree, (5) strongly disagree. We hope that you picked (1).

Literature review This is a section of a research report in which the previous research that has been done in the area is reviewed and related to the present problem being studied.

Matching In a study, subjects may be assigned to their groups using matching or random assignment. In matching in a two-group study, pairs of similar 'matched' subjects are formed and then one member of the pair is randomly assigned to one group and the other member to the other group. This ensures that the two groups have similar characteristics.

Maturation The phenomenon where participants in a study change spontaneously over time due to natural maturational changes. For example, children may grow older or an infection may spontaneously clear up.

Mean The average of a group of scores. For example, the mean of the scores 7, 8 and 9 is $(7 + 8 + 9) \div 3 = 8$. In statistical notation the mean of a sample is represented by the symbol $\overline{X}$. The mean of a population is represented by the symbol μ.

Measurement A procedure where qualities or quantities are attributed to characteristics of objects, persons or events. Weighing a patient involves a measurement process, as does a clinical judgement about whether a symptom is present or not.

Median The 'middle' score of a group of scores. For example, the median of the scores 7, 8 and 9 is 8. The median is the 50th percentile. The median is often used in preference to the mean when a group of scores contains a small number of extremely small or large scores because it is less sensitive to extreme values.

Meta-analysis Statistical approach to combining the results extracted from several related studies. The overall, pooled statistic represents the best estimate of the effect of a factor on health-related outcomes.

Mixed methods Refers to the combined use of both quantitative and qualitative methods for conducting a research project. The advantage of mixed methods is that the data produced by the study includes both objective facts and the subjective experiences of the participants.

Mode The mode is the most frequently occurring score in a group of scores. For example, the mode of the scores 7, 8, 8, 9, 10 is 8.

Mortality Used to describe a situation where some participants in a study are unable to continue in a study. This might be because they died or because they refuse to continue. If there is high mortality in a group in a study this can jeopardize the internal validity of the study, because differences between the groups may be caused by differential mortality.

Multiple group time series A type of research design where two groups or cases are repeatedly measured over time to produce a series of measurements. One group or case receives an intervention and the other does not. The effects of the intervention may then be studied by comparing the two series.

n The symbol used to represent the number of cases in a sample.

N The symbol used to represent the number of cases in a population.

n = 1 design A research design in which one subject, rather than a group of subjects, is studied.

Natural comparison study A type of study in which naturally occurring groups are compared with one another. For example, the health status of smokers versus non-smokers may be studied in a natural comparison study. The researcher does not assign the participants to the groups. These are naturally occurring. Studies of gender differences are natural comparisons.

Natural setting The normal setting of the phenomenon or people under study. Studies performed under laboratory conditions may sometimes have diminished external validity.

Negative correlation A correlation is a measure of the strength and direction of the association between two variables. A negative correlation between two variables implies that, as one variable gets bigger, the value of the other variable becomes smaller.

Negative skew A frequency distribution where there is a long tail towards the negative end of the x-axis. Figure G.1 represents both positively and negatively skewed samples. The position of the 'tail' of the distribution determines whether the skew is positive or negative.

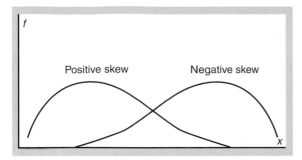

Figure G.1 • Positive and negative skew.

Nominal scale Measurement scales may be nominal, ordinal, interval or ratio. A nominal scale (often called a categorical scale) is one in which the values are distinct categories, e.g. male or female, Catholic or Protestant, or Jewish or Muslim. It has the property of distinctiveness of values, but not ordering, equidistant intervals or an absolute zero.

Non-directional hypothesis This asserts that there are differences between groups in the data but with no direction specified. For example, the hypothesis 'smokers and non-smokers have different life expectancies' is a non-directional hypothesis.

Non-experimental study A study in which the researcher observes a situation but does not systematically manipulate or experiment with it. This may also be called a descriptive design.

Non-parametric test Statistical tests are chosen on the basis of the type of scales that are being analysed. Tests that are suitable for the analysis of ordinal or nominal data are termed non-parametric.

Normal curve A bell-shaped curve, as shown in Figure G.2. The normal curve is symmetrical and unimodal (has one peak).

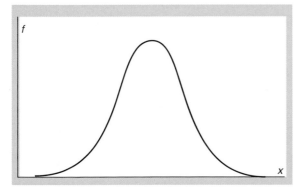

Figure G.2 • Normal curve.

Null hypothesis The hypothesis in a study that asserts there is no difference between groups or relationship between variables. The statistician normally poses the null hypothesis and then tests it statistically. If it is rejected, the alternative hypothesis (that there is a difference between two groups or a relationship between variables) is accepted. The null hypothesis is represented by the symbol H_0.

Objective measures Measures derived from a mechanical measuring process involving a minimum amount of human interpretation, e.g. weight measurements.

Observation A situation where the researcher studies the phenomenon without deliberate intervention.

Observed frequency The actual number of occurrences of an event observed by a researcher. For example, the observed frequency of females who passed the exam in a group of students might be 37 students. See also *Expected frequency*.

Observer as participant Where the researcher studies the behaviour of a group by actively participating in the group's activities and situation.

Odds ratio (OR) An index of effect size suitable for nominal scale data. The OR provides a comparison of the magnitude risk or therapeutic benefits between an experimental and a control group.

One-tailed test A statistical test where a difference between two groups is expected to occur in a particular direction. For example, it may be hypothesized that smokers will have more health problems than non-smokers. This would be tested by applying a one-tailed test of significance.

Open-ended question If a question is asked without a predefined set of responses it is an open-ended question. For example, the question 'What did you think about the program?' is an open-ended question.

Operational definition The specific way in which a concept or variable has been measured in a study. For example, the operational definition of anxiety in a study might be scores from the Spielberger State–Trait Anxiety Inventory or a self-rating on a 1–10 scale.

Ordinal scale Measurement scales may be nominal, ordinal, interval or ratio. An ordinal scale has the following properties: (i) the values are distinguishable; (ii) they are ordered but the intervals between the points are not equidistant, nor is there a meaningful zero point. The values of an ordinal scale are often ranked, e.g. 1st, 3rd.

Paradigm A general world view of health by the researcher. In the present book we argued for a 'post-positivist' paradigm, which includes the use of both quantitative and qualitative methods.

Parametric test Statistical tests are chosen on the basis of the type of data being analysed. Statistical tests that are suitable for the analysis of interval or ratio data are termed parametric.

Participation A situation where the researcher studies the phenomenon by actively participating.

Percentile The position of a score on a frequency distribution expressed in standard score units such that the 50th percentile is the median and all scores fall below the 100th percentile.

Phenomenology Phenomenology has its origins in both philosophy and psychology. In health science research, phenomenology is one of the methods used by qualitative researchers to study the way in which persons consciously experience health and illness in their lives.

Pie diagram A graphical method of representing the frequency distribution of a set of categorical data in the shape of a pie.

Pilot study A preliminary study where the procedures and protocols are tested or 'piloted'.

Placebo effect The phenomenon where an otherwise worthless intervention in a study nevertheless induces an improvement in the patient's condition or perception of the condition, perhaps due to the expectations of the participants in the study.

Population A group of people, institutions, cases or objects defined as that under study by the researcher. Samples are drawn from populations. Examples of populations are all coronary heart disease cases in the UK, all Australian men, and all 'not-for-profit' hospitals in Canada.

Population parameter A value derived from a population. For example, the average age of all the patients in a population defined by the researcher is a population parameter. In statistical notation, population parameters are represented by Greek letters.

Population validity The extent to which a sample reflects the characteristics of a population from which it is drawn.

Positive correlation A correlation is a measure of the strength and direction of the association between two variables. A positive correlation between two variables implies that, as the values of one variable get bigger, so do the values of the other variable.

Positive skew A frequency distribution where there is a long tail towards the positive end of the x-axis.

Post-test only design A type of experimental study in which measurements of the groups are taken only after an intervention has occurred. This is generally done to avoid the effects of measurement upon people's response to the interventions.

Power The probability of rejecting the null hypothesis when the alternative hypothesis is true, i.e. correctly identifying an effect when it is there.

Pre-test/post-test design A type of experimental study in which measurements of the groups are taken both prior to and following an intervention. This allows the direct comparison of pre-intervention and post-intervention results for individual subjects and groups of subjects.

Predictive validity The extent to which a test or measure can validly predict a future event. For example, a clinical test may have high predictive validity with respect to 5-year mortality of people with cancer. It is often expressed in the form of a correlation coefficient.

Prevalence The overall occurrence of a particular disease in a specific population at a specific point in time.

Probability The chance or likelihood of an event. The probability of flipping a 'heads' with a fair coin is 0.5 or ½. Probabilities may vary in value from 0 ('no chance') to 1 (certain).

Procedure A section in a research report that describes the protocol or procedure followed for the collection of data.

Proportion The ratio of one value to another expressed as a fraction of 1. For example, the proportion of women in the adult population is about 0.5.

Protocol deviation A deviation from the ideal procedure described as having been followed in a study by the researcher.

Qualitative methods An approach to research that emphasizes the non-numerical and interpretive analysis of social phenomena.

Quantitative methods An approach to research that emphasizes the collection of numerical data and the statistical analysis of hypotheses proposed by the researcher.

Quasi-experimental design A structured research design that is experiment-like but does not involve its full characteristics such as a control group and random assignment of subjects to treatment groups.

Questionnaire A means of collecting data from people where they provide written responses to a set of questions, either in their own words or by selecting predefined answers.

Quota sample The result of a sampling procedure in which the researcher sets quotas for the number of cases in particular categories to be included in the sample. For example, a sample of 100 might have quotas of 50 men and 50 women. The cases, however, are still selected on the basis of convenience rather than randomly. See also *Stratified random sample*.

Random assignment In an experiment, subjects are assigned to their groups by using a random assignment method. In random assignment, subjects are assigned to their groups using a random procedure. For example, in a two-group study the tossing of a coin to assign subjects to groups would be a random assignment procedure.

Random sample A group of cases drawn from a population such that each member of the population has had an equal chance of selection.

Random sampling The process of selecting cases from a population such that each member of the population has had an equal chance of selection.

Range In a group of scores the range is the difference between the maximum and minimum scores.

Ratio scale Measurement scales may be nominal, ordinal, interval or ratio. A ratio scale has the following properties: the values are distinctive, ordered and equidistant, and the zero point represents an absence of the quantity rather than being an arbitrary zero. Metres and kilograms are examples of ratio scales.

Refereed journal A journal in which the articles are vetted by independent referees for quality and interest. Refereed journals generally carry more highly regarded articles.

Regression to the mean The phenomenon where an individual who is measured on a test and obtains an extreme (very high or low) score and then upon re-measurement tends to move towards (regress) the average score (mean). Regression to the mean may be misinterpreted as representing a real change in score.

Relationships Associations between variables.

Reliability The extent to which a test or measurement result is reproducible.

Repeated measures The situation where a group of cases are measured on more than one occasion, for example prior to and following an intervention.

Representative sample A sample that accurately reflects the characteristics of the population from which it is drawn. Sometimes termed an 'unbiased' sample.

Reversal Reversal of the order of interventions is often used in experimental studies to control for the effects of order of administration. For example, intervention B preceded by intervention A may have a different effect than B followed by A.

Risk factors In epidemiology, a risk factor is an agent that is believed to increase the probability of a certain outcome or illness. For example, smoking may be a risk factor for the onset of coronary heart disease.

Rosenthal effect The phenomenon where the expectations of the researchers in a study influence the outcome. For example, if an observer believes that a particular intervention is effective, he/she may under-report or discount symptoms inconsistent with this belief.

Sample A group of cases selected from a population.

Sampling error Because a sample is smaller than the population from which it is drawn, there is often a discrepancy between the values obtained for the sample and those that apply to the population. For example, the average age of a sample might be 22 years and the average age of the population might be 28 years. This discrepancy is termed the sampling error.

Sampling method The method by which a sample is drawn from a population. Broadly, there are two approaches: random, in which every case in the population has an equal chance of selection, and non-random, in which cases have different chances of selection.

Scattergram A graph displaying the relationship between a set of paired scores on two variables. Also referred to as a scatterplot.

Semi-interquartile range A measure of the spread of a frequency distribution, being the distance between the first and third quartiles.

Semiotics A method of interpretation aiming to uncover the hidden, implicit meanings in texts.

Sensitivity This is a statistic used to analyse the accuracy of diagnostic or screening test for a disease. It represents the ratio of true positives and true negatives. A high degree of sensitivity indicates that the test is accurate in that it identifies the people who actually have the disease or condition. See also *Specificity*.

Shared variance In the examination of relationships between variables, researchers are concerned about the extent to which when one variable changes the other also changes. Shared variance refers to the extent to which this occurs.

Skewness A characteristic of the shape of a frequency distribution. See also *Negative skew*, *Positive skew*.

Specificity This is a static relevant to analysing the accuracy of a diagnostic or screening tests for a disease. It represents the ratio of true negatives divided by the number of true negatives and false positives. A high degree of specificity indicates that the test is accurate; it correctly identifies those who do not have the disease or condition. See also *Sensitivity*.

Standard deviation A measure of the dispersion or variability of a group of scores. The standard deviation of a sample is represented by the symbol s and by the symbol σ for a population.

Standard error of the mean If a number of samples were taken from the same population and the mean calculated for each sample, the standard deviation of this distribution of means is known as the standard error of the mean. The standard error of the mean is used in statistical inferences about population means.

Standard normal curve An idealized normal or bell-shaped frequency distribution with a mean of 0 and a standard deviation of 1 unit.

Standardized test A standardized test is one that has known characteristics, especially known levels of reliability and validity. Researchers use standardized tests wherever possible in preference to unstandardized tests.

Statistic A statistic is a number with known properties derived from sample data. There are two types of statistics: inferential statistics, which are used to apply statistical tests, and descriptive statistics, which are used to describe characteristics of the sample.

Statistical significance When researchers have demonstrated statistical significance through the application of a statistical test, they have demonstrated that the result obtained is probably not due to chance but is 'real'. This does not mean the result is important or interesting. See also *Clinical significance*.

Stratified random sample A type of sample in which the researcher wishes to ensure that important subgroups and their representation are preserved in the sample. For example, if a researcher randomly selected a subsample of 50 men and then 50 women, the sample has been stratified with respect to gender. See also *Quota sample*.

Structured interview An interview in which the questions are generally predefined, i.e. asked in a fixed order with the answers recorded by the researcher on a response sheet.

Subjective measures Measures derived from a measurement process involving a substantial degree of human interpretation, e.g. subjective ratings of pain, clinical ratings of social skills.

Subjects Participants in a study.

Surveys A type of research design in which characteristics of the cases under study are systematically recorded without the researcher attempting actively to change the situation. A non-experimental type of study.

Systematic sample A method of drawing a sample from a population where, for example, every 10th case is selected from a population list.

Systematic review A principled approach to summarizing research in a specific area of health care. The system used is parallel to the methodology for conducting empirical research.

Test–retest reliability When a test or assessment procedure is administered twice to the same group of people, the correlation between the first score and the second score is termed the test–retest reliability. This is a measure of the reproducibility of an assessment procedure.

Time series A series of measurements taken repeatedly from the same person, or group of people, over time.

Transcript A verbatim written version of an interview.

Transformed score A score that has been altered by an arithmetic manipulation, such as a z score.

True negative The situation that occurs when a diagnostic test indicates the person being assessed does not have a disease when he/she really does not.

True positive The situation that occurs when a diagnostic test indicates the person being assessed does have a disease when he/she does.

Two–tailed test A statistical test where a difference between two groups is tested without reference to the expected direction of the difference.

Type I error When researchers, on the basis of a statistical test applied to a sample of data, wrongly conclude that there is evidence of an association between variables or difference between groups in the population, they have committed a type I error. The probability of a type I error is represented by the symbol α.

Type II error A 'miss'. When researchers, on the basis of a statistical test applied to a sample of data, wrongly conclude that there is no evidence of an association between variables or difference between groups in the population, they have committed a type II error. The probability of a type II error is represented by the symbol β.

Unstructured interview An interview in which there may be no pre-planned questions or fixed agenda. The dialogue is usually recorded in a transcript or field notes which are subsequently analysed.

Utilitarian ethics A form of consequentialism which holds that the morally correct action is the one which maximizes benefits for all the people involved. For example, immunizing children against diseases such as mumps may be mildly painful to a child, but it is the right action because it will protect the individual child and the community from the disease.

Validity The extent to which a test measures what it is intended to measure.

Variability The extent to which a group of scores varies or is spread out. This is usually measured by a descriptive statistic such as the standard deviation range or semi-interquartile range.

Variable A property or attribute that varies. For example, gender, age, weight are all variables.

Variance A measure of the dispersion or variability of a group of scores. The variance of a sample is represented by the symbol s^2 and the symbol σ^2 for a population. See also *Standard deviation*.

z scores Transformed scores which express how many standard deviations a specific score is above or below the mean. For instance, a corresponding z score of 22 implies that a given score is two standard deviations below the mean.

Zero correlation Correlation is used to measure the strength and direction of an association between two variables. A zero correlation implies that two variables are unrelated to one another.

References and further reading

Baggini J, Fosl PS 2010 The philosopher's toolkit: a compendium of philosophical concepts and methods, 2nd edn. Wiley-Blackwell, Oxford

Beecher H 1959 Measurement of subjective responses. Oxford University Press, Oxford

Bloom BS 2005 Effects of continuing medical education on improving physician clinical care and patient health: A review of systematic reviews. International Journal of Technol Assess Health Care 21(3): 380–5

Bonita R, Beaglehole R, Kjellström T 2006 Basic epidemiology, 2nd edn. World Health Organization, Geneva

Chalmers A 2007 What is this thing called science. University of Queensland Press, St Lucia

Coates S, Steed L 2003 SPSS: Analysis without anguish. John Wiley & Sons Australia Ltd, Sydney

Cochrane A 1972 Effectiveness and efficiency. Random reflections on health services. Nuffield Provincial Hospitals Trust, London

Cohen J 1988 Statistical power analysis for the behavioural sciences, 2nd edn. Routledge, London

Daly J, Kellehear A, Glikman M 1997 The health researcher: a methodological guide. Oxford University Press, Melbourne

Dawes M, Davies P, Gray A, et al 2005 Evidence-based practice: a primer for health care professionals. Elsevier/Churchill Livingstone, Edinburgh

Denzin NK, Lincoln YS 2011 The SAGE handbook of qualitative research. Sage: Thousand Oaks, California

Dooley D 2001 Social research methods. Prentice Hall, New Jersey

Doyle J, Thomas SA 2000 Capturing policy in hearing-aid decisions by audiologists. In: Conolly T, Arkes J, Hammond K (eds) Judgement and decision making, 2nd edn. Cambridge University Press, Cambridge, pp 245–258

Duncan P 2010. Values, ethics and healthcare. Sage, London

Ellis P 2010 The essential guide to effect sizes: statistical power, meta-analysis, and the interpretation of research results. Cambridge University Press, Cambridge

Emanuel E, Wendler D, Grady C 2000. What makes clinical research ethical? Journal of the American Medical Association 283(20): 2701–2711

Engel GL 2003 The clinical application of the biopsychosocial model. In: Frankel R, Quill T, McDaniel S (eds) The biopsychosocial approach: past, present and future. University of Rochester Press, New York

Epstein L, Ogden J 2005 A qualitative study of GPs' views of treating obesity. British Journal of General Practice 55(519): 750–754

Evans WP 2012 Breast cancer screening. CA: A Cancer Journal for Clinicians 62: 5–9

Fara P 2009 Science: a four thousand year history. Oxford University Press, New York

Gerrig RJ, Zimbardo PG, Campbell AJ, et al 2009 Psychology and life (Australian edn). Pearson, Frenchs Forest, NSW, Australia

Guba EG, Lincoln YS 1982 Epistemological and methodological bases of naturalistic inquiry Educational Communications and Technology Journal 30: 233–252

Guba EG, Lincoln YS 1994 Competing paradigms in qualitative research. In: Denzin NK, Lincoln YS (eds) Handbook of qualitative research. SAGE, London, pp 105–117

Hay D, Oken D 1977 The psychological stress of intensive care unit nursing. In: Monat A, Lazarus R S (eds) Stress and coping. Columbia University Press, New York, pp 118–131

Hicks CM 2009 Research methods for clinical therapists: applied project design and analysis. Elsevier Health Sciences, London

Hossain P, Kawar B, El Nahas M 2007 Obesity and diabetes in the developing world – a growing challenge. New England Journal of Medicine 356(1): 213–215

Huck SW, Cormier WH, Bounds WG 1974 Reading statistics and research. Harper & Row, New York

Kindon S, Pain R, Kesby M 2007 Participatory action research approaches and methods: connecting people. Routledge, New York

Laing RD, Esterson A 1970 Sanity, madness and the family. Penguin, London

Liamputtong P 2009 Qualitative research methods, 3rd edn. Oxford University Press, Melbourne

Lincoln YS, Guba EG 1985 Naturalistic inquiry. Sage, London

Lu A, Jia H, Xiao C, Lu Q 2004 Theory of tradition Chinese medicine and therapeutic method of diseases, World Journal of Gastroenterology 10(13): 1854–1856

McGartland M, Polgar S 1994 Paradigm collapse in psychology: the necessity for a 'two methods' approach. Australian Psychologist 29(1): 21–28

McGinn F 1996 The plight of rural parents caring for adult children with HIV. Families in Society. Journal of Contemporary Human Services 77: 269–278

Miles MB, Huberman AM 1984 Analysing qualitative data: a source book for new methods. Sage, Beverly Hills, California

Minichiello V, Aroni R, Hays T 2008 In-depth interviewing: principles, techniques, analysis. Pearson Education Australia, Sydney

Morgan D, Morgan R 2009 Single-case research methods for the behavioral and health sciences. SAGE, Los Angeles

Morse JM, Field PA 2003 Nursing research: the application of qualitative approaches, 2nd edn. Nelson Thornes, Cheltenham

Mostofsky E, Burger M, Schlaug G 2010 Alcohol and acute ischemic stroke onset. The stroke onset study. Stroke 41: 1845

Muir Gray JA 2009 Evidence-based health care and public health: how to make decisions about health services and public health, 3rd edn. Churchill Livingstone, London

Olanow C, Goetz C, Kordower J 2003 A double-blind controlled trial of bilateral fetal nigral transplantation in Parkinson's disease. Annals of Neurology 54: 403–414

Olanow CW 2004 The scientific basis for the current treatment of Parkinson's disease. Annual Review of Medicine 55: 41–60

Patton MQ 1990 Qualitative evaluation and research methods, 2nd edn. Sage, Newbury Park, California

Polgar S, Morris ME, Reilly S, et al 2003 Reconstructive neurosurgery for Parkinson's disease: a systematic review and preliminary meta-analysis. Brain Research Bulletin 60: 1-24

Polgar S, Ng J 2005 Ethics, methodology and the use of placebo controls in surgical trials. Brain Research Bulletin 67: 290–297

Polgar S, Swerissen H 2000 Research methods in health 2. La Trobe University, Bundoora, Victoria, Australia

Rice PL 2009 Qualitative data analysis: conceptual and practical considerations. Health Promotion Journal of Australia 20(2): 133

Rice PL, Ezzy D 1999 Qualitative research methods: a health focus. Oxford University Press, Oxford

Rosehan DL 1975 On being sane in insane places. In: Krupat E (ed.) Psychology is social. Scott Foresman, Glenview, Illinois, pp 189–200

Sackett D, Strauss S, Richardson W, et al 2000 Evidence based medicine: how to practice and teach EBM, 2nd edn. Churchill Livingstone, Edinburgh

Schwartz M, Polgar S 2003 Statistics for evidence based health care. Tertiary Press, Croydon, Australia

Soares-Weiser K, Thomas S, Gail T, Garner P 2010 Ribavirin for Crimean-Congo hemorrhagic fever: systematic review and meta-analysis. BMC Infectious Diseases 10: 207

Strauss A, Corbin J 1990 Basics of qualitative research: techniques and procedures for developing grounded theory, 2nd edn. Sage, Newbury Park, California

Tashakkori A, Teddlie C 2003 Handbook of mixed methods in social and behavioral research. Sage, Thousand Oaks, California

Taylor R 1979 Medicine out of control. Sun Books, Melbourne

Thomas SA, Steven I, Browning C, et al 1992 Focus groups in health research: a methodological review. Annual Review of Health Social Sciences 2: 7–20

Thomas S, Steven I, Browning C, et al 1993 Patient knowledge, opinions, satisfaction and choices in primary health care provision: a progress report. In: Dossel DP (ed.) The general practice evaluation program: the 1992 work-in progress conference. Australian Government Publishing Service, Canberra

Van Lith T, Fenner P, Schofield P 2011. The lived experience of art making as a companion to the mental health recovery process. Disability and Rehabilitation 33: 652–660

Walker Q, Langlands A 1986 The nurse of mammography in the management of breast cancer. Medical Journal of Australia 1435: 185–187

WHO 2010 Traditional medicine strategy 2002–2005. World Health Organization, Geneva

World Medical Association 2008 Medical association declaration of Helsinki: ethical principles for medical research involving human subjects. 52nd WMA General Assembly, Edinburgh

Appendix A

z scores and associated areas between z and mean and beyond

z	Area between mean and z	Area beyond z	z	Area between mean and z	Area beyond z	z	Area between mean and z	Area beyond z
0.00	0.0000	0.5000	0.23	0.0910	0.4090	0.46	0.1772	0.3228
0.01	0.0040	0.4960	0.24	0.0948	0.4052	0.47	0.1808	0.3192
0.02	0.0080	0.4920	0.25	0.0987	0.4013	0.48	0.1844	0.3156
0.03	0.0120	0.4880	0.26	0.1026	0.3974	0.49	0.1879	0.3121
0.04	0.0160	0.4840	0.27	0.1064	0.3936	0.50	0.1915	0.3085
0.05	0.0199	0.4801	0.28	0.1103	0.3897	0.51	0.1950	0.3050
0.06	0.0239	0.4761	0.29	0.1141	0.3859	0.52	0.1985	0.3015
0.07	0.0279	0.4721	0.30	0.1179	0.3821	0.53	0.2019	0.2981
0.08	0.0319	0.4681	0.31	0.1217	0.3783	0.54	0.2054	0.2946
0.09	0.0359	0.4641	0.32	0.1255	0.3745	0.55	0.2088	0.2912
0.10	0.0398	0.4602	0.33	0.1293	0.3707	0.56	0.2123	0.2877
0.11	0.0438	0.4562	0.34	0.1331	0.3669	0.57	0.2157	0.2843
0.12	0.0478	0.4522	0.35	0.1368	0.3632	0.58	0.2190	0.2810
0.13	0.0517	0.4483	0.36	0.1406	0.3594	0.59	0.2224	0.2776
0.14	0.0557	0.4443	0.37	0.1443	0.3557	0.60	0.2257	0.2743
0.15	0.0596	0.4404	0.38	0.1480	0.3520	0.61	0.2291	0.2709
0.16	0.0636	0.4364	0.39	0.1517	0.3483	0.62	0.2324	0.2676
0.17	0.0675	0.4325	0.40	0.1554	0.3446	0.63	0.2357	0.2643
0.18	0.0714	0.4286	0.41	0.1591	0.3409	0.64	0.2389	0.2611
0.19	0.0753	0.4247	0.42	0.1628	0.3372	0.65	0.2422	0.2578
0.20	0.0793	0.4207	0.43	0.1664	0.3336	0.66	0.2454	0.2546
0.21	0.0832	0.4168	0.44	0.1700	0.3300	0.67	0.2486	0.2514
0.22	0.0871	0.4129	0.45	0.1736	0.3264	0.68	0.2517	0.2483

Continued

z	Area between mean and z	Area beyond z	z	Area between mean and z	Area beyond z	z	Area between mean and z	Area beyond z
0.69	0.2549	0.2451	1.03	0.3485	0.1515	1.37	0.4147	0.0853
0.70	0.2580	0.2420	1.04	0.3508	0.1492	1.38	0.4162	0.0838
0.71	0.2611	0.2389	1.05	0.3531	0.1469	1.39	0.4177	0.0823
0.72	0.2642	0.2358	1.06	0.3554	0.1446	1.40	0.4192	0.0808
0.73	0.2673	0.2327	1.07	0.3577	0.1423	1.41	0.4207	0.0793
0.74	0.2704	0.2296	1.08	0.3599	0.1401	1.42	0.4222	0.0778
0.75	0.2734	0.2266	1.09	0.3621	0.1379	1.43	0.4236	0.0764
0.76	0.2764	0.2236	1.10	0.3643	0.1357	1.44	0.4251	0.0749
0.77	0.2794	0.2206	1.11	0.3665	0.1335	1.45	0.4265	0.0735
0.78	0.2823	0.2177	1.12	0.3686	0.1314	1.46	0.4279	0.0721
0.79	0.2852	0.2148	1.13	0.3708	0.1292	1.47	0.4292	0.0708
0.80	0.2881	0.2119	1.14	0.3729	0.1271	1.48	0.4306	0.0694
0.81	0.2910	0.2090	1.15	0.3749	0.1251	1.49	0.4319	0.0681
0.82	0.2939	0.2061	1.16	0.3770	0.1230	1.50	0.4332	0.0668
0.83	0.2967	0.2033	1.17	0.3790	0.1210	1.51	0.4345	0.0655
0.84	0.2995	0.2005	1.18	0.3810	0.1190	1.52	0.4357	0.0643
0.85	0.3023	0.1977	1.19	0.3830	0.1170	1.53	0.4370	0.0630
0.86	0.3051	0.1949	1.20	0.3849	0.1151	1.54	0.4382	0.0618
0.87	0.3078	0.1922	1.21	0.3869	0.1131	1.55	0.4394	0.0606
0.88	0.3106	0.1894	1.22	0.3888	0.1112	1.56	0.4406	0.0594
0.89	0.3133	0.1867	1.23	0.3907	0.1093	1.57	0.4418	0.0582
0.90	0.3159	0.1841	1.24	0.3925	0.1075	1.58	0.4429	0.0571
0.91	0.3186	0.1814	1.25	0.3944	0.1056	1.59	0.4441	0.0559
0.92	0.3212	0.1788	1.26	0.3962	0.1038	1.60	0.4452	0.0548
0.93	0.3238	0.1762	1.27	0.3980	0.1020	1.61	0.4463	0.0537
0.94	0.3264	0.1736	1.28	0.3997	0.1003	1.62	0.4474	0.0526
0.95	0.3289	0.1711	1.29	0.4015	0.0985	1.63	0.4484	0.0516
0.96	0.3315	0.1685	1.30	0.4032	0.0968	1.64	0.4495	0.0505
0.97	0.3340	0.1660	1.31	0.4049	0.0951	1.65	0.4505	0.0495
0.98	0.3365	0.1635	1.32	0.4066	0.0934	1.66	0.4515	0.0485
0.99	0.3389	0.1611	1.33	0.4082	0.0918	1.67	0.4525	0.0475
1.00	0.3413	0.1587	1.34	0.4099	0.0901	1.68	0.4535	0.0465
1.01	0.3438	0.1562	1.35	0.4115	0.0885	1.69	0.4545	0.0455
1.02	0.3461	0.1539	1.36	0.4131	0.0869	1.70	0.4554	0.0446

z	Area between mean and z	Area beyond z	z	Area between mean and z	Area beyond z	z	Area between mean and z	Area beyond z
1.71	0.4564	0.0436	2.05	0.4798	0.0202	2.39	0.4916	0.0084
1.72	0.4573	0.0427	2.06	0.4803	0.0197	2.40	0.4918	0.0082
1.73	0.4582	0.0418	2.07	0.4808	0.0192	2.41	0.4920	0.0080
1.74	0.4591	0.0409	2.08	0.4812	0.0188	2.42	0.4922	0.0078
1.75	0.4599	0.0401	2.09	0.4817	0.0183	2.43	0.4925	0.0075
1.76	0.4608	0.0392	2.10	0.4821	0.0179	2.44	0.4927	0.0073
1.77	0.4616	0.0384	2.11	0.4826	0.0174	2.45	0.4929	0.0071
1.78	0.4625	0.0375	2.12	0.4830	0.0170	2.46	0.4931	0.0069
1.79	0.4633	0.0367	2.13	0.4834	0.0166	2.47	0.4932	0.0068
1.80	0.4641	0.0359	2.14	0.4838	0.0162	2.48	0.4934	0.0066
1.81	0.4649	0.0351	2.15	0.4842	0.0158	2.49	0.4936	0.0064
1.82	0.4656	0.0344	2.16	0.4846	0.0154	2.50	0.4938	0.0062
1.83	0.4664	0.0336	2.17	0.4850	0.0150	2.51	0.4940	0.0060
1.84	0.4671	0.0329	2.18	0.4854	0.0146	2.52	0.4941	0.0059
1.85	0.4678	0.0322	2.19	0.4857	0.0143	2.53	0.4943	0.0057
1.86	0.4686	0.0314	2.20	0.4861	0.0139	2.54	0,4945	0.0055
1.87	0.4693	0.0307	2.21	0.4864	0.0136	2.55	0.4946	0.0054
1.88	0.4699	0.0301	2.22	0.4868	0.0132	2.56	0.4948	0.0052
1.89	0.4706	0.0294	2.23	0.4871	0.0129	2.57	0.4949	0.0051
1.90	0.4713	0.0287	2.24	0.4875	0.0125	2.58	0.4951	0.0049
1.91	0.4719	0.0281	2.25	0.4878	0.0122	2.59	0.4952	0.0048
1.92	0.4726	0.0274	2.26	0.4881	0.0119	2.60	0.4953	0.0047
1.93	0.4732	0.0268	2.27	0.4884	0.0116	2.61	0.4955	0.0045
1.94	0.4738	0.0262	2.28	0.4887	0.0113	2.62	0.4956	0.0044
1.95	0.4744	0.0256	2.29	0.4890	0.0110	2.63	0.4957	0.0043
1.96	0.4750	0.0250	2.30	0.4893	0.0107	2.64	0.4959	0.0041
1.97	0.4756	0.0244	2.31	0.4896	0.0104	2.65	0.4960	0.0040
1.98	0.4761	0.0239	2.32	0.4898	0.0102	2.66	0.4961	0.0039
1.99	0.4767	0.0233	2.33	0.4901	0.0099	2.67	0.4962	0.0038
2.00	0.4772	0.0228	2.34	0.4904	0.0096	2.68	0.4963	0.0037
2.01	0.4778	0.0222	2.35	0.4906	0.0094	2.69	0.4964	0.0036
2.02	0.4783	0.0217	2.36	0.4909	0.0091	2.70	0.4965	0.0035
2.03	0.4788	0.0212	2.37	0.4911	0.0089	2.71	0.4966	0.0034
2.04	0.4793	0.0207	2.38	0.4913	0.0087	2.72	0.4967	0.0033

Continued

z	Area between mean and z	Area beyond z	z	Area between mean and z	Area beyond z	z	Area between mean and z	Area beyond z
2.73	0.4968	0.0032	2.94	0.4984	0.0016	3.15	0.4992	0.0008
2.74	0.4969	0.0031	2.95	0.4984	0.0016	3.16	0.4992	0.0008
2.75	0.4970	0.0030	2.96	0.4985	0.0015	3.17	0.4992	0.0008
2.76	0.4971	0.0029	2.97	0.4985	0.0015	3.18	0.4993	0.0007
2.77	0.4972	0.0028	2.98	0.4986	0.0014	3.19	0.4993	0.0007
2.78	0.4973	0.0027	2.99	0.4986	0.0014	3.20	0.4993	0.0007
2.79	0.4974	0.0026	3.00	0.4987	0.0013	3.21	0.4993	0.0007
2.80	0.4974	0.0026	3.01	0.4987	0.0013	3.22	0.4994	0.0006
2.81	0.4975	0.0025	3.02	0.4987	0.0013	3.23	0.4994	0.0006
2.82	0.4976	0.0024	3.03	0.4988	0.0012	3.24	0.4994	0.0006
2.83	0.4977	0.0023	3.04	0.4988	0.0012	3.25	0.4994	0.0006
2.84	0.4977	0.0023	3.05	0.4989	0.0011	3.30	0.4995	0.0005
2.85	0.4978	0.0022	3.06	0.4989	0.0011	3.35	0.4996	0.0004
2.86	0.4979	0.0021	3.07	0.4989	0.0011	3.40	0.4997	0.0003
2.87	0.4979	0.0021	3.08	0.4990	0.0010	3.45	0.4997	0.0003
2.88	0.4980	0.0020	3.09	0.4990	0.0010	3.50	0.4998	0.0002
2.89	0.4981	0.0019	3.10	0.4990	0.0010	3.60	0.4998	0.0002
2.90	0.4981	0.0019	3.11	0.4991	0.0009	3.70	0.4999	0.0001
2.91	0.4982	0.0018	3.12	0.4991	0.0009	3.80	0.4999	0.0001
2.92	0.4982	0.0018	3.13	0.4991	0.0009	3.90	0.49995	0.00005
2.93	0.4983	0.0017	3.14	0.4992	0.0008	4.00	0.49997	0.00003

Appendix B

t distribution

Directional p	0.4	0.25	0.1	0.05	0.025	0.01	0.005	0.001
Non-directional p	0.8	0.5	0.2	0.1	0.05	0.02	0.01	0.002
Degrees of freedom								
1	0.325	1.000	3.078	6.314	12.706	31.821	63.657	318.31
2	0.289	0.816	1.886	2.920	4.303	6.965	9.925	22.326
3	0.277	0.765	1.638	2.353	3.182	4.541	5.841	10.213
4	0.271	0.741	1.533	2.132	2.776	3.747	4.604	7.173
5	0.267	0.727	1.476	2.015	2.571	3.365	4.032	5.893
6	0.265	0.718	1.440	1.943	2.447	3.143	3.707	5.208
7	0.263	0.711	1.415	1.895	2.365	2.998	3.499	4.785
8	0.262	0.706	1.397	1.860	2.306	2.896	3.355	4.501
9	0.261	0.703	1.383	1.833	2.262	2.821	3.250	4.297
10	0.260	0.700	1.372	1.812	2.228	2.764	3.169	4.144
11	0.260	0.697	1.363	1.796	2.201	2.718	3.106	4.025
12	0.259	0.695	1.356	1.782	2.179	2.681	3.055	3.930
13	0.259	0.694	1.350	1.771	2.160	2.650	3.012	3.852
14	0.258	0.692	1.345	1.761	2.145	2.624	2.977	3.787
15	0.258	0.691	1.341	1.753	2.131	2.602	2.947	3.733
16	0.258	0.690	1.337	1.746	2.120	2.583	2.921	3.686
17	0.257	0.689	1.333	1.740	2.110	2.567	2.898	3.646
18	0.257	0.688	1.330	1.734	2.101	2.552	2.878	3.610
19	0.257	0.688	1.328	1.729	2.093	2.539	2.861	3.579
20	0.257	0.687	1.325	1.725	2.086	2.528	2.845	3.552
21	0.257	0.686	1.323	1.721	2.080	2.518	2.831	3.527

Directional p	0.4	0.25	0.1	0.05	0.025	0.01	0.005	0.001
Non-directional p	0.8	0.5	0.2	0.1	0.05	0.02	0.01	0.002
Degrees of freedom								
22	0.256	0.686	1.321	1.717	2.074	2.508	2.819	3.505
23	0.256	0.685	1.319	1.714	2.069	2.500	2.807	3.485
24	0.256	0.685	1.318	1.711	2.064	2.492	2.797	3.467
25	0.256	0.684	1.316	1.708	2.060	2.485	2.787	3.450
26	0.256	0.684	1.315	1.706	2.056	2.479	2.779	3.435
27	0.256	0.684	1.314	1.703	2.052	2.473	2.771	3.421
28	0.256	0.683	1.313	1.701	2.048	2.467	2.763	3.408
29	0.256	0.683	1.311	1.699	2.045	2.462	2.756	3.396
30	0.256	0.683	1.310	1.697	2.042	2.457	2.750	3.385
40	0.255	0.681	1.303	1.684	2.021	2.423	2.704	3.307
60	0.254	0.679	1.296	1.671	2.000	2.390	2.660	3.232
120	0.254	0.677	1.289	1.658	1.980	2.358	2.617	3.160
∞	0.253	0.674	1.282	1.645	1.960	2.326	2.576	3.090

Appendix C

Chi-square (χ^2)

df	0.99	0.98	0.95	0.90	0.80	0.70	0.50	0.30	0.20	0.10	0.05	0.02	0.01	0.001
1	0.00016	0.00063	0.0039	0.016	0.064	0.15	0.46	1.07	1.64	2.71	3.84	5.41	6.64	10.83
2	0.02	0.04	0.10	0.21	0.45	0.71	1.39	2.41	3.22	4.60	5.99	7.82	9.21	13.82
3	0.12	0.18	0.35	0.58	1.00	1.42	2.37	3.66	4.64	6.25	7.82	9.84	11.34	16.27
4	0.30	0.43	0.71	1.06	1.65	2.20	3.36	4.88	5.99	7.78	9.49	11.67	13.28	18.46
5	0.55	0.75	1.14	1.61	2.34	3.00	4.35	6.06	7.29	9.24	11.07	13.39	15.09	20.52
6	0.87	1.13	1.64	2.20	3.07	3.83	5.35	7.23	8.56	10.64	12.59	15.03	16.81	22.46
7	1.24	1.56	2.17	2.83	3.82	4.67	6.35	8.38	9.80	12.02	14.07	16.62	18.48	24.32
8	1.65	2.03	2.73	3.49	4.59	5.53	7.34	9.52	11.03	13.36	15.51	18.17	20.09	26.12
9	2.09	2.53	3.32	4.17	5.38	6.39	8.34	10.66	12.24	14.68	16.92	19.68	21.67	27.88
10	2.56	3.06	3.94	4.86	6.18	7.27	9.34	11.78	13.44	15.99	18.31	21.16	23.21	29.59
11	3.05	3.61	4.58	5.58	6.99	8.15	10.34	12.90	14.63	17.28	19.68	22.62	24.72	31.26
12	3.57	4.18	5.23	6.30	7.81	9.03	11.34	14.01	15.81	18.55	21.03	24.05	26.22	32.91
13	4.11	4.76	5.89	7.04	8.63	9.93	12.34	15.12	16.98	19.81	22.36	25.47	27.69	34.53
14	4.66	5.37	6.57	7.79	9.47	10.82	13.34	16.22	18.15	21.06	23.68	26.87	29.14	36.12
15	5.23	5.98	7.26	8.55	10.31	11.72	14.34	17.32	19.31	22.31	25.00	28.26	30.58	37.70
16	5.81	6.61	7.96	9.31	11.15	12.62	15.34	18.42	20.46	23.54	26.30	29.63	32.00	39.29
17	6.41	7.26	8.67	10.08	12.00	13.53	16.34	19.51	21.62	24.77	27.59	31.00	33.41	40.75
18	7.02	7.91	9.39	10.86	12.86	14.44	17.34	20.60	22.76	25.99	28.87	32.35	34.80	42.31
19	7.63	8.57	10.12	11.65	13.72	15.35	18.34	21.69	23.90	27.20	30.14	33.69	36.19	43.82
20	8.26	9.24	10.85	12.44	14.58	16.27	19.34	22.78	25.04	28.41	31.41	35.02	37.57	45.32
21	8.90	9.92	11.59	13.24	15.44	17.18	20.34	23.86	26.17	29.62	32.67	36.34	38.93	46.80
df	0.99	0.98	0.95	0.90	0.80	0.70	0.50	0.30	0.20	0.10	0.05	0.02	0.01	0.001
22	9.54	10.60	12.34	14.04	16.31	18.10	21.34	24.94	27.30	30.81	33.92	37.66	40.29	48.27
23	10.20	11.29	13.09	14.85	17.19	19.02	22.34	26.02	28.43	32.01	35.17	38.97	41.64	49.73
24	10.86	11.99	13.85	15.66	18.06	19.94	23.34	27.10	29.55	33.20	36.42	40.27	42.98	51.18

Continued

df	0.99	0.98	0.95	0.90	0.80	0.70	0.50	0.30	0.20	0.10	0.05	0.02	0.01	0.001
25	11.52	12.70	14.61	16.47	18.94	20.87	24.34	28.17	30.68	34.38	37.65	41.57	44.31	52.62
26	12.20	13.41	15.38	17.29	19.82	21.79	25.34	29.25	31.80	35.56	38.88	42.86	45.64	54.05
27	12.88	14.12	16.15	18.11	20.70	22.72	26.34	30.32	32.91	36.74	40.11	44.14	46.96	55.48
28	13.56	14.85	16.93	18.94	21.59	23.65	27.34	31.39	34.03	37.92	41.34	45.42	48.28	56.89
29	14.26	15.57	17.71	19.77	22.48	24.58	28.34	32.46	35.14	39.09	42.56	46.69	49.59	58.30
30	14.95	16.31	18.49	20.60	23.36	25.51	29.34	33.53	36.25	40.26	43.77	47.96	50.89	59.70

Index

A

AB designs, 71–72, 72f, 209
ABAB designs, 72–73, 73f, 209
   baselines, 72
   features, 72
   uses, 72–73
absolute risk reduction, 173
abstracts, 20, 209
acquiescent response mode, 209
aims of research *see* research
α (alpha) level, 160, 165
   rejecting null hypothesis, 160
alternative hypothesis, 160, 165, 209
analytical epidemiology, 65
anonymity, 45
apparatus and tools (research), 21, 209
   critical evaluation of published research, 194–195
appendices, research publications, 21
appraisal of published research *see* critical evaluation of published research
area sampling, 37, 209
area under normal curve, 135–136, 136f
   worked example, 135
assignment, 195, 209
   critical evaluation of published research, 195
   errors, 209
   independent groups, 54f, 56
   matched groups, 56
   matching, 212
   randomized-controlled trial (RCT), 59
audio recording, 94
auditability, 187
authority, 209
average deviation, 128–129

B

bar graph, 117, 117f, 209
baselines, 75, 209
   ABAB designs, 72
   multiple baseline designs, 73, 73f
   $n = 1$ designs, 72f
'before–after' design, 54, 54f
bell-shaped curve, 134, 134f, 209
benefits of research, 47–48
   bias, 209 *see also* confounding and bias
binomial theorem, 152–153, 161
bioethics, 43–44
biopsychosocial model, 8–9
blinding, 60
bracketing, 78

C

case-control designs, 66, 209
case studies *see* single case ($n = 1$) designs
categorical scales, 87–88 *see also* nominal scales
causality, 54, 209
   correlation and, 145–146
   criteria, 54
census, 64
census studies, 33
centile rank *see* percentiles
central limit theorem, 153
central tendency, 125–127, 128f, 209
   mean, 126–127
   median, 125–127, 126f, 126t
   mode, 125, 126t–127t, 127
chain sampling, 39, 40t
chi-square test (χ^2), 163–165, 169, 209–210, 225t–226t
   appropriate usage, 164
   assumptions, 167

chi-square test *(Continued)*
   contingency tables *see* contingency tables
   worked example, 164–165, 165t
clinical decision making, 174f–175f, 177–178
   type I error, 177, 177t
   type II error, 174f, 177, 177t
clinical significance, 173, 176–177, 177t, 210
closed questions, 87–88, 87t, 210
closing statements, 90
Cochrane Collaboration, 191, 207–208
   Database of Systematic Reviews, 207
   evidence-based practice, 207–208
   hierarchy of evidence, 207
coding, 210
   systematic reviews *see* systematic reviews
coding of data, 97, 182–183
   predetermined coding, 182
   thematic analysis, 182–183
   units of analysis, 182
      concepts, 182
      sentences, 182
      themes, 182–183
      words, 182
coefficient of determination, 145
Cohen's *d*, 174, 178
cohort study, 67, 210
column graph *see* bar graph
combined methods, 96, 212
complete observer, 102, 210
complete participant, 102, 210
computer-assisted data analysis, 183–184
   meta-analysis, 203
   statistical packages, 168, 168t
conclusions (research publications), 21
confidence intervals, 154–155, 210
   calculating, 174
   meta-analysis interpretation of results, 205

Page numbers followed by f indicate figures; t, tables; b, boxes.

confidence intervals *(Continued)*
  sample sizes and, 174
  significance and, 174, 174f
  use in health research, 157
  using *t* distribution, 155–157,
    156f–157f
  worked examples, 154, 155f, 157 *see*
    also effect size
confidentiality, 45
confounding and bias, 54–55
  'before–after' design, 54, 54f
  history, 55, 211
  internal validity, 55
  maturation, 55, 212
  observer bias, 55
  placebo effects, 55
  qualitative research, 80
consent, informed *see* informed
  consent
construct validity, 108–109
content analysis, 183–184
  example, 183
content validity, 108, 210
contingency tables, 165–167, 166t
  2 × 2 contingency table, 166, 166t
continuous data, 210
  effect size *see* effect size
  organization and presentation,
    118–120
  grouped frequency distributions,
    118, 119t
  probability and, 157–158
control, 210
control groups, 55–56, 210
  assignment of participants *see*
    assignment
  critical evaluation of published
    research, 195
  definition, 55
  internal validity, 55
  internal validity and, 56
  no intervention control group, 59
  placebo effect and, 55, 60
    randomized-controlled trial (RCT),
      in, 58 *see also* randomized-
      controlled trial (RCT)
  types, 59 *see also* placebo effect
control variables, 53
  naturalistic comparison studies, 65
controlled observation, 7
convenience sampling, 40t
correlation, 139–141
  associations between variables,
    143–144, 144f
  causation and, 145–146
  correlation coefficient, 140–143, 210
    curvilinear, 210
    inter-observer (inter-rater)
      reliability, 144, 144t
    Pearson's *r see* Pearson's *r*
    predictive validity, 145
    reliability, 144–145
    selection, 141, 141t
    shared variance, estimation of, 145
    Spearman's ρ, 143, 143t
    test–retest reliability, 144

correlation *(Continued)*
  line of 'best-fit', 140, 140f
  linear correlation, 140, 140f
  negative correlation, 140f, 141, 212
  non-linear correlation, 140, 140f
  path analysis, 145–146
  positive correlation, 140f, 141
  scattergram/scatterplot, 140, 140f
  use in health research, 143–145
  zero correlation, 216
correlational designs, 66–67, 67t, 210
counterbalanced design, 57
credibility, 187
critical evaluation of published
  research, 192–194
  apparatus and tools, 194–195
    validity and reliability, 195
  discussion, 196–197
    generalization of results, 196–197
    inferences, 196
    interpretations, 196
    research protocol deviations, 196
    statistical and clinical significance,
      197
    theoretical significance, 197
  guidelines, 192
    problems, 193t
    quantitative approaches, 192
    websites, 192
  hypotheses and aims, 192–194
  literature review, 192
  methods section, 194–195
  participants, 194
    demographic information, 194
    sample size, 194
    sampling, 194
  procedure, 195
    assignment, 195
    control groups, 195
    research design, 195
    settings, 195
    treatments/interventions, 195
  research design, 194
  results section, 196
    qualitative analysis, 196
    statistics, 196
    tables and graphs, 196
  systematic reviews, 202
critical theory, 210
critical values, 136, 136f, 210
  worked example, 136
cultural differences, qualitative
  research on, 77–78
cumulative frequency, 126
curvilinear correlation coefficient, 210

D

data, 210
  analysis, 19, 178
    coding of data *see* coding of data
    computer-assisted data analysis *see*
      computer-assisted data analysis
    critical evaluation *see* critical
      evaluation of published research

data *(Continued)*
  descriptive statistics *see*
    descriptive statistics
  encoding raw data, 167
  inferential *see* inferential statistics
  interviews, 96–97
  qualitative *see* qualitative research
  quantitative *see* inferential statistics
  coding *see* coding of data
  collection methods, 18
    combined, 96, 212
    focus groups *see* focus groups
    interviews *see* interviews
    observation *see* observation
    qualitative research, 81
    questionnaires *see* questionnaires
    recording information, 94–96, 95t
    retrospective, 66
  interpretation *see* interpretation of
    data
  organization and presentation *see*
    organization and presentation
    of data
  qualitative methods, 14
  quantitative methods, 13–14
  saturation, 187
  types
    continuous *see* continuous data
    discontinuous data *see*
      discontinuous data
    discrete *see* discrete data
    interval data, 118–120
    nominal data *see* nominal data
    ordinal data *see* ordinal data
    qualitative data, 13–14
    ratio data, 118–120
decision level, α (alpha) *see* α (alpha)
  level
decision making *see* clinical decision
  making
Declaration of Helsinki (1964, WMA),
  44
deduction, 6, 210
degrees of freedom, 155–156, 165
demographic questions, 90
deontological ethics, 44, 210
dependent variables, 53
  multiple dependent variables, 58
description, of phenomena, 5–6
descriptive epidemiology, 65
descriptive statistics, 19, 162, 178, 210
  discontinuous data, 120–123
    odds, 122–123, 122t
    percentages, 121
    proportions, 121
    rates *see* rates
    ratios, 120
  inferential and, relationship between,
    160–163
  mean, 126–127
  median, 125–127, 126f, 126t
  mode, 125, 126t–127t, 127
  normal distribution *see* normal
    distribution
  standard scores *see* standard scores
    (*z* scores)

descriptive statistics *(Continued)*
  using statistical packages, 168, 168t
  variability *see* variability
determinism, 5, 210
deviant case sampling, 40t
deviations
  average, 128–129
  standard, 129, 215
directional hypothesis, 210
discontinuous data, 210
  descriptive statistics *see* descriptive
    statistics
  effect size *see* effect size
  probability and, 157–158 *see also*
    discrete data
discrete data, 115–116
  graphing, 116–117, 117f, 117t
  nominal data *see* nominal data
  ordinal data *see* ordinal data
  organization, 116
discussion (research publications), 19,
  21, 210
  critical evaluation *see* critical
    evaluation of published research
dispersion, 210
  dissemination, 19 *see also* research
    publications
distribution, normal *see* normal
  distribution
double-barrelled questions, 89
double-blind design, 60

E

ecological designs, 66–67
ecological validity, 41, 210
  setting of research and, 195
effect size, 171–173, 176, 177t, 178–
  179, 210
  absolute risk reduction, 173
  Cohen's *d*, 174, 178
  confidence intervals *see* confidence
    intervals
  continuous data, 172–173
    test–retest reliability – worked
      example, 172, 172t
    two treatment groups – worked
      example, 172–173, 172t
  discontinuous data, 173
    odds ratio, 173
    randomized-controlled trial (RCT)
      – worked example, 173
  meta-analysis, 204–205
  single case (*n* = 1) designs, 75
empathy, 210
empiricism, 5
endemic pattern, 65
epidemic pattern, 65
epidemiology, 64–65, 68, 210
  analytical epidemiology, 65
  correlational designs, 66–67, 67t
  descriptive epidemiology, 65
  incidence, 65
  prevalence, 65
  risk factors, 215

epistemology, 4–5
equivalence, 110
errors
  assignment, 209
  sample size *(n)* and, 41
  sampling, 37–38, 38f
  type I *see* type I error
  type II *see* type II error
ethical considerations in health
    research, 31, 43–50
  anonymity, 45
  benefits of the research, 47–48
  clinical research, 86
  confidentiality and right to privacy,
    45
  conflict of interest, 45–46
  Declaration of Helsinki (1964,
    WMA), 44
  history, 44
  independent review, 46
  informed consent *see* informed
    consent
  key principles and concepts, 44–46
  no intervention control group, 59
  non-experimental designs, 63–64
  Nuremberg Code (1947), 44
  placebo effect, 60
  qualitative research, 80
  questionnaires, 86
  research
    design and, 48
    funding bodies, 46
    proposals *see* research
    question, 48
    resources, 46–48
  risk and harm minimization, 45
  scientific excellence and quality, 45
ethics, 210–211
  bioethics, 43–44
  history, 43–44
  medical ethics, 43–44
  philosophical principles, 43–46
    deontology, 44
    utilitarianism, 44
ethics committees, 48, 211
  members, 48
ethnography, 97, 211
ethnomethodology, 79, 211
evidence-based practice, 22–23, 191,
  211
  Cochrane Collaboration, 207–208
  confidence intervals, 157
  systematic reviews, 207
expectancy effects, 59, 195
expected frequency, 211
experimental designs, 51–62, 211
  confounding and bias *see*
    confounding and bias
  control groups *see* control
  double-blind design, 60
  epidemiology *see* epidemiology
  factorial design *see* factorial
    design
  non-experimental designs *vs.*, 64
  post-test only design, 56–57
  pre-test/post-test design, 57

experimental designs *(Continued)*
  randomized-controlled trial (RCT)
    see randomized-controlled trial
    (RCT)
  repeated measures design, 57
  types, 56–58
  variables
    control variables, 53
    dependent variable, 53
    independent variable, 53
    multiple dependent variables, 58
    see also non-experimental
      designs
external validity, 33–42, 61, 109, 211
  ecological validity, 41
  naturalistic designs, 69–70
  population validity, 40–41
  randomized-controlled trial (RCT),
    61
extraneous variables, 65, 73–75, 210
extreme case sampling, 40t
extreme response mode, 211

F

face-to-face interviews, 92–93
face validity, 108
facilitator, focus groups, 95
factorial design, 57–58, 58t, 211
  independent groups, 57–58, 58f
factual questions, 90
false negative, 211
false positive, 211
falsification, 7–8
  process, 7–8
field notes, 14, 216
focus groups, 95–96
  advantages, 95–96
  disadvantages, 96
  facilitator, 95
  participants, 95
follow-up, interviews, 94
forced-choice response format, 88,
  89t, 211
forest plot, 211
frequency distributions, 177, 177f,
  211
  graphing *see* graphing
  grouped, 118, 119t
  negative skew, 212–213, 213f
  positive skew, 214
frequency polygons, 119–120, 120f,
  211
Friedman two-way analysis of variance,
  163t
fully crossed design, 57
funding bodies, research, 46

G

Gaussian curve, 134
generalization, 6
  critical evaluation of published
    research, 196–197

graphing, 178
    bar graph, 117, 117f
    discrete data, 117f, 117t
    frequency distributions, 118–120
        frequency polygons, 119–120,
            120f
        histograms, 118–119, 119f, 211
    pie chart, 117, 117f, 117t
grounded theory, 79, 97, 184–185, 211
    example, 184 see also thematic
        analysis
group interview see focus groups
grouped frequency distributions, 118,
    119t
    worked example, 118
groups, assignment into see assignment

H

harm see risk and harm minimization
Hawthorn effect, 211 see also placebo
    effect
health care
    clinical decision making see clinical
        decision making
    evidence-based health care, 22–23
    narrative reviews of research
        evidence, 200
    positivist paradigm, contributions, 7
    qualitative evidence, application,
        15, 77
    quantitative evidence, application, 15
    research problems relating to see
        research
    theories, role, 6
health research, 1–10
    clinical decision making see clinical
        decision making
    confidence intervals, use, 157
    correlations, use, 143–145
    effect size and, 176, 177t
    evidence-based medicine and, 22–23
    method, 3–4
    methodology, 3
    qualitative topics, 77
    research problems see research
    scientific methods see scientific
        method
    social context see social context
hermeneutics, 211
histograms, 118–119, 119f, 211
history, 211
holistic perspective, 13
homogeneous sampling, 40t
hypotheses, 5f, 6, 31, 151–152, 159, 211
    critical evaluation of published
        research, 192–194
    directional hypothesis, 210
    generation in quantitative research,
        13
    non-directional hypothesis, 213
    one-tailed test, 213
hypothesis testing, 159–170
    alternative hypothesis, 160
    decision level, α (alpha), 160

hypothesis testing (Continued)
    examples, 160–162, 162f
    null hypothesis, 160
    probability, 160–162, 163t
    sampling distribution, 160
    steps, 160
    type I error see type I error
    type II error see type II error

I

immersion, 188
incidence rates, 65, 121, 122f, 211
incidental samples, 35–36, 211
    incidental sampling, 35
    quota sampling, 35–36, 36t
inclusion criteria, 36, 202
independent variable, 53, 211
    design, 57–58, 58f
induction, 6, 211
inferential statistics, 19, 162–163, 178
    aim, 163
    alternative hypothesis, 165
    chi-square test (χ^2) see chi-square
        test (χ^2)
    confidence intervals see confidence
        intervals
    degrees of freedom, 155–156, 165
    descriptive statistics and, relationship
        between, 160–163
    hypothesis testing see hypothesis
        testing
    non-parametric tests, 164
    not required, 163
    null hypothesis, 165
    parametric tests, 164
    probability see probability
    statistical decisions, 176, 176t
    statistical packages see statistics
    test selection, 163–164, 163t, 169
        examples, 164
    type I error see type I error
    type II error see type II error
    using statistical packages, 167, 168t,
        169 see also data
informed consent, 44–45, 211
    plain language statements, 45
instrumentation, 211
    in observation, 101, 101t
inter-observer (inter-rater) reliability,
    107, 107t, 144, 144t, 211–212
internal consistency, 107
internal validity, 55, 61, 109, 211
    control groups and, 56
    multiple-group time-series designs,
        69
    natural recovery, 55
    naturalistic designs, 69–70
interpolation, 119
interpretation of data, 19
    critical evaluation of published
        research, 196
    meta-analysis see meta-analysis
    $n = 1$ designs see single case ($n = 1$)
        designs

interpretation of data (Continued)
    qualitative data see qualitative
        research
    randomized-controlled trial (RCT),
        59
    statistical decisions, 176, 176t
    systematic reviews, 203
    type I error see type I error
    type II error see type II error
    using statistical packages, 60,
        168t
interquartile range, 130
interrupted time series, 211–212
interval data, organization and
    presentation, 118–120
interval scales, 111–112, 111t–112t,
    212
interviews, 92, 212
    analysis of data, 96–97
        coding, 97
        ethnography, 97
        grounded theory, 97
        qualitative, 97
        quantitative, 97
        thematic analysis, 97
    focus groups see focus groups
    method, 92–93
        face-to-face, 92–93
        remote, 92–93
    models, 91–92, 92t
        non-schedule standardized
            interview, 91–92
        schedule standardized interview,
            91–92
        structure/formality, 91–92
    process, 93–94
        follow-up, 94
        free-form (unstructured) notes, 94
        participants, 93
        response schedules/answer
            checklists, 93–94
    questionnaires, compared with,
        86–87, 86t
    recording information, 94–96
        audio taping, 94
        comparison of techniques, 94–95,
            95t
        video recording, 94
    structured interview, 216
    techniques, 91–98
    transcript, 96
    unstructured interview, 216
intra-observer reliability, 107, 212
introduction (research publications),
    20
    critical evaluation see critical
        evaluation of published research
        see also literature review

K

knowledge, 4
    advances in, 7
    epistemology, 4
    ontology, 4

knowledge *(Continued)*
  perspectives, 11–12
  theories *see* theories *see also*
    scientific method
Kruskal–Wallis *H* test, 163t

L

laboratory observations, 100–101, 101t
  laws, 6 *see also* hypotheses
Likert scales, 88, 89t, 212
line of 'best-fit', 140, 140f
linear correlation, 140, 140f
literature review, 29, 212
  critical evaluation of published
    research, 192
  literature searching, 29
  PICO approach, 29
  synthesis of research, 199–200

M

McNemar's test, 163t
mammography, case study of test
    validity, 109
Mann–Whitney test, 163t
matched group, 56
matching, 212
maturation, 212
maximum variation sampling, 40t
McNemar's test, 163t
mean, 126–127, 212
  sampling distribtions *see* sampling
  z score and, 219t–222t
measurement, 5–6, 105–112, 212
  definition, 105
  objective and subjective measures,
    106
  operationalization, 106
  reliability *see* reliability
  standardized measures and tests *see*
    standardized measures and tests
  tools and procedures, 106–109
measurement scale types, 110–112, 112t
  interval scales, 111–112, 111t–112t
    nominal scales, 110, 111t *see also*
      nominal data
    ordinal scales, 111, 111t *see also*
      ordinal data
  ratio scales, 111–112, 111t–112t
median, 125–127, 126f, 126t, 212
medical ethics, 43–44
medical model, 8
meta-analysis, 203–206, 212
  combining data from diverse studies,
    204, 204t
  extracting data from individual
    studies, 204
    effect size, 204
  forest plot, 211
  interpretation of results, 204–206,
    205f–206f
    confidence intervals, 205
    effect size, 205

meta-analysis *(Continued)*
    odds ratio, 205
    sample sizes, 205
    studies, 205
    weights and totals, 205–206
  strategies, 203
    qualitative, 203
    quantitative, 203
    software packages, 203
method(s) (health research), 3–4
  methodology *vs.*, 3
  scientific *see* scientific method
method(s) section (research
    publications), 20–21, 30
  apparatus and tools, 21
  choice, 30
  critical evaluation *see* critical
    evaluation of published research
  definition, 3
  history of scientific method, 4–5
  participants, 20
  procedure, 21
methodology, method *vs.*, 3
mixed designs, 75, 187, 194
mixed methods, 212
mode, 125, 126t–127t, 127, 212
models, 8–9
  biopsychosocial model, 8–9
  medical model, 8
  psychosocial model, 8–9
moral conduct, 43–44
moral principles, 43–44, 47
mortality, 212
multiple baseline designs, 73, 73f
  baselines, 73f
  features, 73
multiple dependent variables, 58
multiple-group time-series design,
    68–69, 69f, 212
Murphy's Law, 47

N

n, 212 *see also* sample
N, 212 *see also* population
n = 1 designs, 72f, 75
narrative review, 200–201
  quality, 201
  role in health care, 200
natural setting, 212
naturalistic comparison studies, 212
  control variables, 65
negative correlation, 140f, 141, 212
negative skew, 212–213, 213f
nominal data
  organization and presentation, 116,
    116t
  worked example, 116, 116t
nominal scales, 110, 111t–112t, 213
non-directional hypothesis, 213
non-directional probability, 156
non-equivalence, 110
non-experimental designs, 63–64, 213
  case-control designs, 66
  cohort study, 67

non-experimental designs *(Continued)*
  correlational designs, 66–67, 67t
  epidemiology *see* epidemiology
  experimental designs *vs.*, 64
  naturalistic comparison studies,
    65–66
  quasi-experimental designs *see* quasi-
    experimental designs
  reasons for use, 63
  surveys, 64, 68f
non-linear correlation, 140, 140f
non-parametric tests, 164, 213
non-schedule standardized interview,
    91–92
non-standardized interview, 91
normal curve *see* normal distribution
normal distribution, 134–135, 134f,
    213f
  calculating area under normal curve,
    135–136, 136f
    worked example, 135
  critical values, 136, 136f
  standard normal curve, 135, 213
    for comparison of distributions,
      136–138, 137f, 137t
    worked examples, 136–137
  worked example, 135
note-taking, 94, 102–103
null hypothesis, 160, 165, 213
  null results, reasons for, 175
null results, 175
Nuremberg Code (1947), 44

O

objective measures, 213
observation, 5–6, 5f, 99–104, 213
  AB design, in, 72
  advantages, 99
  approaches, 99–101
  controlled, 7
  data collection, 100f, 104
  instrumentation, 101, 101t
  observers *see* observer(s)
  qualitative research, 102–104
    focus of observation (behaviours
      and settings), 103
    principles, 102
  quantitative research, 104
    definition of relevant variables,
      104
    observation and structure, 104
    observer roles, 104
  settings, 100–101, 101t
    laboratory observations, 100–101,
      101t
  single case (*n* = 1) designs, 75
  theories and, 8
observed frequency, 213
observer(s), 99–100, 100f, 100t
  bias, 55
  inter-observer (inter-rater) reliability,
    107, 107t
  outside observers, 99–100, 100f,
    100t

observer(s) (Continued)
  roles, 101–102
    complete observer, 102
    complete participant, 102
    observer as participant, 102
    participant as observer, 102
    quantitative observation, 104
  self-observations, 99–100, 100f,
    100t
observer as participant, 102, 213
odds ratio (OR), 122–123, 122t,
  173–174, 213
  meta-analysis interpretation of
    results, 205
one-tailed test, 213
ontological realism, 5
ontology, 4
open questions, 87–88, 87t, 213
operational construct sampling, 40t
operational definition, 106, 213
operationalization, operational
  definition, 106
opinion questions, 90
opportunistic sampling, 40t
ordinal data
  organization and presentation, 116,
    116t
  worked example, 116, 116t
ordinal scales, 111, 111t–112t, 213
organization and presentation of data,
  19, 113–124
  continuous data see continuous data
  discrete data see discrete data
  interval data, 118–120
  nominal data see nominal data
  ordinal data see ordinal data
  ratio data, 118–120
outcomes, measurement, 110

P

p value see probability
pain management, example of n = 1
  design, 74–75, 75t
pandemic pattern, 65
paradigm, 5, 213
parametric tests, 164, 213
participant as observer, 102
participants, 20, 213
  assignment into groups see
    assignment
  availability, 47
  critical evaluation of published
    research see critical evaluation of
    published research
  ethical considerations see ethical
    considerations in health research
  expectations, 8
  focus groups, 95
  human, 60
  hypotheses and, 30
  interviews, 93
  participant observer, 48
  placebo effect see placebo effect
  population definition, 58

participants (Continued)
  randomized-controlled trial (RCT),
    in, 58
  rights and benefits from research,
    47–48
  standardized measures and tests, 110
    see also sampling
path analysis, 145–146
Pearson's r, 141–143, 142f, 142t
  assumptions, 142–143
percentages, 121
percentiles, 130, 130f, 135–136,
  213–214
personal meaning, 79
phenomenology, 78, 214
PICO approach to literature reviews,
  29
pie chart, 117, 117f, 117t, 214
pilot studies, 31, 214
  questionnaires, 85–86
placebo effect, 55, 214
  control groups and, 55, 60
  double-blind design, 60
  ethical considerations, 60
  mechanism, 60
population, 214
  definition, 58
  health indicators, 65
  parameter, 214
population validity, 40–41, 214
positioning of researcher, 13
positive correlation, 140f, 141, 214
positive skew, 214
positivist paradigm, 5–7
  contributions to health care, 7
  controlled observation, 7
  deduction, 6
  generalization and induction, 6
  hypotheses and laws, 6
  observations, description and
    measurement, 5–6
  theories see theories
  verification and falsification, 7
post-positivist paradigms, 7–9
  falsification see falsification
  qualitative methods, 9
  quantitative methods, 9
  theory-dependence of observation, 8
post-test only design, 56–57, 214
power, 214
  analysis, 176–177
    definition, 176
    type II error, 176
pragmatism, 9
  qualitative methods, 9
  quantitative methods, 9
pre-test/post-test design, 57, 214
predictive validity, 108, 108t, 145, 214
prevalence rates, 65, 121, 214
probability, 149–158, 214
  continuous data and, 157–158
  discontinuous data and, 157–158
  hypothesis testing see hypothesis
    testing
  non-directional probability, 156
  sampling distributions see sampling

probability (Continued)
  two-tail probability, 156
  worked examples, 150, 150f–151f,
    150t see also effect size
procedure (research publications), 214
  critical evaluation see critical
    evaluation of published research
professional publication, 19–20
proportions, 121, 214
protocol deviation, 214
psychosocial model, 8–9
publication see research publications
purposive sampling, 39–40, 40t
  strategies, 39
    extreme or deviant case sampling,
      39
    maximum variation sampling, 39
    snowball or chain sampling, 39,
      40t
    theory-based sampling, 39–40

Q

qualitative research, 9, 11–16, 214
  aims, 77
  analysis of data, 97, 181–188
    accuracy, 187–188
    an example, 81
    coding see coding of data
    computer-assisted data analysis,
      183–184
    content analysis see content
      analysis
    critical evaluation, 196
    thematic analysis see thematic
      analysis
    worked example, 186
  applications in health care, 15, 77
  approaches to, 78–79
    ethnomethodology, 79
    grounded theory, 79
    phenomenology, 78
    symbolic interactionism, 78–79
  auditability, 187
  characteristics, 79–80
  coding of data see coding of data
  confounding and bias, 80
  contrasted with quantitative
    methods, 12–15, 12t
  credibility, 187
  on cultural differences, 77–78
  data, 13–14
  data saturation, 187
  ethnography, 97, 211
  example, 80–81
  grounded theory see grounded theory
  holistic perspective, 13
  immersion, 188
  interpretation of data, 182, 185–187
    semiotics, 185
    worked example, 186
  interviews see interviews
  meta-analysis strategy, 203
  observation see observation
  planning, 80

qualitative research *(Continued)*
  problems and questions, 77–78
  quantitative methods
    contrasted with, 5–6
    integration with, 15
  questionnaires *see* questionnaires
  sampling, 38–39, 80
    purposive *see* purposive sampling
  social context, 5, 185–187
  subjectivity of researcher, 13
  thematic analysis *see* thematic
    analysis
  theories, 14–15
  triangulation, 187, 187f
quantitative research, 9, 11–16, 97,
    214
  analysis of data *see* inferential
    statistics
  applications in health care, 15
  hypothesis generation, 13
  inferential statistics *see* inferential
    statistics
  interviews, 92, 97
  meta-analysis strategy, 203
  objectivity of researcher, 13
  observation *see* observation
  qualitative methods
    contrasted with, 5–6, 12–15, 12t
    integration with, 15
  questionnaires *see* questionnaires
  randomized-controlled trial (RCT),
    30–31
  reductionism, 12–13
  statistics *see* statistics
  theories, 14
quartile deviation, 130
quasi-experimental designs, 63–70, 214
  multiple-group time-series designs,
    68–69, 69f
  time-series designs, 67–68, 68f
questionnaires, 83–90, 214
  acquiescent response mode, 209
  administration, 86
    interviewers, 86–87
  clinical research, use of in, 86
  construction, 85–86
  ethical considerations, 86
  extreme response mode, 211
  interviews, compared with, 86–87,
    86t
  Likert scales, 88, 89t
  missing data, 87
  pilot study, 85–86
  question format, 86–89, 88t
    ambiguous questions, 89
    bias and leading questions, 89
    closed questions, 87–88, 87t, 210
    double-barrelled questions, 89
    forced-choice response, 88, 89t
    level of wording, 89
    open questions, 87–88, 87t
  structure, 90
    closing statements and return
      instructions, 90
    demographic questions, 90
    factual questions, 90

questionnaires *(Continued)*
    introductory statement, 90
    opinion questions, 90
questions
  questionnaires *see* questionnaires
  research questions *see* research
quota sampling, 35–36, 36t, 214

R

random assignment, 59
random purposive sampling, 40t
random sampling, 214
  advantages, 36
  disadvantages, 36
  list method, 36
  procedure, 36
  raffle method, 36
  stratified random sampling *see*
    stratified random sampling
randomized-controlled trial (RCT),
    30–31, 51–62, 58f
  assignment, 59
  control groups, 58
    types, 59
  double-blind design, 60
  efficacy, 59
  external validity, 61
  outcome measurement, 59
  process, 58
  statistical analysis and interpretation,
    59
range, 128, 214
rank-ordering of scores, 143t
rates, 121–122
  incidence rates, 121, 122f
  prevalence rates, 121
ratio data, organization and
    presentation, 118–120
ratio scales, 111–112, 111t–112t,
    214–215
ratios, 120
raw scores, 133, 135
reasoning, 4
recording information, 94–96, 95t
  observation, 100f, 104
reductionism, 12–13
refereed journal, 215
references (research publications), 21
regression to the mean, 215
relationships, 215
reliability, 107, 215
  correlation, 144–145
  critical evaluation of published
    research, 195
  inter-observer (inter-rater) reliability,
    107, 107t, 144, 144t
  internal consistency, 107
  intra-observer reliability, 107
  standardized measures and tests *see*
    standardized measures and tests
  test–retest reliability, 107, 144, 172,
    172t
remote interviews, 92–93
repeated measures design, 57, 215

representative samples, 34–37, 35f,
    215
research
  aims, 18, 31
    critical evaluation of published
      research, 192–194
  design, 18, 30–31
    'before–after' design, 54, 54f
    confounding and bias *see*
      confounding and bias
    critical evaluation of published
      research, 195
    ethical considerations and, 48
    experimental *see* experimental
      designs
    interrupted time series, 211–212
    multiple group time series, 212
    non-experimental *see* non-
      experimental designs
    qualitative research, an example,
      81 *see also* experimental
      designs
  funding bodies, ethics and, 46
  hypotheses *see* hypotheses
  planning, 18
    economic issues, 47
    qualitative research, 80
    qualitative research, an example,
      80
  problems, 18, 27–29
    cost-effectiveness of health
      services, 28–29
    demographic changes, 28
    environmental and social changes,
      27–28
    qualitative research, an example,
      80
    scientific and technological
      advances, 28
    types, 27
  process, 17–24
    algorithm, 17–19, 18f
    data analysis *see* data
    data collection *see* data
    data organization *see* organization
      and presentation of data
    data presentation *see* organization
      and presentation of data
    dissemination, 19 *see also* research
      publications
    evaluation and dissemination, 19
    interpretation of data *see*
      interpretation of data
    literature review *see* literature
      review
  proposals, 31
    content, 31
  protocol deviations, critical
    evaluation of published research,
    196
  publications *see* research publications
  questions, 18
    ethical considerations and, 48
    formulation of, 25–32, 28f
    methodological considerations,
      30–31

research *(Continued)*
　qualitative research, an example, 80
　systematic reviews, 201
research publications, 19–21, 19t
　conclusions, 21
　critical evaluation *see* critical evaluation of published research
　discussion, 19, 21, 210
　introduction, 20
　meta-analysis *see* meta-analysis
　method section *see* methods section (research publications)
　publication process, 22
　refereed journal, 215
　references and appendices, 21
　results section, 21
　style, 21–22
　systematic reviews *see* systematic reviews
　title and abstract, 20
resources available, 46–48
results (research publications), 21
　analysis of data *see* data
　critical evaluation of results section *see* critical evaluation of published research
　organization and presentation *see* organization and presentation of data
return instructions, 90
reversal, 215
risk and harm minimization, 45, 47
risk factors, 215
Rosenthal effect, 215

S

sample, 215
　bias, 209
　selection, 58
　size *(n)*, 37–38, 151
　　confidence intervals and, 174
　　critical evaluation of published research, 194
　　error and, 41
　　meta-analysis interpretation of results, 205
sampling
　critical evaluation of published research, 194
　distributions, 151–152
　　central limit theorem, 153
　　hypothesis testing and *see* hypothesis testing
　　of the mean, 152–154, 154f
　　worked example, 151, 151f–152f
　error, 37–38, 38f, 215
　qualitative research, 80
　strategies, 33–42, 215
　　aim, 41
　　area sampling, 37
　　basic issues, 34, 34t
　　incidental sampling *see* incidental samples

sampling *(Continued)*
　purposive sampling *see* purposive sampling
　in qualitative research *see* qualitative research
　random sampling *see* random sampling
　representative samples, 34–37, 35f
　stratified random sampling *see* stratified random sampling
　systematic sampling, 37, 216
　types, 41
　systematic reviews, 206
scales (of measurement) *see* measurement scale types
scattergram/scatterplot, 140, 140f, 215
scepticism, 5
scientific method, 5f
　determinism, 5
　history, 4–5
　ontological realism, 5
　positivist paradigm, 5–7, 5f
　scepticism, 5
search strategy, systematic reviews, 201–202
self-observations, 99–100, 100f, 100t
semi-interquartile range, 130, 130f, 215
semiotics, 185, 215
sensitivity, 108t, 109, 215
shared variance, estimation of, 145, 215
Sign test, 163t, 164
significance, 215
　clinically/practically, 173, 176–177, 177t, 210
　confidence intervals and, 174, 174f
　critical evaluation of published research, 197
　level, 160, 171 *see also* α (alpha) level
single case (*n* = 1) designs, 71–76, 212
　AB designs, 71–72, 72f, 209
　ABAB designs *see* ABAB designs
　baselines, 72f, 75
　effect size, 75
　interpretation of results, 74–75
　　an example, 74–75, 75t
　multiple baseline designs *see* multiple baseline designs
　uses, 75
　validity, 75
　variability, 74
skewness, 215
snowball sampling, 39, 40t
social context, of research, 8–9
　qualitative research, 5, 185–187
Spearman's ρ, 143, 143t
specificity, 108t, 109, 215
SPSS, 167 *see also* statistics
standard deviation, 129, 215
standard error of the mean, 215
　standard normal curve, 215 *see also* normal distribution
standard scores (z scores), 133–134, 134f, 216, 219t–222t
　worked example, 133

standardized measures and tests, 109–110, 215
　characteristics, 110
　　acceptability to participants/patients, 110
　　accessibility, 110
　　reliability, 110
　　theoretical framework, 110
　　validity, 110
Statistical Package for Social Sciences (SPSS), 167
statistical significance, 215 *see also* significance
statistics, 115, 215
　descriptive statistics *see* descriptive statistics
　inferential statistics *see* inferential statistics
　statistical packages, 167–169
　　descriptive statistics, 168, 168t
　　encoding raw data, 167
　　identifying statistical analysis required, 167
　　inferential statistics, 167, 168t, 169
　　interpretation, 60, 167, 168t
　　printout, 167
　　selection, 167
　　training, 167
stratified purposeful sampling, 40t
stratified random sampling, 36–37, 215–216
　advantages, 37
　disadvantages, 37
structured interview, 216
style guide for research publications, 21–22
subjective measures, 216
subjects, 216 *see also* participants
surveys, 63–70, 68f, 216
symbolic interactionism, 78–79
synthesis of research, 199–208
　basic principles, 200
　literature review, 199–200
　meta-analysis *see* meta-analysis
　narrative reviews of research evidence *see* narrative review
　statistics, 204, 204t
　systematic review *see* systematic reviews
systematic reviews, 208, 216
　appraisal and selection of key papers, 202
　　criteria example, 202
　characteristics, 201
　Cochrane Collaboration *see* Cochrane Collaboration
　coding, 202–203
　　features, 202, 203t
　evidence-based practice, 207
　interpretation of data, 203
　interpretation of research evidence, 203
　research questions, 201
　search strategy, 201–202

systematic reviews *(Continued)*
  theoretical framework, 201
  validity, 206–207
    extracting the data, 207
    sampling, 206 *see also* synthesis of research
systematic sample, 216
systematic sampling, 37

T

t distribution, 155–157, 156f–157f, 223t–224t
tables of results, critical evaluation, 196
tabulating data, conventions, 116
telephone interviews, 92–93
test validity *see* validity
test–retest reliability, 107, 144, 172, 172t, 216
thematic analysis, 97, 182–185
  example, 184
  themes, 184 *see also* grounded theory
theoretical framework, systematic reviews, 201
theories, 5f, 6
  observations and, 8
  qualitative methods, 14
  quantitative methods, 14
  role in health care, 6
theory-based sampling, 40t
theory testing, 14–15
time-series designs, 67–68, 68f, 216
title (research publications), 20
tradition, medical, 4
  traditional Chinese Medicine (TCM), 4
traditional Chinese Medicine (TCM), 4
transcript, 216
transformed score, 216
treatment
  administration, 59
  fidelity, 195
  parameters, 195

triangulation, 187, 187f
true negative, 216
true positive, 216
two-tail probability, 156
two-tailed test, 216
type I error, 161, 172t, 175, 216
  clinical decision making, 177, 177t
  minimize occurrence, 175
  type II error and, 175
type II error, 161, 172t, 174f, 175, 216
  clinical decision making, 177, 177t
  minimize occurrence, 175
  power analysis, 176–177
  type I error and, 175

U

unaided observation, 101, 101t
unstructured interview, 216
utilitarian ethics, 44, 216

V

validity, 108–109, 216
  case study of test validity, 109
  confounding and bias *see* confounding and bias
  critical evaluation of published research, 195
  ecological validity *see* ecological validity
  external *see* external validity
  internal *see* internal validity
  predictive validity, 108, 108t, 145
  single case (*n* = 1) designs, 75
  standardized measures and tests *see* standardized measures and tests
  systematic reviews *see* systematic reviews
  test validity, types, 108–109
    construct validity, 108–109
    content or face validity, 108

validity *(Continued)*
  predictive validity, 108, 108t
  sensitivity and specificity, 108t, 109
variability, 125, 128–130, 210, 216
  percentiles, 130, 130f
  range, 128
    average deviation, 128–129
  semi-interquartile range, 130, 130f
  single case (*n* = 1) designs, 74
  standard deviation, 129 *see also* variance
variables, 216
  control variables, 53
    naturalistic comparison studies, 65
  dependent *see* dependent variables
  independent *see* independent variable
  in quantitative observation, 104
variance, 129, 216
  shared variance, estimation, 145 *see also* variability
verification, 7
'verstehen,' 184–185
video recording, 94
volunteer effect, 36

W

weight of study, 205–206
wording of questions, 89
writing styles, 21

X

χ^2 (chi-square test) *see* chi-square test (χ^2)

Z

z scores (standard scores), 133–134, 134f, 216, 219t–222t
zero correlation, 216